STORY OF A GREAT HOSPITAL

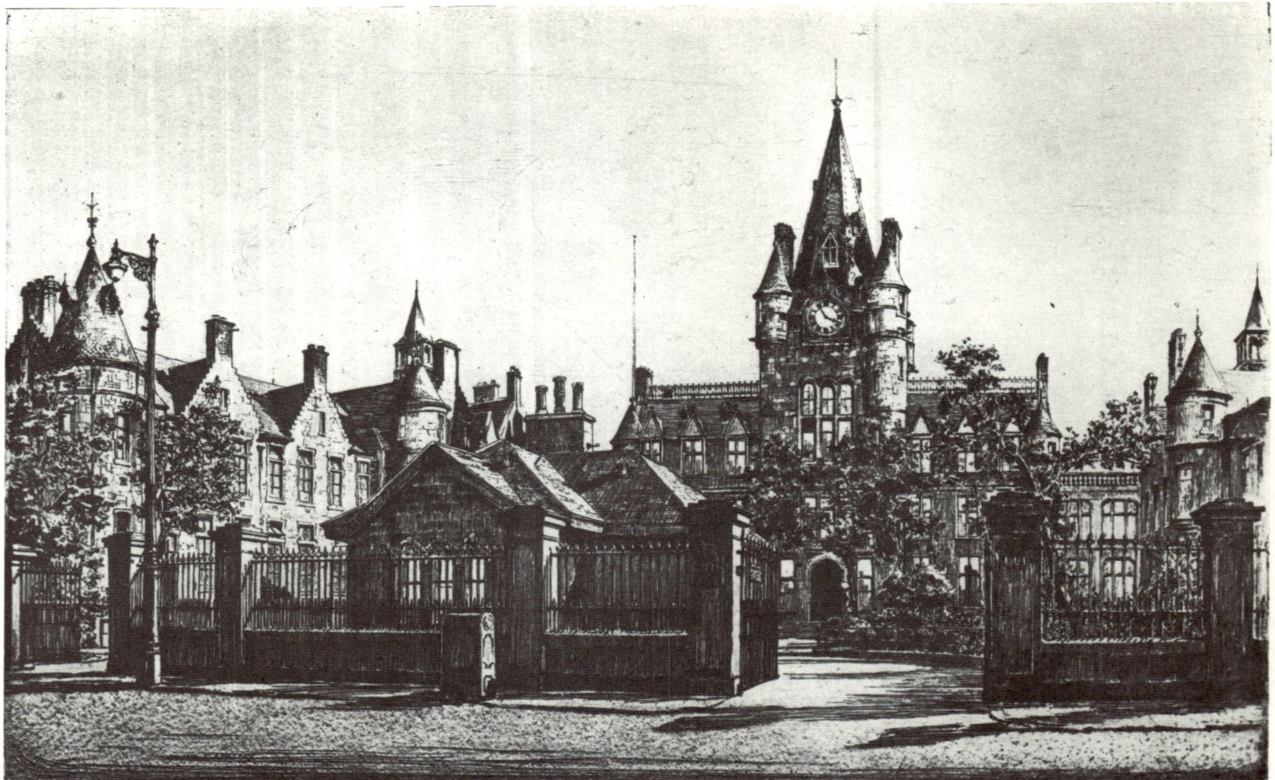

Etching by Wilfred C. Applebey

STORY OF A GREAT HOSPITAL

THE ROYAL INFIRMARY OF EDINBURGH 1729-1929

BY

A. LOGAN TURNER, M.D., LL.D., Hon. F.R.C.P. Edin.

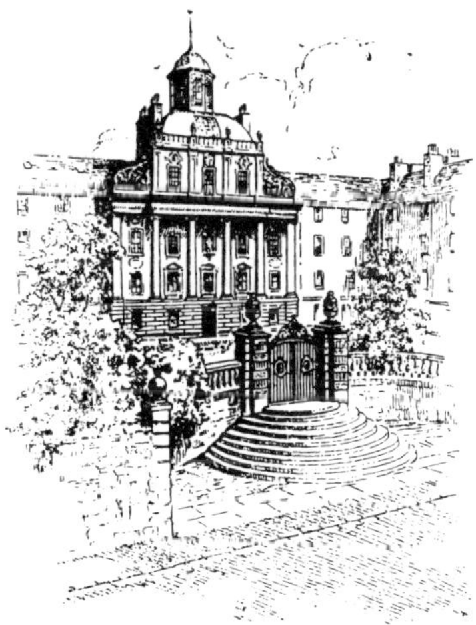

JAMES THIN
1979

THE MERCAT PRESS, EDINBURGH

This is a fascimile of the 1937 edition published by Oliver and Boyd, Ltd., Edinburgh

SBN 0 901824 59 3

Printed by John G Eccles Printers Ltd, Henderson Road, Inverness

TO PAST, PRESENT, AND
FUTURE GENERATIONS OF
STUDENTS OF MEDICINE
AT EDINBURGH

PREFACE TO THE 1979 REPRINT

Dr Logan Turner first outlines the origins and development of the Royal Infirmary of Edinburgh to commemorate its Bicentenary year in 1929 and later amplified it in "Story of a Great Hospital" published in 1937.

Preparations for the commemoration of the 250th Anniversary of the foundation of the hospital and the Centenary of the present building found both volumes out of print. Such a situation called for a remedy and thanks to the good offices of Mr Ainslie Thin and The Mercat Press the larger of the two volumes is again in print.

I would like to record our appreciation of the generosity of Dr John W. A. Turner and Dr Francis Logan Turner, the author's heirs, in waiving all claims of royalties.

I commend the volume to all who hold affectionate memories of a great hospital, be they patients who were cared for in it or nurses and doctors who owe their skills to the training they received there.

DONALD McINTOSH
Lately Consultant Surgeon
The Royal Infirmary of Edinburgh

PREFACE

As in recent years the history of more than one of Britain's famous hospitals has been written and published, the time appears opportune to add to the list the story of the Royal Infirmary of Edinburgh, the first of the large voluntary hospitals in Scotland, founded two hundred and eight years ago. In a small book entitled *The Royal Infirmary of Edinburgh, 1729-1929*, I outlined the story of the hospital in connection with the commemoration of its bicentenary year; but with that exception all previous publications deal with only a limited period of its history. These are *An Account of the Rise and Establishment of the Infirmary, or Hospital for Sick Poor, erected at Edinburgh, 1730*; *The History and Statutes of the Royal Infirmary, 1749*; and *The History of the Royal Infirmary, 1778*, to which must be added "The Old Infirmary and Earlier Hospitals," a paper contributed in 1927 by Dr Robert Thin to Volume xv of the *Book of the Old Edinburgh Club*. In Dr John D. Comrie's *History of Scottish Medicine* I found a veritable store-house of information relative to medicine in Edinburgh.

In order to make good the above deficiency a more comprehensive story has now been written. The period covers two centuries, 1729 to 1929. Although during the past eight years the hospital has continued to expand and several important problems affecting its policy have been under consideration, some indeed still unsolved, the events occurring in that brief space of time can hardly be regarded as constituting history. It may well be left, therefore, to some future historian to deal with these recent years in their proper perspective. Nevertheless occasional references have been made both in the text and in footnotes to some of the latest developments.

The opportunity has been taken to sketch very shortly the commencement of the voluntary hospital movement in Great Britain and Ireland. As the Royal Infirmary has been from its inception an essential part of the Edinburgh School of Medicine its history must of necessity be very closely interwoven with that of the School; therefore the narrative contains many interesting facts connected with the rise and progress of the latter. A chapter has also been introduced to show the influence of the medical school at Leiden in the seventeenth and early eighteenth centuries upon the origin of the Infirmary and the foundation of the medical faculty of the University of Edinburgh.

I gladly take this opportunity of acknowledging the assistance given to me by many friends: to the Board of Management for the privilege of making use of the minutes of the Infirmary without which this story could not have been written; and to Mr William S. Caw, the late Treasurer and Clerk, who placed at my disposal his unique knowledge of past events in the life of the hospital and whose carefully compiled index of the old volumes of minutes certainly eased my task. I am greatly indebted also to members of the various administrative departments for help willingly given: to Colonel Alexander Dron Stewart, the Superintendent; to Mr Henry Maw, Secretary and Treasurer; Mr James Williamson, Cashier; Mr Duncan McNeil, Registrar; Mr Andrew Whyte, Steward; Mr Thomas W. Turnbull, Architect and Master of Works, especially for the drawings of the Plans illustrating two of the schemes of extension, and to Mr Russell Paton, the Organising Secretary for Subscriptions. Miss Elizabeth D. Smaill, Lady Superintendent of Nurses, has given me much useful information concerning the Nursing Department, for which I am grateful.

My thanks are also extended to Professor Sir John Fraser who kindly read my manuscript and offered some valuable suggestions ; to Miss Marguerite Wood, Keeper of the City Records ; to Mr Thomas H. Graham, Librarian, Royal College of Physicians of Edinburgh ; to Miss Margaret Lorrain Smith, my secretary, for her careful reading of the proof sheets and the preparation of the Index ; and to my sister for her unfailing interest and ever ready assistance.

Finally, I gratefully acknowledge the courtesy of Mr Wilfred C. Appleby in permitting me to reproduce his etching of the main entrance of the Royal Infirmary as the *Frontispiece*, and the care bestowed by the publishers upon the production of the volume and illustrations.

A. LOGAN TURNER

EDINBURGH, *October* 1937

CONTENTS

CONTENTS

CONTENTS

CONTENTS

ILLUSTRATIONS

ILLUSTRATIONS

" It is good occasionally to unroll the pages of the past and to endeavour to discover the successive steps by which the existing state of things has been brought about."—*The Early History of the Medical Profession in Edinburgh*, by Dr John Gairdner, 1864.

" The saving and restoring to health members of society, whose labours are indispensable in a State, may well be ranked among the more important services done to the community. Hence, in all well-regulated societies, public funds and private charities have been devoted to the use of the poor."—*The History of the Royal Infirmary, 1778.*

CHAPTER I

THE BEGINNINGS OF MEDICINE

EGYPTIAN, ASSYRIAN AND BABYLONIAN MEDICINE—GREEK MEDICINE—ÆSCULAPIUS AND HIPPOCRATES—THE MEDICAL SCHOOL OF COS—THE SCHOOL AT ALEXANDRIA—GALEN AND ROMAN MEDICINE—THE SCHOOL AT SALERNO — BYZANTINE AND ARABIC MEDICINE — THE MEDIEVAL UNIVERSITIES IN EUROPE AND THE RENAISSANCE—THE SCHOOLS AT BOLOGNA AND PADUA.

A brief sketch of the main centres of learning which, throughout the ages, have influenced the progress of Medicine, and in which can be traced through more than twenty centuries the unbroken thread of the old Greek spirit of enquiry into the nature of things, appears a fitting prelude to the story of the Royal Infirmary and of the Edinburgh School of Medicine, one and indivisible, founded coincidentally more than two hundred years ago.[1] But, centuries before Greek civilisation lifted the veil of Nature and sowed the seeds of scientific enquiry, a long age existed in which mysticism, magic and superstition dominated the minds of the dwellers on the banks of the Nile and on the fertile plains watered by the Tigris and Euphrates. Even today magic and superstition still prevail amongst primitive races, nor have they entirely disappeared under the influence of modern civilisation !

The ancient Egyptians, Assyrians and Babylonians sought in the supernatural the explanation of many of the phenomena of life. They believed that disease and death were due to some malign influence, of a god or an evil spirit, and the business of the physician was to discover its true nature and then to attack and exorcise it by powerful magic. Hence the

[1] In the preparation of this chapter the writer has made use of the following publications :—" Medicine among the Assyrians and Egyptians in 1500 B.C.," by John D. Comrie, *Edin. Med. Journ.*, New Series II, 1919 ; *Greek Medicine in Rome* (Sir Clifford Allbutt) ; *History of Medicine* (Max Neuburger) ; *The Evolution of Modern Medicine* (Sir William Osler) ; *The Evolution of Anatomy* (Charles Singer) ; *Universities of Europe in the Middle Ages* (H. Rashdall) ; *Interpreters of Nature* (Sir George Newman).

employment of incantations and prayers and the use of armlets and charms to propitiate the spirit, followed by the administration of drugs and appropriate diet. The treatment of disease was thus mainly empirical and the records preserved on the Egyptian papyri disclose the possession of a rich pharmacopœia derived from the animal, vegetable and mineral kingdoms ; and gargles and snuffs, emetics and diaphoretics, poultices and plasters formed part of their therapeutic equipment, as they do in the practice of the modern physician. The Egyptian practitioners had a great reputation, the most renowned amongst them being Imhotep ; and specialism in medicine was highly developed.

Among the Assyrians and Babylonians, linked with Egypt along the great caravan routes through Syria, Medicine attained a higher standard. In the famous Babylonian Code of Laws medical practice was regulated, a scale of fees was laid down and penalties exacted for malpraxis. Ancient Nineveh was the seat of a university and celebrated as a school of medicine.

In Egypt and Babylonia the physician had evolved from the priest. The Greeks, however, broke away from belief in the efficacy of magic and in the influence of the supernatural, and in the writings of their philosophers are to be found the beginnings of scientific medicine. But the Greeks also worshipped their gods ; and as Imhotep, once a famous physician, came to be recognised by the Egyptians of old as their God of Medicine, so Æsculapius, the reputed son of Apollo, became one of the most popular of the Greek Gods, the healer of the sons of men. To him were dedicated the magnificent temples which flourished as natural health resorts, restoring the sick in body and mind and, like the modern hospitals, providing a rich field for clinical research. Today, Æsculapius, shorn of his divine attributes, remains the patron saint of medicine ; and the serpent, by reason of its mystical character and regarded throughout the ages as a symbol of supernatural power, endures as an emblem of the art of healing.

Hippocrates, the most renowned of all their early physicians, whose name is associated with the foundation of Greek Medicine, was born in 460 B.C. in the Ægean island of Cos. In its medical school he taught that medicine was a science founded on observation and experience and on the evidences of the senses. It demanded from the physician careful observation and the accurate recording of Nature's manifestations; and, from the facts ascertained, conclusions must be drawn by inductive reasoning. Disease was to be regarded as one of the processes of Nature and Nature was the source of healing—the *vis medicatrix naturæ*. In her power of healing she was not to be thwarted by artificial means, but to be assisted by personal hygiene, by suitable diet and by the patient's proper conduct of life, simplicity being the key-note of the therapeutic measures then taught. The Greek spirit was that of enquiry, of moderation, of reason and of freedom. But in the school of Cos no human anatomy was taught and physiology was dominated by the philosophies. Hippocrates died in 370 B.C. and following this event little progress was made in medicine prior to the rise of the Alexandrian School.

With the conquest of Egypt and the overthrow of the Persian rule by Alexander the Great in 332 B.C. the centre of learning and of Greek scientific thought passed to Alexandria during the dynasty of the Ptolemies. As enlightened patrons of learning they established a great school of literature, science and the arts which flourished for nearly three hundred years. Around its museum and vast library were founded the laboratories and clinics of its medical school, a school that acquired the distinction of founding the study of human anatomy and where, for the first time, the structure of man's body was investigated by dissection.

During the later years of the Ptolemaic rule, however, the position of Alexandria as a scientific school declined, and its disciples, emigrating to the East, founded new schools in the cities of Asia Minor. Amongst these, Pergamos, founded by the Greeks, occupied a special place as a school of medicine and as the birthplace, in 129 A.D., of Claudius Galen who, after Hippocrates, was one of the greatest of the ancient Greek physicians. Following a period of study in his native city and in the schools of Smyrna and Alexandria, Galen practised in Athens, but later sought his fortune in imperial Rome, as other Greek physicians had done before him. With access to the Hippocratic writings and imbued with the Hippocratic tradition he believed in the search after facts and in the employment of inductive reasoning. As an anatomist he was a descriptive writer, although his knowledge was not gained by human dissection; as a physiologist he used experimental methods, in some respects resembling the technique of modern research; as a physician he placed reliance on treatment by drugs rather than on the resources of Nature. Galen founded no school of medicine but his dogmatic teaching was accepted as infallible: it dominated medical thought down to the time of the Renaissance, when the anatomists of Bologna and Padua proved that the structure of the human body was not altogether as he had propounded it.

In the early Middle Ages following "the glory that was Greece and the grandeur that was Rome" the Barbarian hordes swept over Italy, laying waste an early civilisation. The primitive theories regarding disease were revived and, with the demolition of important centres of learning, the Greek spirit and influence became submerged. But, although thus checked and the flame reduced to a dull glow it was never entirely extinguished. In Southern Italy there survived through early medieval times "the one centre of pure Greek inspiration in Europe," which has earned a reputation in medical history somewhat comparable with that of Alexandria in bygone days.

Thirty miles south-east of Naples lies the little seaboard town of Salerno, its shores washed by the placid waters of the blue Tyrrhenian Sea; and a few miles to the south, across the bay, rise the majestic columns of the three Doric Temples of Pæstum—the ruined monuments of the vanished splendours of the once prosperous colony of *Magna Grecia*. Salerno, fortunate in its situation, was once an important commercial port trading with the cities of the Eastern Mediterranean, the mild character of its climate giving the district the reputation of a salubrious health resort ; and in the eleventh century its medical school and the fame of its physicians were already well established.

> Then at every season of the year
> There are crowds of guests and travellers here :
> Pilgrims and mendicant friars, and traders
> From the Levant with figs and wine,
> And bands of wounded and sick crusaders
> Coming back from Palestine.[1]

There, Duke Robert Guiscard of Normandy, returning from the East, was healed of his wounds and, making Salerno his capital, he built its cathedral, despoiling the temples of Pæstum in order to beautify it.

The origin of the medical school at Salerno remains wrapped in obscurity, but in the ninth century a flourishing lay College of Medicine already existed which deservedly acquired the title of *Civitas Hippocraticum.* Founded independently of ecclesiastical and civic control, education was in the hands of lay teachers and, throughout the tenth and eleventh centuries, it enjoyed a reputation which attracted to its classrooms students from many parts of Europe. Regulations were laid down for preliminary study : anatomy was taught by dissection on swine : the physiology was on Galenian lines : in therapeutics the value of hygiene and diet and the conduct of the patient's mode of life were insisted upon ; and in the famous *Regimen Sanitatis* was embodied its cyclopedia of medicine. Practical instruction in physic and surgery was given in the hospitals, and the student was taught the importance of bedside observation. The course of training extended over five years, and women, as well as men, were admitted to the curriculum of study. In those days women taught and practised medicine, and specialism was not unknown. At a later date the State instituted regulations against unlicensed practitioners.

[1] Longfellow's " The Golden Legend."

In many respects, therefore, the medical school of Salerno was the prototype of the school of medicine of the twentieth century, the forerunner in Europe of the Edinburgh School. Although stimulating and maintaining a high standard of education for four centuries it added no great names to the history of medicine; but in an age of superstition and empiricism it kept alive the true spirit of medicine. With the inevitable ebb and flow of human progress, however, the school began to decline in the thirteenth century. The old spirit was awakening elsewhere and, with the birth and growth of the medieval universities and the foundation of their medical faculties, the status of the Salernitan School became undermined until eventually it was no longer recognised as an educational institution.

In the Eastern Empire, also, the Byzantine physicians of the early Christian Era "conserved the all pervasive Greek spirit and kept the lamp alight." In Syria and Persia, and even farther east, the Christian Nestorians founded medical schools and hospitals of which those at Edessa were the most celebrated. They translated Greek manuscripts into Syriac and later into Arabic and, after the fall of Constantinople in 1453, many of these precious manuscripts were recovered and brought back to Europe.

When in the seventh century the hosts of Islam spread through the Græco-Roman world, overcoming Egypt, continuing their triumphant progress through Syria and Persia, the whole of northern Africa and thence through Spain into Western Europe, the intellectual leadership passed to those of Arabic speech. Having founded their empire, the Arabians applied themselves to the study of the sciences and, with the assistance of the Nestorian translators, they became acquainted with the writings of the Greek philosophers and physicians; and in course of time they produced their own great men in medicine. The Græco-Arabic amalgam undoubtedly suffered by reason of its successive translations—Syriac, Arabic, Latin—and from the many commentaries superadded by its several compilers, confusing and concealing much of the original Greek thought. Nevertheless, Arabian medicine had a stimulating effect, energising Western thought, and was not without its influence upon the rise of the universities in Europe.

During the darkest period of the Middle Ages, therefore, the flame of scientific enquiry had not been wholly quenched : it remained in the isolated centre at Salerno and in the Eastern Empire, and, through Arabian influence, it acquired a greater brilliance. Although in that epoch the Church remained the education authority, in Italy the monastic schools had never enjoyed a complete monopoly ; and with the commencement of the struggle for political and civil independence in the Italian cities in the twelfth century, the revival was initiated in the secular schools from which developed the university system. There was a demand for "fruitful knowledge, for science applied to the regulation of social life, for civilisation in the strictest sense of the word." The study of Roman jurisprudence became a necessity and, at Bologna, a law school was established, its university becoming in course of time the most important centre of legal training in Europe, instruction in medicine being a somewhat later development.

Of the universities north of the Alps, that of Montpellier, constituted towards the end of the thirteenth century, was of special importance. Unlike Bologna it derived its earliest recognition, not so much as a school of law, as one of medicine. From its geographical position near the frontier of Spain, it probably owed its origin to the influence of the Arabic and Jewish schools in that country, although, through its close proximity to the Mediterranean and its contact with the trade from the East, it may have absorbed some of the leaven of the ancient Greek tradition. The University of Paris, on the other hand, in the medieval period failed as a medical school to reach the position attained by Salerno and Montpellier.

The desire for self-expression and for freedom of thought, the revolt against the barrenness and dogmatism of medievalism and the authority of the Church, ideals which had already found expression in the thirteenth century, gained both in strength and in volume during the succeeding two hundred years. With the study of the *Literæ Humaniores*, a new standard of culture and a fresh view of life were substituted for the former traditional limitations, and in this movement philosophy, science, art and religion were participators. The scientific spirit of enquiry gradually displaced the old docile submission to authority.

In Italy, the nursing mother of the Renaissance, with the classical literature of Greece now studied direct through Latin translations and no longer from Arabic sources, medicine shared in the new intellectual movement, as many of the Humanists were also physicians. Amongst the northern Italian cities, medieval Padua, standing in the fertile plains of Venezia, became, in the period of the Revival of Learning, the most important centre of scientific enquiry. In its University, established on the model of Bologna, mathematicians, astronomers, naturalists and physicians probed the secrets of Nature to place Padua in the forefront of learning. Granted full university privileges and coming under the protection of the Venetian Republic, outside the Papal State, the University offered attractions to teachers and students of Protestant countries and gave greater facilities for the study of anatomy and medicine.

Within its walls there gathered men from all the countries of Europe. Like Lucentio they had the great desire—

> To see fair Padua, nursery of arts
> . . . for I have Pisa left,
> And am to Padua come, as he that leaves
> A shallow plash, to plunge him in the deep
> And with satiety seeks to quench his thirst.[1]

These men grouped themselves in "nations," they elected their own officials and ordained their own statutes. Many braved the difficulties and dangers of a long trans-alpine journey and, living under Spartan conditions, willingly suffered much physical discomfort in their thirst for knowledge.

[1] *The Taming of the Shrew.*

In the middle of the sixteenth century Andreas Vesalius brought a new spirit into the teaching of anatomy. His father was apothecary at the Court of Charles v, his mother a lady of English extraction. While still a boy and during his early classical studies at the University of Louvain young Vesalius displayed great zeal for anatomical study by dissecting such animals as he could acquire. Turning to medicine as a profession he proceeded to Paris but he crossed the Alps, in 1537, to seek at Padua what he had failed to obtain in the northern capital. Having graduated doctor of medicine at Padua he was appointed, at the age of twenty-three, to the chair of surgery and anatomy. In his anatomical theatre the teaching of anatomy was revolutionised : the study of the human body by dissection supplanted the written word and nothing was regarded as a fact unless it was actually observed. For five years Vesalius laboured incessantly : he corrected the long established errors, he systematised anatomical study and, in 1543, produced his great work on *The Fabric of the Human Body*. As the reformer of anatomy he founded a school.

In the hands of his pupils and successors Padua retained its reputation throughout the sixteenth century. With the appointment, in 1565, of Hieronymus Fabricius of Aquapendente to the chair of surgery and anatomy, the school for nearly fifty years had the services of the last of the great Paduan figures. William Harvey, a graduate of Padua in 1602, studied under him and no doubt he listened to the master's description of the valves of the veins, learning his views on the circulation of the blood and laying the foundation of his own future immortal work.

After the retirement of Fabricius, in 1613, the teaching of human anatomy at Padua lost the attraction which the earlier anatomists in the school had given to the subject. The swing of the pendulum once more carried Bologna into the ascendant, where Malpighi for twenty-five years occupied the chair of medicine. He was the first to describe the delicate network of capillary blood vessels connecting the arteries and the veins, finding the missing link to complete the chain of Harvey's discovery of the circulation.

Thus the science and art of medicine had emerged from the mists of superstition into the light of a real and accepted philosophy. North of the Alps old schools of medicine became invigorated and new schools came to life. The students who had studied in Italy carried back the Paduan tradition to the land of their birth where they helped to found new centres of education. Harvey brought the conception of scientific enquiry to England and the seventeenth century became the era of the first great English physicians, Thomas Sydenham and his followers, men who learnt the art of medicine by their system of careful notes and by constant observation of symptoms and signs at the bedside of the patient. How the New Learning came later in the century to Edinburgh, and by a less direct route, will be told in another chapter.[1]

[1] Chapter III.

CHAPTER II

THE RISE OF THE VOLUNTARY HOSPITAL MOVEMENT IN BRITAIN

THE MONASTIC HOSPITAL—THE REFORMATION—DISSOLUTION OF THE MONASTERIES AND DISAPPEARANCE OF THE MONASTIC HOSPITALS—THE ROYAL HOSPITAL MOVEMENT—THE VOLUNTARY HOSPITAL MOVEMENT.

To trace the origin of the voluntary hospital movement in Britain it is necessary to recall the part taken by the religious orders of the early Christian Church and to recognise the spiritual motive which impelled them to accept the burden of the poor and the sick and thus inspire the world with the hospital spirit. When St Augustine and his monks landed on the Kentish coast in the sixth century, bringing Christianity to Anglo-Saxon England, they founded at Canterbury the first Benedictine Monastery with its hospital, supplying the means to succour the destitute and appointing the " infirmarius " whose duty it was to attend to the sick. " The Church then held the gates of learning and they who entered were bidden to tread her path and hers alone."

The monasteries thus became centres of education, and medicine passed increasingly under the influence of the monks who read the medical treatises and other precious manuscripts preserved in their libraries; but for the time being medicine appears to have lost its progressive and inquisitorial character. They learnt the properties of herbs and the mixing and dispensing of drugs and, as clerical physicians, many of them attained a high reputation for experience and skill. The surgery of the monastery was in the hands of the barbers. Medical practice ceased to be based on independent observation and was conducted largely by rule. Along with this was blended the spiritual means of acquiring health, as the hospital attached to the monastery was " an ecclesiastical not a medical institution. It was care rather than cure : for the relief of the body, when possible, but pre-eminently for the refreshment of the soul." [1] Moreover, the practice of physic, hampered by superstition, often consisted in the use of potions and charms : these were the days of belief in the efficacy of relics, and pilgrimages were made to the shrines containing them. Treatment was probably considered more effective because it was practised by priests and administered on consecrated ground.

The inmates of the monastic hospitals, unlike those of the hospitals of modern times, were mainly the aged and the disabled, unfit for work and for taking an active part in the life of the community. Many suffered from chronic and often incurable diseases, the acute type of illness rarely coming under treatment. The hospitals were frequently used also as places of refuge, as rest-houses for travellers, as temporary lodgings for the able-bodied and as billets for soldiers. They provided accommodation for old retainers and pensioners : they were, in effect, hostels as well as hospitals. In many cases abuses began to creep into their methods of administration.

Of such a type was the Pre-Reformation hospital in Britain, and with its disappearance along with the monastery the people were deprived of much that was helpful alike to body and soul. Further, as considerable employers of labour their dissolution largely increased the number of the unemployed class, thus adding to the vagrant population of the country. The monastic hospitals, therefore, undoubtedly performed a duty which no other organisation, save the State, could have satisfactorily fulfilled.

The action of Henry VIII, in the later years of his reign, in bringing about the dissolution of the monasteries and the secularisation of their property, was directed to free the nation and the Church from the papal supremacy. It was not his intention, nor indeed his wish, to destroy the hospitals as such, but rather to suppress all those under the supervision of the monastic houses. Thus the Hospital of St Cross at Winchester

[1] *Medieval Hospitals of England*, by Miss R. M. Clay.

survived but under a reformed system of administration. Throughout his life his attitude had not been unsympathetic towards an improvement in medical education and to him the profession was indebted for more than one progressive measure. The new intellectual movement had reached England in the later years of the fifteenth century before his accession to the throne and, as a patron of the Revival of Letters, Henry attracted to his Court the scholars who had brought from Italy the new spirit and a fresh interest in the study of Greek literature and of scientific medicine. William Grocyn, John Colet and Thomas Linacre, with their pupils and friends, Dutch Erasmus and Sir Thomas More, were amongst the learned men to whom he extended his favours. Science began again to influence medicine and Greek methods once more became the subject of careful first-hand study.

Amongst the earliest of the English Medical Humanists to restore Greek thought in England was Thomas Linacre, a classical student at Oxford. After visiting Bologna, Florence and Rome, he finally reached Padua where he studied medicine and took his doctor's degree. On his return to his native land he taught at Oxford, translated the writings of Aristotle and Galen, revealing to his fellow-countrymen the true sources of natural knowledge. In 1509, he became physician to Henry VIII and, through his influence, the monarch, in 1518, granted the charter of foundation of the Royal College of Physicians of London to which Linacre was elected as the first president. Henry founded also the Regius Professorships of Medicine at Cambridge (1540) and Oxford (1545); and by an Act of 1540 he united the incorporated company of barbers with the guild of pure or military surgeons, a union which, at first sight, might appear to be a retrograde step, but which nevertheless was the means of establishing an active educational and licensing body.

In London, the hospitals of St Bartholomew and St Thomas, as Church property, had suffered in the debacle, their rents and revenues being confiscated to the King. But the citizens raised their voices in protest against this suppression. So great were the sufferings of the poor, thus bereft of the means of obtaining charitable relief, that the Lord Mayor found it necessary, in 1538, to petition the King to restore these institutions for the benefit of the community. In reponse to this appeal he reapplied a portion of their revenues for this purpose and established them under secular control. Thus endowed and assisted by the contributions of the people of London, St Bartholomew's and St Thomas's were able to continue their work as hospitals available for medical and surgical aid to the sick poor. St Mary of Bethlehem—the notorious " Bedlam "—also survived the Reformation as an asylum for lunatics. Two new foundations, as a further part of the restoration scheme in the reign of Edward VI, Bridewell and Christ's Hospital—the former a House of Correction, the latter " the Blue Coat School " for education—completed the Royal Foundations.[1]

No organised attempt, however, was made to replace the monastic hospitals. Even the various Poor Laws enacted in the reign of Queen Elizabeth and the inauguration of the workhouse system for the aged and infirm with hospital wards attached, while marking a step forward in social organisation, failed to supply the skilled medical aid justly due to the sick poor of the nation.

The Royal Hospitals in London certainly helped to bridge the gap between the old monastic hospital system and the voluntary subscription movement of the eighteenth century, but their inadequacy to meet the needs of the nation requires no emphasis. During the visitations of the plague, which from time to time ravaged the country, the people had learnt from bitter experience the need of hospital accommodation and of suitable provision for the sick. In the years that had elapsed since the Reformation the State had not shouldered its responsibility, and even as late as 1700 it remained indifferent to the question of national hygiene : the Parliaments of the day had taken no steps to meet the situation. Accordingly when the demand for a hospital service became clamant at the end of the seventeenth century it was met by " the rekindling of the smouldering spirit of charity " in a spontaneous and

[1] Chelsea and Greenwich Hospitals were foundations of the seventeenth century.

voluntary movement on the part of those who were genuinely interested in the health of the nation, and charitably disposed towards the establishment of such a service.[1]

Broadly stated, the principle underlying the voluntary hospital system consisted in free-will subscriptions towards the construction of hospital buildings and their annual upkeep and maintenance; in their administration by voluntary management; and in the service of an honorary visiting staff of physicians and surgeons giving their skill gratuitously to the care of the patients who, in turn, received treatment without the exaction of payment. The voluntary hospitals were subject to no organised control from without, nor to any periodic inspection by State or other authority. In the course of time and through force of circumstances certain changes have been introduced, but the fundamental principle of the voluntary system has not been radically altered.

The voluntary hospital movement, once started, developed rapidly. Public appeals for raising subscriptions were anticipated, in a few instances, in the form of bequests and endowments from certain philanthropic persons. Examples of such private beneficence are supplied in the case of one or two hospitals in Ireland. Thus, Dr Steevens, in 1710, bequeathed his estate for the erection of a hospital near the city of Dublin, which, however, was not opened till 1734. The bequest of Miss Mercer of Dublin in the latter year had a similar destination. Again John Radcliffe, who died in 1714, left a portion of his fortune to found an Infirmary at Oxford, and John Addenbrooke of Cambridge, in 1719, acted in the same way, though years elapsed before these two schemes were realised. Thomas Guy in his lifetime declared his intention to build and equip a hospital which he planned for the accommodation of 435 patients, and Guy's Hospital was opened in London, in 1725, with 60 patients, shortly after his death.

In the foundation of the Westminster Hospital, however, there was established the first voluntary hospital raised by general subscription for the reception, without payment, of

[1] *The Romance of the British Voluntary Hospital Movement*, by A. Delbert Evans and L. G. Redmond Howard. (London: Hutchinson & Co., Ltd.)

the sick poor. Small premises were acquired in "Petty France," in 1719, and the first patient was admitted in the following year. Lanesborough House at Hyde Park Corner was converted into St George's Hospital and opened as such in 1734. The London Hospital in Whitechapel Fields (1741), and the Middlesex in Soho (1745) completed for the time being the most important of the voluntary institutions in London.[1]

The erection of hospitals, however, was not confined to the metropolis. The movement spread throughout provincial England. In the first half of the century hospitals were erected at Bristol and at York, Exeter and Bath, and in 1753 the Infirmary at Newcastle-upon-Tyne was opened.

At the time of the Reformation in Scotland—a quarter of a century later than in England—many of the Church lands and revenues were confiscated to the Crown. Some of the more important religious houses had already suffered either in the natural process of decay or during preceding English invasions. Amongst the latter were the Abbeys of Kelso, Dryburgh and Melrose; and, in Edinburgh, the Collegiate Buildings of St Mary-in-the-Fields and the Monastery of the Black Friars. The Black Friars' buildings along with those of the Grey Friars were finally destroyed by the mob at the Reformation in 1559, the hospitals attached to them suffering the same fate. Later on, a Charter of 1567 placed their properties and their endowments at the disposal of the Town Council, and the use to which they were applied will be told in another chapter. But Trinity Church and Hospital, standing at the foot of Leith Wynd beneath the south-western face of the Calton crags, remained, and the provost and prebendaries, with easy conscience, renouncing the old faith and adopting the new, continued for many years to enjoy the income of their benefices.[2] Founded by Queen Mary of Gueldres in 1460, the Trinity Hospital was gifted, in 1567, to the Town Council after the Reformation by the Regent Moray, to be administered by them

[1] The hospitals of Charing Cross, University College, King's College and St Mary were founded in the early part of the nineteenth century as part of the movement in medical education.

[2] *Edinburgh, 1329-1929*. (Oliver & Boyd, Edinburgh, 1929.)

"for honest poor and impotent persons and advanced in years." Owing to its ruinous condition, however, it was then rebuilt on the west side of the Leith Wynd in close proximity to the Church and on its new site continued to serve its purpose till the nineteenth century.[1]

The voluntary movement developed more slowly in Scotland than it had done south of the Border. The little hospital in Robertson's Close, Edinburgh, the nucleus of the Royal Infirmary, was opened in 1729; in Glasgow the Town's Hospital was erected in 1733 by public subscription, in response to the demand for some provision for the destitute poor, the members of the Faculty of Physicians and Surgeons giving their services gratuitously; the Royal Infirmary in Glasgow was opened in 1749. The original Aberdeen Infirmary containing six beds was ready for occupation in 1742 and was visited daily by the professor of medicine and his pupils. Dumfries and Galloway Infirmary was built in 1778, Montrose Infirmary in 1782 and that at Dundee in the closing decade of the century.

The voluntary hospital movement was, therefore, the response of the people to a widespread desire to see the poor of the nation provided with suitable accommodation and with skilled medical and surgical service in time of sickness and injury. Throughout the length and breadth of the land the revival of the spirit of charity expressed itself in the building of hospitals with that single purpose in view. It was the reawakening of a spiritual movement which in medieval times was exemplified in the monastic hospitals. But in Edinburgh, as a future chapter will reveal, the appeal was made on a broader basis. Through the enthusiasm and far-sighted vision of a small group of men, inspired by the example of the town of Leiden in Holland, the hospital was founded not only for the care of the sick poor but as an essential and integral part of the new medical school developing in association with the university. Although the old Universities of Oxford and

[1] The buildings were demolished in 1848 when the Waverley Station was built. The funds of the old endowment are still administered by the Town Council for aged beneficiaries. Many of the stones of Trinity Church were preserved and used in the construction of Trinity College Church in Jeffrey Street.

Cambridge conferred degrees in medicine and their regius professors delivered occasional lectures on physic, they were content to regard that instruction merely as part of the equipment of the well-educated scholar. In Glasgow, the University in 1714 revived the old chair of medicine, created in 1637, and founded a chair of anatomy and botany in 1720, appointments to which were of a purely titular character. But in none of these university centres was a hospital at the same time founded to provide the clinical teaching necessary to complete the education of the medical student. Twenty-six years elapsed before any real progress was made in establishing a medical faculty at Glasgow, and faculties of medicine at Aberdeen and St Andrews were creations of the nineteenth century.

CHAPTER III

THE MEDICAL SCHOOL AT LEIDEN, 1575-1738

HOLLAND AND THE MEDICAL SCHOOL AT LEIDEN IN THE SEVENTEENTH CENTURY—IN THE EIGHTEENTH CENTURY DURING THE PERIOD OF BOERHAAVE.

In the closing years of the sixteenth century peace had settled upon the Northern Netherlands. The Dutch under the leadership of William the Silent, Prince of Orange, had freed these provinces from the Spanish yoke, Philip II of Spain having failed to impose his will upon those who had fought for national independence and liberty of conscience. For twelve weary months, during a period of intense hardship and suffering the citizens of Leiden under their heroic burgomaster, Adrian van der Werf, had successfully defended the town and thereafter received the thanks and reward of a grateful leader. When offered by the Prince the temporary remission of taxation or the gift of a university, in recognition of their stern resistance, the citizens wisely chose the latter. Thus, in 1575, the University of Leiden was founded, the first of the universities of Holland: it antedated by seven years the creation of the College of Edinburgh, on which Leiden was destined, more than a century later, to exercise such important and far-reaching influences.

In industry, in agriculture, in the arts and sciences, Holland flourished during the greater part of the seventeenth century. The period was her golden age, a century remarkable for such men as Grotius, the lawyer, and Spinoza, the philosopher; the brothers de Witt, the statesmen; the admirals, van Tromp and de Ruyter; Tasman, the navigator and explorer; Rembrandt and Jan Steen of Leiden and Vermeer of Delft, Frans Hals and Hobbema, the painters; the Elzevirs, the printers; and in science, Huygens, the physicist, van Leeuwenhoek, the microscopist, Swammerdam, the entomologist, and

Boerhaave, the physician. Leiden soon became an industrious and thriving provincial city, and the University, not long after its creation, attained an outstanding position amongst the universities of northern Europe, attracting to its several faculties the young men of many countries. With its Protestant foundation it placed no ban upon the enrolment of students of any religious faith and it selected its professors without distinction of nationality from those who had proved themselves most worthy of choice. But unlike the College of Edinburgh, Leiden at its creation included a faculty of medicine as an integral part of its *studium generale* and, within a very few years, the city became famous as a centre of medical education.

The earliest teachers in the faculty had been students at the great school of Padua and, imbued with its traditions, the young Dutchmen brought back to Holland the Hippocratic ideals of medicine and founded a school at Leiden. The locus indeed had changed from the sunlit plains south of the Alps, where the heat was tempered by the soft breezes of the Adriatic, to the cold bleak shores of the grey North Sea. But the spirit of scientific enquiry flourished in this new environment amongst a virile and industrious people and all the essentials then required for a medical curriculum were soon provided : chairs of botany, chemistry, anatomy, and medicine were founded, and a physic garden was planted in the large and airy courtyard of the Convent Infirmary. Pieter Paauw in the chair of anatomy built, in 1597, an anatomical theatre and furnished his museum ; and human dissection became a routine practice.

The teaching of anatomy was reflected in contemporary Dutch art and formed a popular and frequent subject on the canvases of some of the great painters of the seventeenth century. It is represented at Amsterdam in Rembrandt's "Dissection Scene" in which Tulpius, a pupil of Pieter Paauw, having removed the skull cap, has exposed the convolutions of the brain ; and again, in the same artist's famous "School of Anatomy" at the Hague. Portraits of physicians and governors of hospitals, dignified figures with their high ruffed collars and pointed beards, are also illustrations of the interest taken in the profession of medicine by the painters of that period.

The members of the young faculty at Leiden were men of vision, and from the inception of the movement they planned a coordinated scheme of study which combined university and hospital tuition. They introduced bedside instruction on lines similar to those employed in the hospital at Padua. For this purpose they claimed the privilege of apportioning a certain number of beds in the Convent Infirmary for clinical teaching and secured permission to make *post-mortem* examinations, when these were deemed necessary. Thus the medical school was created and, prior to 1600, although still in its infancy, it enrolled 128 students, of whom 13 entered from England: it was not till after 1600 that Scottish students of medicine enrolled in the medical faculty.[1]

The geographical position of Scotland played an important part in bringing the Scottish people in contact with the nations dwelling on the eastern shores of the North Sea, from the Scandinavian countries southwards to the English Channel. Although their relations were mainly of a commercial and industrial character they extended into other fields of human activity, relations strengthened by the soldier of fortune in war time and by the philosopher as the man of peace. From the East Coast ports of Scotland wool, coal and fish were the chief exports, and the old Burgh Records of Edinburgh contain numerous references to international business transactions and to the regulations enacted to control the amount of export from the country. In 1601, Dutch weavers were brought to Edinburgh to instruct the apprentices in the art of weaving and dyeing, and a woollen factory was established in the vicinity of Paul's Work at the north end of the Leith Wynd, and another in the Canongate.

A period of foreign education had long been part of the recognised training of such Scotsmen as were able to indulge

[1] *English-Speaking Students of Medicine at the University of Leiden*, by R. W. Innes Smith, M.D. Edin. (Oliver & Boyd, Edinburgh, 1932.)

in it. It became a European movement made possible through the common use of the more or less universal Latin speech. The Scot abroad was a familiar figure and proof of the high estimation in which many of them were held is seen in their appointment as teachers in foreign schools. Scottish scholars filled university chairs and sometimes administrative posts in a number of the universities of Western Europe, especially in France where, on completing their training, they were retained as professors of philosophy, of divinity and law. In medicine too, similar distinctions were conferred until the time arrived when the medical schools in Scotland were in the position to retain their distinguished sons.

In the seventeenth century Holland, with its pre-eminent repute in learning and scholarship, was a powerful attraction to both English and Scots. Students of law, desirous of seeking at the fountainhead the means of acquiring the knowledge that was not available at home, repaired to Leiden, Utrecht and Groningen, made famous by the writings of Grotius, as their predecessors in former years had gone to Paris and Orléans. The Scottish Presbyterians sought in Holland an asylum for that freedom of thought which they could not obtain in their own country. Refugee covenanters settled in Rotterdam which became their home, and Scots colonies and kirks were founded in more than one of the Dutch towns. With these well-established and generally friendly relations between the two countries it is not surprising that, when the medical school at Leiden became recognised as a valuable educational centre, the young Scotsmen should proceed thither to improve their professional training.

In the library of the University of Leiden the *Album Studiosorum*,[1] published in 1875, the tercentenary year of the University, is an encyclopædia of information from which can be gleaned many interesting facts relative to those who studied there during that long period. It does not, however, supply a perfectly accurate statement of the total number of students matriculating in each of the faculties: hence

[1] *Album Studiosorum Academiæ Lugduno Batavia.* (The Hague, 1875.)

the figures in this chapter purporting to give the number of students in the faculty of medicine are only *approximately* correct and must be so interpreted in the light of that knowledge. Amongst them also are the names of graduates in other schools who repaired to Leiden for a further course of study.[1]

With the beginning of the seventeenth century the number of students of medicine showed a definite and progressive increase, and in its first fifty years the English-speaking members amongst them comprised 9·6 per cent. of the total matriculating in the faculty. The Scotsmen were still few in number, but five of them were signatories of the Patent of 1656, when the physicians in Edinburgh made their third unsuccessful attempt, in the time of Cromwell, to found a College of Physicians in the city.

After the election of Franciscus Sylvius—to give him his Latin name—to the chair of medicine at Leiden, in 1658, a fresh impetus was given to the teaching of medicine and the reputation of the school became more widespread. During his tenure of the chair Sylvius more than justified the wisdom displayed by the curators in their selection. An enthusiastic teacher, he inspired his pupils: as a physiologist he studied the digestive processes: as a chemist he expounded the chemical basis of the physiological phenomena of the body. As a physician and as a teacher of clinical medicine Sylvius developed and extended the system of bedside instruction and insisted upon the regular attendance of his pupils in the wards: "I led my students by the very hand into the practice of medicine," he wrote. "I took them daily into the hospital for the purpose of seeing the sick, to whose complaints and other notable symptoms I directed attention, asking immediately afterwards what they had observed, their views as to the cause and proper treatment. . . . I pitted against each other those students holding different opinions."

During his professorship of nearly fifteen years, 1109 students enrolled in the faculty of medicine, the highest number in any single year being 110. Of English-speaking

[1] R. W. Innes Smith, *op. cit.*

students during this period there were 90, of whom 58 were Englishmen and 32 from Scotland, figures which clearly show that the popularity of Leiden as a medical school had considerably increased. Among his Scottish pupils was Archibald Stevensone—afterwards Sir Archibald—a Lothian Scot, who graduated at Leiden in 1659. One of the founders of the Royal College of Physicians of Edinburgh, in 1681, he was its first president. In the following year Sir Robert Sibbald was at Leiden. Of the twenty-one physicians who signed the Patent of Foundation of the Royal College of Physicians, nine had been students at Leiden and five of them during the professorship of Sylvius.

On the roll of the teaching staff of the University of Leiden is the name of Archibald Pitcairne, born in Edinburgh, the son of a bailie of the city and the proprietor of Pitcairne in Fife. Young Pitcairne graduated Master of Arts at Edinburgh and Doctor of Medicine at Rheims. A scholar, a man of pungent wit and an ardent Jacobite, he established his reputation as a physician of great ability and learning in his profession so that his name became well known beyond the confines of Scotland. In the autumn of 1691, the curators of the University of Leiden, faced with a vacancy in the chair of practice of physic and anxious to maintain the high standard of instruction, extended an invitation to Pitcairne. Having accepted the position he delivered his inaugural lecture on 26th April 1692. But the tenure of his professorship was brief. In the following year, after the close of the session, he was again in Edinburgh, and writing to the curators in December he tendered his resignation as an "unexpected obstacle"—his approaching marriage with the daughter of Sir Archibald Stevensone—prevented his return to Leiden. As Pitcairne had come to Scotland without permission, he was dismissed from his professorship on account of this "improper conduct." During the twelve months in which he occupied the chair, sixty-seven men enrolled in the faculty of medicine, amongst whom were John Monro, the father of Alexander Monro, *primus*; Richard Mead, a future physician to St Thomas's Hospital and a pioneer in the creation of Preventive State Medicine in England; and the young Dutchman, Hermann Boerhaave, destined in due course to occupy with such conspicuous success the chair of practice of physic at Leiden.

The commencement of the eighteenth century found the school of medicine approaching the zenith of its reputation as the chief centre of medical education in Europe. On the road to Haarlem between Leiden and the sea lies the little village of Voorhout, its church spire a conspicuous landmark in the flat polderland. In the village "manse" Hermann Boerhaave was born on the last day of December 1668, the son of the pastor of the Reformed Church, a man well versed in Greek, Latin and Hebrew. Both by family tradition and early education young Hermann was intended for the ministry, but, while still a boy, he developed an interest in natural science and, when engaged in his theological and philosophical studies at the University of Leiden, he read books on botany and chemistry and practised dissection on the vermin in his father's garden. He followed his own inclinations, studied medicine and, in order to graduate, went to the University of Harderwijk to receive his degree.[1]

During the years of waiting for practice at Leiden he studied mathematics, read the classics and the writings of Hippocrates, became proficient in a number of European languages and continued his scientific studies. With his perseverance and industry time never hung heavily on his hands: there were few idle hours in the daily life of this studious young Dutchman. His appointment to the lectureship in the institutes of medicine in 1701 gave him his first opportunity of showing his capabilities as a teacher and in 1709, on the death of Hotton, he was elected professor of the institutes and of botany. As curator of the botanic garden he was able to gratify his taste for flowers, adding to the collection of plants, many of them brought from different parts of the world: classifying and cataloguing them he compiled

[1] *Life and Writings of Hermann Boerhaave*, by William Burton, M.D., and articles in *Janus*, December, 1918, by E. C. van Leersum.

his *Index Plantarum*, a treatise which paved the way for the work of Linnæus who, several years later, spent a year at Leiden with Boerhaave from whom he received both help and encouragement. In those days the scientific subjects in the curriculum were considerably more circumscribed than they are today and dual professorships were not uncommon. For some men the teaching of physiology and botany and the supervision of the botanic garden might prove a sufficient tax upon their time and capacity. It was otherwise, however, with Boerhaave whose dynamic energy seemed equal to any task. In 1714, on the death of Bidloo, he accepted the chair of practice of physic and, two years later, added the professorship of chemistry to his other duties.[1]

In the chair of practice of physic and in the wards of the hospital his genius as a teacher found its fullest expression: in the rôle of an interpreter of Nature, rather than in that of a discoverer, the claim can be made that he was "the great preceptor of medicine" in the early part of the eighteenth century. As such, he made Leiden a Mecca especially for the English-speaking students of medicine who attended the school in greater numbers than at any previous time in its history; although during the fifteen years of the professorship of Franciscus Sylvius the total number of students from all countries was larger in proportion than in the period of Boerhaave.

In Edinburgh, at the dawn of the eighteenth century, the facilities for medical training were obviously inadequate. The University, nearly one hundred and fifty years old, had no medical faculty and was doing little to advance the study of medicine: three professors of medicine had been elected but none of them engaged in teaching. At old Surgeons' Hall, close by the High School Yards, anatomy was being taught, and the physicians conducted a dispensary at their Hall in Fountain Close at the foot of the High Street. But there was no hospital in the modern sense of the word, either in Edinburgh or elsewhere in Scotland. Coordinated effort did not exist: there was no real creative force at work, and the young

[1] In 1729 he resigned the chairs of botany and chemistry.

Scotsmen were disappointed with the insufficient means of training provided. So they turned their eyes longingly across the North Sea to the friendly country of Holland in which the university city of Leiden had already established a wide reputation.

The sea voyage to Holland in those days was uncertain, slow, often hazardous and, as a rule, uncomfortable. If the decision were taken to cross the sea from the Thames, a favourite route, the journey from Edinburgh to London was made by stage-coach, or on horseback which, if more rapid, was certainly more expensive. The voyage from the Thames was normally one of forty-eight hours, but the venture might occupy many days when unfavourable conditions of weather prevailed. Fishing smacks, in which cabin accommodation scarcely existed, sailing from Leith were a popular means of transit, and the ship's progress was often delayed. But on reaching port the Scots felt at home amongst a people with whom they had much in common.

To the young Edinburgh men, Holland with its low-lying, flat landscape, traversed by rivers and intersected by a network of canals, must have presented in its physical features a striking contrast to the hilly and mountainous land of their birth :

> While the pent ocean, rising o'er the pile,
> Sees an amphibious world beneath him smile ;
> The slow canal, the yellow blossom'd vale,
> The willow-tufted bank, the gliding sail,
> The crowded mart, the cultivated plain,
> A new creation rescued from his reign.[1]

Perchance in their daily walks they missed that vista of distant hills and sea with which their eyes had become so familiar at home.

At Leiden they found a hive of industry, with a busy anatomical department, a well-equipped chemical laboratory, a richly-stocked physic garden and a library ; and, what was so very important, a hospital in which, for nearly a hundred years, bedside instruction had been regularly carried

[1] *The Traveller* by Oliver Goldsmith, published 1764.

on. The Scots found themselves, too, amongst the youth of many nationalities: English—their old enemies—and Irish; Norwegians, Swedes, Danes and Dutch; French, Germans and Austrians; Russians, Poles and Turks; Dutch colonists from the East Indies and the Cape of Good Hope; British colonists from the West Indies and the North American continent. Truly a peaceful League of Nations assembled for a common purpose, and in the Latin language they possessed a common tongue for friendly intercourse.

The magnet that drew all these men to Leiden in those days was the personality of Hermann Boerhaave. While his manner was simple, unassuming, courteous and amiable, his appearance somewhat belied the real greatness of the man: well built, with a slight tendency to corpulence, his florid complexion and negligence in dress, almost amounting to shabbiness, suggested the rustic rather than the academic figure. But these externals were redeemed by his well-developed head and his piercing eyes, a distinctive feature expressing the keen intelligence which lay behind them. Conversing fluently in English, French and German, he lectured with facility in Latin. A brilliant expositor, clear and logical, he held the attention of his audience in the classroom and inspired his pupils; and grafted upon the scientific subjects in the curriculum was bedside instruction in the hospital. There Boerhaave was at his best. He taught the importance of symptoms and of careful enquiry into the case history, the accurate observation of clinical signs and the drawing of conclusions only from the facts thus ascertained. He revived the teaching of Hippocrates—the return to the study of Nature—a method so familiar to the student of today, but to the men of those far-off times a new experience, a revelation, something to be copied and emulated. It was the pattern upon which the teaching of medicine in the Edinburgh School was founded.

When the pages of the *Album Studiosorum* are studied from 1709 to 1738, a period of almost thirty years covering Boerhaave's professorships, they reveal how greatly he attracted the men from the English-speaking countries. The total number enrolled in the faculty of medicine from all countries during the Boerhaavian era reached approximately 1919: of these, 659—or more than one-third of the whole—were English-speaking, of whom 340 entered from England and Wales, 205 from Scotland, 107 from Ireland, and 7 from the British Colonies in the New World. Among those who sat on the benches in Boerhaave's classroom in the autumn of 1718 were three young men who retained a very vivid memory of their experience and who, before many years had elapsed, were to play their part in making the history of medical education. One of them was the Dutchman, Gerhard van Swieten, who was called by the Empress Maria Theresa from Leiden to Vienna, where he established clinical teaching, then unknown in that city. The other two youths were Alexander Monro, the son of John Monro who had studied under Pitcairne when the latter was at Leiden, and John Rutherford, a brother Scot. The part they were destined to take in the creation and progress of the School of Medicine in Edinburgh along with Andrew St Clair, Andrew Plummer and John Innes, pupils of Boerhaave two years later, will form the theme of another chapter.

Boerhaave described no new disease: his name is not associated with any new method of diagnosis nor with the discovery of any particular clinical phenomenon. His chief contributions to medical literature were his *Aphorismi* and the *Institutiones Medicæ* which represented the medical knowledge of the period and which guided and controlled medical teaching at Edinburgh for nearly fifty years. They have long lost their value and are but dusty volumes on the topmost shelves of academic libraries. Even the name of their author remains unknown to most of the younger generations; but of the many thousands who have qualified in the Edinburgh school in the years which have since elapsed, all have been, unconsciously perhaps, influenced by the traditions of Leiden, handed down by their teachers from one generation to another.

Upon his death in 1738, at the age of sixty-nine, honoured by his fellow-countrymen, a Fellow of the Royal Society, London, and of *L'Académie Royale des Sciences*, Paris, the supreme attraction of the Leiden school passed away. Notwithstanding the reputation of Albinus, as anatomist and surgeon, and of Gaubius, the chemist, who continued to draw many English-speaking students to Holland, the matriculation roll during the years following Boerhaave's decease all too clearly tells this tale. And when the five closing years of the eighteenth century were reached, the matriculates in medicine averaged annually twenty-six in number, among whom appear the names of a solitary Englishman and of one American.

Thus, through the school at Leiden, the Hippocratic tradition came to Edinburgh, handed on to the first teachers in its medical school by an inspiring figure who imbued them with his enthusiasm and with the desire to follow in his footsteps. At Leiden, too, they learnt the value of a combination of university and hospital education, correlating the study of clinical medicine with the other branches of medical learning ; and they were taught to recognise that accurate observation and experience at the bedside were the basic principles of all medical practice.

CHAPTER IV

THE FOUNDATION OF THE EDINBURGH SCHOOL OF MEDICINE

THE PHYSIC GARDEN, 1676—THE ROYAL COLLEGE OF PHYSICIANS OF EDINBURGH, 1681—SIR ROBERT SIBBALD AND SIR ANDREW BALFOUR—THE FIRST PROFESSORS OF MEDICINE, 1685—THE ANATOMICAL THEATRE AT SURGEONS' HALL, 1697—JOHN AND ALEXANDER MONRO—THE FOUNDATION OF THE FACULTY OF MEDICINE, 1726.

DURING the second half of the seventeenth century, when some of the events just recorded were making the school of medicine at Leiden famous, a number of the physicians and surgeons in Edinburgh, impressed by what they had seen and learnt during continental travel and study, determined to raise the status of the profession in the city and to introduce some reform in the measures employed in educating the student of medicine.

Since the incorporation of the Barber-Surgeons in Edinburgh in 1505, and their enrolment among the Incorporated Crafts of the Burgh, instruction in surgery and the license to practise in the city and suburbs had become the privilege of that body. The apprentices had to show evidence that they could read and write: they acquired a superficial knowledge of anatomy and they gained their clinical experience in the practice of their masters. Other classes of practitioner developed in the country: the apothecaries who received a civic status through alliance with the surgeons; the military surgeons who served with the army; and the physicians, many of them men of considerable attainments who, as a rule, had been trained on the Continent and received their degrees from foreign universities. There remained, in addition, the innumerable body of quacks and charlatans.

About the year 1670 two physicians in Edinburgh, Robert Sibbald and Andrew Balfour, keenly interested in the study of botany, were successful in establishing a Physic Garden, securing a plot of ground close to the Abbey of Holyroodhouse where many medicinal plants were grown. But five years later the garden was transferred to Trinity Hospital, a lease of the ground being granted by the Town Council for nineteen years. In 1676 the Council appointed as keeper James Sutherland, a herbalist, who had been in charge of the physic garden at the Abbey, granting him a yearly salary of £20 and "joining his profession of botany with the other professions taught in the Town's College."[1] Thus a distinct step forward was made in effecting some improvement in medical education.

During the same century the physicians in the city had made three abortive attempts to found a College of Physicians, but it was not till 1681 that success finally crowned their efforts when a Patent was obtained from Charles II for the erection of a Royal College. The Charter granted them authority to examine and license those desirous of practising physic in Edinburgh and the suburbs and, in a special clause, it prevented the magistrates from permitting anyone to open an apothecary's shop until the College, by examination, was satisfied that the applicant possessed the necessary knowledge of drugs. But the Charter contained a further important clause, which prohibited the College from founding a school in which to teach the Art of Medicine, an enactment in all probability postponing for a number of years the creation of the Edinburgh Medical School.

Robert Sibbald, who was the mainspring of the movement which resulted in the successful foundation of the College of Physicians, was a man of enterprise and energy, a member of the family of the Sibbalds of Balgonie in Fife. He received part of his medical education at Leiden and Paris and graduated at the University of Angers. His literary and

[1] The Town's College was the original designation of the University of Edinburgh. The year 1676 has been accepted as the date of the foundation of the chair of botany in the University; but Mr John Macqueen Cowan, in *Notes from the Royal Botanic Garden* (Edinburgh, 1933), produces evidence to show that it was not till 1st February 1695 that the Town Council actually elected James Sutherland as professor of botany.

scientific contributions were numerous and varied, ranging from historical descriptions of the Kingdom of Scotland, geographical, antiquarian, ecclesiastical and political, to his memoirs on the natural history of the whales frequenting the Scottish waters, including that of *Balænoptera Sibbaldi*, appropriately named after him. Andrew Balfour, his friend and senior in years, also claimed connection with the county of Fife. Studying in London, Paris and Padua, he ultimately graduated at the University of Caen. Both men were knighted and each in turn was elected president of the Royal College of Physicians.

Four years after the foundation of the Royal College, the Town Council, in 1685, at the instigation of the physicians, elected three of the Fellows as professors of medicine in the Town's College—Sir Robert Sibbald, James Halket and Archibald Pitcairne, joint professors of the theory and practice of medicine;[1] but, beyond assigning them convenient rooms for their accommodation, the appointments remained purely titular: there was no salary attached to the chairs nor apparently was any instruction imparted.

So far so good! But something much more concrete was necessary before a teaching school was established in the city. Ten years after the appointment of the three professors of medicine a fresh impetus was given to this laudable movement which, in the interval, seemed to suffer from the lack of properly directed control. On this occasion the impetus came from the Incorporation of Surgeons which, being granted a Patent from William and Mary, ratified by an Act of the Scots Parliament in 1695, was empowered to license qualified surgeons and apothecaries to practise throughout the whole south-eastern area of Scotland instead of, as formerly, merely within the city and suburbs of Edinburgh.[2] This extension necessitated the provision of a greater supply of anatomical material for purposes of instruction. Accordingly

[1] The Town Council, as the patrons of the Town's College by the Charter of James VI, had the sole right of creating professorships in the city until the Universities (Scotland) Act, 1858.

[2] The Medical Act of 1858 finally removed the old territorial restrictions confining licenses to practise within certain areas.

the Incorporation petitioned the Town Council for bodies for dissection: this was granted on the condition that the surgeons provided an anatomical theatre before the term of Michaelmas, 1697, a condition duly fulfilled. Surgeons' Hall with its anatomical theatre, which became the cradle of the Edinburgh School of Anatomy, was erected in the south-east corner of the old Black Friars' property just within the boundary formed by the Flodden Wall. When the theatre was first opened, dissections were conducted by several members of the Incorporation in turn, but in 1705 a new system was introduced whereby the entire duty was assigned to one of their number. On application to the Town Council for pecuniary assistance, a yearly payment of £15 was granted and the first lecturer and his successors were designated by the Town Council as "Professors of Anatomy in this City and College."

The name of Monro will always be inseparably linked with the story of the foundation of the medical school of Edinburgh and with the early days of the Infirmary, and "to John Monro belongs by right the honourable title of 'Father of the Edinburgh Medical School.'" Born in 1670, the third son of Sir Alexander Monro, of Bearcrofts, in the county of Stirling, John Monro became apprenticed to William Borthwick, surgeon in Edinburgh; and later, following the example of other young men of the period he went to Leiden where, as already related, he studied under Pitcairne who occupied the chair of practice of physic. Accepting a commission as surgeon in the army Monro served for a time in Belgium with the Forces commanded by William III. During leave of absence he married his cousin and, in 1697, his son Alexander was born in London. Having resigned his commission, at the age of thirty, John Monro returned to Edinburgh in 1700, joined the Incorporation of Surgeons—of which he was made Deacon in 1712-13—and commenced practice as a surgeon-apothecary in a house in Bailie Fyfe's Close, off the High Street. Impressed by what he had seen in Holland and Italy he constantly pondered over a scheme to establish a "medical seminary" in Scotland.[1]

Recognising the talents of his son Alexander, who early showed evidence of exceptional ability and industry, John Monro gave him an education to fit him to participate in the project so near his heart. After attending the Arts classes in the University young Alexander was apprenticed to his father and received such instruction in anatomy and botany as was then available in Edinburgh. In 1717, he worked under William Cheselden, the anatomist and surgeon in London, and showed considerable skill as a dissector. In Paris he studied surgery and then proceeded to Leiden, where he became a favourite pupil of Boerhaave. Returning home in the autumn of 1719, he was examined and admitted a member of the Incorporation of Surgeons and, in the following January, was unanimously recommended by his brethren of the Incorporation as the teacher of anatomy at Surgeons' Hall. The Town Council then appointed him "Professor of Anatomy in the City and College." Thus at the age of twenty-two, Alexander Monro commenced his lectures in October, 1720, with a class of fifty-seven students.[2]

During the first five years of his professorship 313 students attended his class. In 1725, there was a repetition of the rumours, circulated a few years earlier, that the graves in the Grey Friars' Churchyard were being violated and the bodies removed to Surgeons' Hall, an act which so aroused the indignation of the populace that the building was threatened with destruction. To safeguard the contents of his museum Monro petitioned the Town Council for appropriate accommodation within the University and, the request being readily granted, anatomy was taught for the first time in the city within academic walls.

Meanwhile the physicians, refusing to be daunted by the lack of response to their previous efforts, petitioned the Town Council to appoint in 1713 James Crawford, a graduate of

[1] *The Monros of Auchinbowie*, by John Alexander Inglis. (T. & A. Constable, Edinburgh, 1911.)

[2] *The Edinburgh School of Anatomy*, by John Struthers.

Leiden, and a Fellow of the Royal College, to the chair of chemistry and medicine in the University; and in 1724 they obtained the election of William Porterfield, another of their Fellows, to the professorship of the institutes and practice of physic. But again there is little or no evidence to show that either of them discharged the duties of his office. It is clear, however, from the records of the University that Crawford was recognised as a member of the Senatus. He accompanied the students to the Kirk and, along with his colleagues, he signed the Commission appointing Principal William Wishart as the representative of the University at the General Assembly of the Church of Scotland.

The closing act of this somewhat protracted drama was now to be staged. Four other pupils of Boerhaave had recently returned from Leiden—John Rutherford, Andrew St Clair, Andrew Plummer and John Innes. Licensed to practise by the Royal College of Physicians and admitted as Fellows in 1724, they proceeded to purchase, as a chemical laboratory, a house adjacent to the College Garden, an open space which had been part of the old Kirk-o'-Field on the east side of the College buildings. With the consent of the Town Council they planted medicinal herbs in the garden and, in the laboratory, they taught some of the branches of medicine.[1]

Following the translation of Alexander Monro to the University, these four physicians petitioned the Town Council to institute the Profession of Medicine within the College of Edinburgh and, in response to this appeal, the Council on 9th February 1726 " did unanimously constitute, nominate and appoint Andrew St Clair and John Rutherford, Professors of the Theory and Practice of Medicine, and Andrew Plummer and John Innes, Professors of Medicine and Chemistry in the College of Edinburgh with full powers to profess and teach and to examine candidates, and to do every other thing requisite and necessary to the graduation of doctors of

[1] Part of the College Garden had been previously used as a Physic Garden, but had become neglected by James Sutherland, the professor of botany, and by his successors, Charles and George Preston.

medicine."[1] This action was confirmed by the Senatus of the University on 12th October 1726, when it "accepted the Act of the Town Council and appointed these gentlemen 'Professors of Medicine' and the several branches thereof in the University, and conferred on them the right to deliberate and vote on College affairs with the other Professors."[2] So at long last an organised school of medicine and the medical faculty of the University were founded. Fifty years had elapsed since Sibbald and Balfour had planted the Physic Garden at Trinity Hospital in which James Sutherland instructed his pupils and "Botany was joined to the other professions taught in the Town's College."

It is difficult today to arrive at the true explanation of the long delay in promoting the interests of medicine as a part of the university system, when all the bodies concerned were favourably disposed towards effecting improvement in the methods of higher education. The Fellows of the Royal College of Physicians of Edinburgh, imbued with the willing spirit, but debarred by the terms of the Charter of 1681 from establishing a medical school, were seeking the help of the Town Council in the furtherance of their legitimate aims to advance the teaching of medicine; while the latter body, as patrons of the Town's College, with the sole right of creating professorships in the City and College, readily responded to the several appeals of the physicians by appointing professors. The Incorporation of Surgeons with its long-established privilege of instructing the surgeon-apothecaries was taking definite steps to improve its methods of teaching anatomy and was successful in obtaining from the Town Council professorships for its teachers. The Town's College which, by the terms of the Charter granted by James VI in 1582, was free to add the profession of medicine to the other liberal professions to be taught in the College, nevertheless maintained a passive attitude towards the several

[1] Records of Town Council, Edinburgh, 9th February 1726. On the same date Mr Joseph Gibson was elected professor of midwifery in the city. Although this date is accepted as that of the foundation of the chair in the University, Joseph Gibson did not teach students, confining his instruction to midwives.

[2] Minutes of Senatus of the University, 12th October 1726.

medical professorial appointments which the Town Council were then making.

This *laissez-faire* policy on the part of the University becomes more difficult to understand when it is recalled that during part of that period—1703 to 1716—it had at its head William Carstares, the broad-minded statesman under whose guiding hand the College was expanding and had come to acquire the status of a University. During his tenure of office as Principal, Carstares laboured to raise the standard of learning in the College, modelling the system on the methods of the universities of Holland, of which he had intimate personal knowledge; and, through his influence, the faculty of arts was founded and new chairs were added in the subjects of divinity and law. But medicine, with so many of Boerhaave's pupils back from Leiden, received no encouragement from the University which was improving its standard of learning in the other faculties. Its records are silent concerning the duties of the several professors of medicine: the Senatus merely confirmed the appointment of Sibbald, Halket and Pitcairne in 1685 and, in 1726, accepted the Act of the Town Council in electing four professors with full powers. Even the appointment of Alexander Monro to the chair of anatomy is not mentioned in the minutes of the Senatus.

It was not till the teaching of medicine had become definitely organised outside the University that any action was taken; only then were Monro and the four physicians brought within its walls and the faculty of medicine was founded in 1726. It is more than probable that in this final step may be seen the powerful influence of George Drummond, the personal friend of John and Alexander Monro, and the Lord Provost of the City, for the first time, in 1725-26.

There still remained the erection of a hospital to crown the efforts of John Monro to create a complete medical school.

CHAPTER V

THE FOUNDATION OF THE INFIRMARY, 1729

THE APPEAL OF JOHN MONRO — EDINBURGH IN THE EARLY EIGHTEENTH CENTURY—THE APPEAL BY THE ROYAL COLLEGE OF PHYSICIANS—GEORGE DRUMMOND, LORD PROVOST—THE HOSPITAL IN ROBERTSON'S CLOSE—THE PHYSICIANS AND SURGEONS TO THE HOSPITAL—CLINICAL INSTRUCTION—THE FIRST BOARD OF MANAGEMENT—THE SURGEONS' HOSPITAL.

AFTER John Monro had seen his son launched on his career as a teacher of anatomy in Surgeons' Hall, he proceeded to arouse the interest of his fellow-citizens in the establishment of a hospital in which the practice of physic and surgery might be studied. For this purpose he issued, in 1721, an appeal in the form of a pamphlet in which he set forth the necessity for such an institution along with proposals for raising a fund to build and equip it.[1] Although published anonymously, there seems little doubt that the pamphlet was inspired by the elder Monro and that in all probability it was written by young Alexander.[2] In the first report of the managers of the Infirmary, printed in the autumn of 1730 and prepared at their request by Alexander Monro, then one of their number, this pamphlet is not only referred to but is actually quoted :[3]—

As Men and Christians we have the strongest Inducements, and even obligations to this sort of Charity, as it is warmly recommended and injoyned in the Gospel as one of the greatest Christian Duties : That Humanity and Compassion naturally prompt us to relieve our

[1] Notwithstanding a careful search, the writer has been unable to find a copy of this pamphlet.

[2] Bower, in his *History of the University of Edinburgh* (1817), vol. ii, p. 186, ascribes its authorship to Dr Monro : Sir Alexander Grant, in *The Story of the University of Edinburgh* (1884), vol. i, p. 305, also credits Monro with the authorship. In neither instance is the Christian name stated, but from the context probably Alexander is referred to.

[3] *An Account of the Rise and Establishment of the Infirmary*, etc. (1730.)

Fellow Creatures when in such deplorable Circumstances as many are reduced to, Naked, Starving, and in the outmost Distress from Pain and Trouble of Body and Anguish of Soul ; That as the Relief of these is a Duty, so it is no less Advantage to a Nation, for as many as are recovered in an *Infirmary* are so many working Hands gained to the Country : That students in Physic and Surgery might hereby have rather a better and easier Opportunity of Experience, than they have hitherto had by studying abroad, where such Hospitals are, at a great charge to themselves, and a yearly loss to the Nation : And as a Proof of the whole, they appealed to the good effects of the Infirmaries in all other Civilised Nations.

The appeal unfortunately met with no success and this effort on the part of the Monros, having failed to receive the support it deserved, was in consequence abandoned. But the seeds of a great idea had been sown which were to bear fruit at no distant date.

It is perhaps difficult today to visualise Edinburgh at that period. Then and for many years thereafter it presented the features of a medieval town, enclosed within the narrow confines of its engirdling wall. Standing between the hills and the sea, crowning the western half of the rocky ridge on which it was built, the city extended from the Castle Rock down the long slope to the Netherbow Port at the foot of the High Street. Eastwards from the Netherbow, and without the boundary wall, lay the Burgh of Canongate, still a fashionable garden-suburb, reaching to the low ground at the Abbey Close and Palace of Holyroodhouse. From the High Street, with its lofty tenements occupying the crest, the densely packed wynds and closes descended in more or less parallel lines towards the bottom of the valley on either side. On the north, the more precipitous descent, with the marsh-land and the Nor' Loch below, formed Nature's barrier against enemy attack ; but on the south and east the winding Flodden Wall climbing the higher ground beyond the Grass-market and Cowgate partially encircled the city.

Within these circumscribed limits dwelt the twenty-five to thirty thousand inhabitants of the Burgh, occupying the tall " lands " or tenements, " piled deep and massy, close and high," rising to ten or twelve storeys on either side of the narrow wynds, their upper windows commanding a glorious prospect of hill and pasture-land and sea. Insalubrious and overcrowded, these were the homes of nobles and commoners, of wealthy and poor, of those in professions and those in trade, of the rogues and the ne'er-do-weels. The torches of the linkmen illuminated the streets after darkness had fallen. In the houses there was little daylight or ventilation, save in the upper flats: water had to be carried in pitchers from the tap-wells in the High Street: there was no drainage system, the filth and the garbage being evacuated at curfew by discharging it from the windows into the passageway beneath, to the discomfiture of the townsfolk returning to rest and to the gratification of the dogs and pigs that roamed at large on the cobbled causeway.

In these unattractive surroundings, then as now town life had its amusements and pleasures, at least on six days of the week, with Sunday under the watchful eye of the city patrol. There was horse racing on the sands, tennis at the Water Gate Close by Holyroodhouse, golf and archery on the Links of Leith, and cock-fighting in the pits. The coffee-houses and taverns were popular resorts both for business and pleasure, and heavy drinking characterised the convivial meetings. In the absence of a theatre, an occasional travelling company from England, frowned on by the Kirk, purveyed comedy or the drama. Society sought its pleasure too in the dance in the early evening "Assemblies," the ladies hooped, patched and powdered, in their sedan chairs, forgathering with their squires in the West Bow or in the incommodious apartments in Assembly Close.

The newspapers of the day were insignificant sheets issued twice or thrice in the week, containing little information beyond a belated London letter and a few advertisements. With the transference of the Scottish Parliament to Westminster, many of the nobles and commoners with their families resided in London, so that the social life and trade of the town suffered a corresponding loss. The capital still retained the Law Courts in the Parliament House and it remained the meeting place of the General Assembly of the Church of Scotland, the interest in its particular affairs increasing when, after the Union, politics no longer had their former attraction for the people.

For many years the civic authorities had allocated a part of the revenue for the benefit of the poor and had appointed a physician and surgeon to attend them when required. Since 1682, the Royal College of Physicians had also provided medical assistance for necessitous cases in the city and suburbs, and had in that year delegated two of the Fellows to undertake this duty. The practice was regularly maintained and when, in 1704, the College acquired its Hall in Fountain Close, nearby the Netherbow Port, two physicians attended the Dispensary there on three afternoons in the week. That the College regarded the attendance in the light of a serious obligation is evident from the fact that a fine was exacted from those Fellows who failed to be present at the specified hours, the money being utilised in the purchase of medicines for the patients. But the physicians frequently found themselves hampered in their work owing to the prevailing insanitary conditions and the lack of suitable accommodation for, and supervision of, the sick, which so often rendered their efforts unavailing.

In 1725, therefore, they launched the second and successful appeal, enlisting the sympathy of a number of well-disposed persons to whom they made known their desire to see a hospital erected in Edinburgh. Steps were then taken to raise the necessary subscriptions. In the autumn of that year, George Drummond, just elected Lord Provost, gave his support to the scheme and, further, made the proposal that some of the shares of a moribund Fishery Company, of which he was a manager, might be diverted as a nucleus of the fund, the shares to be assigned for this purpose to Mr David Spence, secretary to the Bank of Scotland. The Lord Provost's suggestion was readily adopted.

An interesting sidelight is thrown on this proposal in another anonymous pamphlet printed in Edinburgh in the form of " A Letter from a Gentleman in the Country to his

Friend at Edinburgh." [1] This method of ventilating individual views on current topics was not uncommon at that period and, in the early days of the Infirmary, more than one such letter was circulated concerning its affairs. Letters to the Editors of the news-prints had not then become the vogue they are today. In this instance the writer expressed his pleasure on learning that the proprietors of the Fishery Stock were still so public-spirited as to desire to assign their shares to a charitable purpose. Of the three proposals that had been made, an addition to the stock of the Society for Propagating Christian Knowledge, the erection of a Linen Manufactory, or a Hospital for Sick and Wounded,—in each instance the principal motive being the good of the Country—the last seemed to the writer the most useful, necessary and likely to succeed. To support that object, therefore, he was willing to give up any small share he had in the Fishery Company.

A further method suggested for raising subscriptions was through the issue of a Voluntary Bond, each subscriber making himself responsible for the payment of £5 sterling in the event of the sum of £2000, deemed necessary for the purpose in view, being collected before the succeeding first Monday in June 1727. The contract was expressed in the following terms :[2]—

Da : Spence
Voluntar Bond
for erecting An Infirmiry
1727.

We subscribers considering that the Selling a fund for erecting and maintaining an Infirmary or Hospital for Sick Poor is a most Pious and Charitable Design and that the promoting and establishing of it in this City of Edinburgh will be of great Advantage and Credit to the Nation in General Do therefore hereby bind and oblige Us severally to pay to David Spence Secretary to the Bank of Scotland and his Successors in Office the Sums annexed to our several

[1] *Proposals for Employing the Remaining Stock of the Fishery, so as to be of Universal Use and Advantage to the Nation.* Edinburgh: Printed in the year MDCCXXV. National Library 2/196.

[2] A framed manuscript copy of one of the Voluntary Bonds is preserved in the Board Room of the Royal Infirmary; the Bond, dated 13th March 1729, is signed by Charles Alston, M.D.

Subscriptions And that on or before the first Monday of June next providing that the Sums now obliged for in this Bond and which shall be obliged for in any separate Bond and shall be contributed, appropriated assigned or transferred in Pursuance of this Charitable Design Shall on or before the said Monday of June next amount at least to the Capital Sum of Two Thousand pounds sterling money, which is computed to be the Smallest Original Fund that will be necessary for erecting and maintaining the said Infirmary or Hospital and which Capital Sum is to be secured and managed for the Purpose above mentioned according to such Regulations and Directions as shall be established and determined by a Plurality of Contributors, But if the Sums so to be sign'd for and contributed on or before the said first Monday of June next shall not extend to a Capital Sum of at least Two Thousand pounds sterling money then this present Obligation shall become void and Null, otherways to stand in full force In Witness whereof these Presents (written on stamp paper by James Spence Son to the said David Spence) are subscrived by Us at the Place and of the Dates annexed to our Several Subscriptions :—

Jo : Elphinstone advocate
for five pounds ster.

Will : Carmichael advocate
for five pounds sterling.

Hugh Dalrymple advocate
for five pounds sterling.

R. Hepburne writer to the Signet
for five pounds sterling.

Jo : Russell writer to the Signet
for five pounds sterling.

During the summer of 1727 the success of the appeal was such as to justify the physicians in making it more widely known to the public through the agency of the news-sheets. Accordingly the following advertisement agreed to at a meeting of the Royal College on 1st August 1727, appeared in *The Caledonian Mercury* on the eighth day of that month :—

The Royal College of Physicians having always shown such a particular concern for the sick poor, that for several years two of ye number have attended every week in ye Hall to give advice, and also medicine to some proper objects gratis, and now considering that yr is ane Hospital for the sick poor to be erected at Edinburgh ;

therefore, they for the encouragement of such a pious undertaking oblidge yrselves that ane or more of their number shall attend the said Hospital faithfully and freely, without any prospect of reward or sallary, until the stock of ye sd Hospital shall be so increased that it can afford a reasonable allowance for one or two Physicians for ye proper use, and the Colledge order this advertisement.

Signed, in yr name by ye President to be published.

The closing passage of this advertisement suggests that the physicians anticipated at some future period payment for services rendered to the Institution. Nor were these anticipations at fault. In 1751, when two "ordinary physicians" were appointed to attend the hospital daily, supplementary to those visiting monthly by rotation—as had been the arrangement prior to that year—an annual salary of £30 sterling was voted by the Board of Management to each of the two ordinary physicians.

The Fellows of the Royal College, conscious of the success that had attended their early efforts in promoting the hospital, and recognising that the time had come when they should make known the result of their appeal, summoned a General Meeting of the Contributors by means of another advertisement in the *Caledonian Mercury* of 5th February 1728 :—

The Subscribers or Contributors for erecting an Infirmary or Hospital for Sick Poor at Edinburgh are desired to be at a General Meeting on Monday, the nineteenth instant at 3 o'clock after Noon, at the Burrow-room ; to direct and order what is necessary for carrying on that charitable work. And the subscribers thereto who have not yet paid are intreated to pay up their Donations.

A gentle but evidently a necessary reminder of obligations incurred !

The scene of future operations now shifts from the Physicians' Hall in Fountain Close, where the early deliberations had been held, to the Burgh Room in the south-east corner of Parliament Square frequently used at that period as additional premises for the transaction of the business of the city. Archibald Macaulay, the Lord Provost, occupied the chair, and "the Gentlemen of the Royal College of Physicians then acquainted the meeting that the capital sum of £2000 designed for erecting the Infirmary was now subscribed." So runs the first Minute of the Royal Infirmary, dated 19th February 1728. A small committee of twelve were then appointed with instructions to call in the money already promised, to acquire the necessary accommodation for the patients and to prepare a plan for the direction and management of the hospital; and finally to report to a general meeting of the contributors.

Prominent among the members of this small committee was George Drummond—the second of that name to occupy the Civic Chair in Edinburgh.[1] Born near Blairgowrie in 1687, a member of an old and illustrious Scottish family, George Drummond, from the early age of eighteen till shortly before his death in 1766, was conspicuously associated with the public life of the capital. With his remarkable aptitude for arithmetic and mathematics he was intrusted, during the negotiations with England prior to the Union, with an important series of calculations upon rating and valuation in Scotland: the ability he then displayed led to his appointment as Accountant-General of Excise and, later, to that of Commissioner of Customs. As a staunch Protestant and Anti-Jacobite he raised a Company of Volunteers in the city during the rising of the '15 and marched to Sheriffmuir to take his place on the battlefield.

A man of wide vision, of high ideals and deep religious feeling, and of great business capacity combined with boundless energy, Drummond devoted himself to the public service. As City Treasurer and six times Lord Provost, he was closely identified during his life with nearly every movement for the welfare of Edinburgh—its sanitary and architectural improvements, the foundation of the medical faculty of the University and the Royal Infirmary, and the extension of the city. The drainage of the Nor' Loch and the building of the North Bridge, in spite of opposition, were schemes for which he arduously worked. Although as Past Grand Master he laid the foundation stone of the Bridge in 1763, he did not live to see it completed: when laid to rest in the Canongate

[1] The first, Sir George Drummond, was Lord Provost in 1683-84.

churchyard his fellow-citizens accorded him a public funeral.[1]

Towards the end of the year—on 16th December 1728—the contributors again met in the Burgh Room and proceeded to elect a large and representative committee of twenty-one members.[2] The personnel of this committee is of considerable interest as it constituted the basis on which future Boards of Management were founded. It is obvious that the contributors were desirous of impressing upon their fellow-citizens the importance of the hospital scheme and, in selecting the committee, were careful to choose those whose names not only carried weight and influence but were likely to gain the confidence of prospective subscribers.

The constitution of the committee was as follows :—The Lord President of the Court of Session, the Lord Justice Clerk, the Lord Advocate, the Lord Provost of Edinburgh, Mr Robert Dundas of Arniston, Advocate, Mr Charles Erskine of Barjarg, Advocate, Mr George Drummond, former Lord Provost, Mr James Nimmo, Dean of Guild, Mr Patrick Lindesay, former Dean of Guild; Doctors John Drummond, Francis Pringle, John Clerk, William Cochrane, Robert Lowis, John Innes, Andrew Plummer, John Learmont, and James Dundas, physicians; Deacon John Kennedy, Mr Alexander Monro, and Mr Robert Hope, surgeons; with Mr David Spence, Secretary to the Bank of Scotland, as Treasurer. There were thus represented on the committee such bodies as the Town Council, the Senators of the College of Justice, the Faculty of Advocates, the Royal College of Physicians, the Incorporation of Surgeons and the general body of Contributors, " classes or societies " which have continued to the present day to have representation on the Board of Management.

The committee decided to hold its meetings in John's Coffee House. Situated in the north-east corner of the

[1] *George Drummond, An Edinburgh Lord Provost of the Eighteenth Century*, by William Baird. (Edinburgh, 1912 : T. & A. Constable.)

[2] In the *History and Statutes of the Royal Infirmary*, 1749 and 1778, this is described as an Election of Managers. In the Minutes of the Infirmary this body is always referred to as the Committee, the word Managers never being employed until on and after 2nd February 1730.

Parliament Close, it was a favourite resort of the judges and lawyers of those days and popular too with the writers and clerks of the Parliament House who assembled there to drink the daily "meridian," the "elevenses" of modern times. The Coffee House continued to serve as the "Board Room" of the Infirmary until 1742, after the second hospital had been opened in Infirmary Street.

Not the least important of the duties of this committee was to call in the subscriptions. From the several references in the Minute-book, from time to time, the members were evidently very desirous of receiving the promised donations for the purpose of investment, the expenditure on the hospital being restricted to the current interest of the Stock subscribed. The General Assembly of the Church of Scotland had previously been approached by the physicians to encourage contributions from the congregations, and the Assembly had earnestly recommended that all the Parish Churches in Scotland should set aside a Lord's Day on which the collection should be made.[1] Thus originated "Infirmary Sunday" in the Churches, the practice remaining unbroken to the present day. The committee, however, found it necessary to communicate directly with the several Presbyteries and to remind them of the Act and Recommendation of the General Assembly. All the parishes in Edinburgh and suburbs then responded along with seventy-two others scattered throughout the length and breadth of Scotland, from Evie in Orkney to Wigtown in the south and, in the west country, the parishes of Largs and Dumbarton. Twelve of the Episcopal congregations in Edinburgh also contributed.

The Honourable the Ladies of the "Assembly" were again appealed to and agreed to arrange another "benefit night." When, in November 1730, the managers published the list of the original subscribers to the hospital, 354 names were attached in an appendix to their report, to which they tactfully yet wisely added these words: "Those who have probably

[1] Act and Recommendation for a voluntary Contribution to be applied towards erecting an Infirmary or Hospital for diseased Poor at *Edinburgh*. Edinburgh, May 11, 1728.

forgot their having subscribed or having assigned their shares of the Fishery Stock, will find their names under the proper Letter to remind them of it, the managers having forbore at this time to distinguish those who have not paid."

The choice of a suitable building to serve as the hospital fell finally upon a house in Robertson's Close, one of several steep narrow alleys on the southern slope of the Cowgate gorge. The agreement of leasehold between the committee and the Town Council was formally concluded on 7th April 1729. The house was acquired at an annual rent of £50 Scots or £4, 3s. 4d. sterling, the lease to run for nineteen years with a break every three years.[1] The "Cowgait," once the *via vaccarum* along which the cows wandered to their pasturage outside the old city wall and where trickled a tiny stream in Edinburgh's primitive days, lay at the bottom of the deep gorge or valley on the south side of the high ridge on which the city was built; and it extended from the Grassmarket eastwards to the Cowgate Port opposite the north end of the Pleasance. At one period in Edinburgh's history persons of high position and fashion were resident in the Cowgate district, in dwellings picturesquely outlined with their timber fronts and projecting galleries. The exact position of the little hospital in Robertson's Close is uncertain, but it stood near the head or south end and probably on the west side of the Close. In its vicinity lay the College Garden, the use of which, it is said, the professors of medicine granted to convalescent patients of the hospital.

The necessary alterations in the building were intrusted to Mr McGill, an architect in the city, and the advice of Deacon Wardrope, wright, was taken in connection with the fittings and furniture, all to be of the plainest description. The bedsteads were of wood, the mattresses of straw, and the sheets made of cotton covered with twilts.[2] Some months after the House was opened the Countess of Stair sent eighty ells [3] of Galloway White from which to make blankets. Candles provided the

[1] The value of £1 Scots was one-twelfth of the £1 sterling.
[2] Twilt or Quilt. [3] One Scots Ell = 37.2 inches.

only means of artificial illumination. There were no nurses, attractive in coloured gowns and starched caps, to welcome the patients: the matron and one servant constituted the entire domestic staff.

Early in July 1729 the arrangements were so far advanced that the committee felt justified in opening the "Little House." Consequently on the 24th day of the month the following momentous advertisement appeared in the news-prints; to quote from the *Caledonian Mercury* of that date:—

> The Committee appointed by the General Meeting of the Contributors for erecting a Hospital for Sick Poor at Edinburgh, having now fitted up a House and provided convenient accommodation for a certain number of Sick Persons, conform to the present Stock, Hereby give notice that upon Wednesday, the 6th of August next, a Physician and Surgeon will attend from 3 to 4 after Noon in the Infirmary at the Head of Robertson's Close, near the College, to receive such Persons as shall be judged proper objects of this Charity, and to give Advice and Medicines during their Sickness.

The notice closed with another admonition to those who had failed to respond to the previous request to pay their subscriptions.

On 6th August 1729, without fuss or ceremony the Infirmary of six beds, destined to become the largest voluntary hospital in the United Kingdom, was opened; and, on the same day, Elizabeth Sinclair, suffering from anæmia, and described in the ledger as from a Parish in Caithness, was admitted as the first patient. In the *Monthly Chronicle* of 18th August, appeared the following short sentence:—"An Infirmary or Hospital for the Sick was lately open'd at Edinburgh, being the First Hospital of that kind that ever was in Scotland."

John Monro's dream had at last taken substance—the medical school initiated and the hospital founded. In his peaceful old age, spent at his country home of Carolside, on the banks of the Leader near Earlston in Berwickshire, he was free to meditate with great satisfaction on the success of his scheme and upon the reputation achieved by his son Alexander. John Monro died in 1740, aged seventy years.

The supervision of the hospital and the care of its inmates were placed in the hands of a mistress or house-keeper and one servant, and very definite rules were prescribed for their conduct. Both women were to be free of the burden of children and the care of a separate family; and neither was to remain a night out of the house, or be absent when needed, without first obtaining leave of the visiting physician or surgeon. The word " nurse " finds no place in the rules of management issued in 1730. The nursing profession—the sisters and nuns—organised upon monastic and conventual lines had disappeared with the abolition of the hospitals, although its traditions had never completely died, as some of the regulations of the modern hospitals are founded on early English monastic life. But the nurse had ceased to be a voluntary helper and, in many instances, the equivalent was a badly paid charwoman. Although the mistress administered the medicines prescribed by the physicians, the term house-keeper more accurately expressed her position in the hospital. She bought the provisions and household necessaries and superintended the cleaning of the rooms, submitting her accounts each week to the visiting physician and surgeon so that they might judge of the suitability of the diet provided for the patients.

Mrs Nisbett was engaged as the first mistress at an annual salary of £4 sterling, but, representations having been made to the managers as to her extravagance, she was dismissed after careful enquiry before the hospital had been opened for a year. Mrs Waldie was appointed her successor at the same salary which later was doubled. When she assumed office the duty of comparing the inventory with the furniture in the hospital was intrusted to Andrew Plummer, and George Cunynghame, surgeon, members of the Board of Management, and was found to conform. At the same time there were in stock " 4½ lb. of small candles, 1 lb. great candles containing seven, about 2 carts of coal, 6 pecks of meal and 2 pecks in bread, 4½ of groats, a peck and a half of sowing seeds and 24 chappin bottles of ale." [1]

[1] Chappin or chopin: A Scotch measure = nearly one quart.

In the early days of the hospital the regulations for the admission of patients were of a simple character. Those in authority had no precedent to follow. It was a new adventure, but the underlying principle was the provision of assistance for the necessitous poor. On one point there was complete unanimity : the benefits were not to be restricted to the poor of Edinburgh and its suburbs. Those residing in any county or burgh, or indeed in any country, were to be attended to at the hospital, provided they were true and worthy objects of the charity and could produce, from a responsible person, a certificate of attestation of their honesty and poverty. From the first, therefore, there was a certain defined limitation as to the qualifications of the individual seeking treatment. Although no geographical limitations were prescribed, he or she must be genuinely poor. The suitability of the patient for indoor treatment naturally rested with the physician or surgeon in waiting, as they alone could judge of the appropriateness of the malady for treatment in the wards. During the first twelve months patients were admitted, not only from Edinburgh and its neighbourhood, but from such widely scattered areas in Scotland as Caithness, Peterhead and the Island of Mull.

During the first year in which the Little House was open thirty-five patients were under treatment, of whom nineteen were cured, five recovered sufficiently to attend to their ordinary affairs, five were dismissed either as incurable or for irregularities, and one died : five still remained in the hospital at the end of the year. In addition to these a number of out-patients received attention from the physicians and surgeons who gave advice daily at the hospital. During the second year thirty-seven in-patients were treated and, in 1733, the number had increased to forty-nine. The diseases under treatment included ague, scurvy, consumption, cancer and conditions causing paralysis.

The cost of upkeep during the first year, including repairs, the salaries of the mistress and servant and the maintenance of the patients, amounted to £97, 19s. 7d. and "two third parts of a penny sterling," so accurate was Mr Spence's accounting : the donations paid to the Treasurer had reached the sum of £2129, 17s. 7d., and one-sixth part of a penny sterling. During the second year the disbursements were only £84, 19s. 5⅚d. sterling, and the Capital Stock at Candlemas, 1731, had reached the sum of £2735, 15s. 3d. sterling. The financial position of the hospital, therefore, was sound.

A strong oak " Charity Box " with iron fittings, with two locks and " a hole in the top " was placed in the hospital to encourage patients and their friends to contribute to the funds of the Institution. One key was intrusted to Mr Spence, the Treasurer, the other to one of the physicians, and each was empowered to open the box when he pleased. On the first occasion, three months after its installation, it was found to contain £4, 6s. 6½d. sterling. The managers therefore resolved that it should be opened once weekly in future, " to prevent Rogues from entertaining a notion of valuable cash being in it and so expose the Infirmary to ane attempt of Robery."

The old Charity Box still remains as a relic of the Little House and, placed within the main entrance of the present Infirmary, it serves a similar useful purpose. When, in January 1932, Sir James Barrie, Chancellor of the University of Edinburgh, opened the Health Exhibition in the city in furtherance of the Bicentenary Extension Appeal of the Royal Infirmary he alluded, in the course of his remarks, to this relic of bygone days :—" The last, glorious culminating scene in the raising of the money ought certainly to have for its central figure the little old Charity Box of the Infirmary which, I am told, is still in action. We should be shown the Lord Provost dropping into that box the last of the 500,000 pound notes. By special arrangement with the Prime Minister tomorrow this will not be paper money, but a golden sovereign so that Scotsmen all over the world can listen in and hear the once familiar clink." [1]

That the claims of the Infirmary, this new venture, appealed even to those living at a distance and who could only with

[1] The Charity Box was attached to Stand 17 at the Health Exhibition in 1932, and at the Arts and Crafts Exhibition held for a similar purpose in April 1934 ; on both occasions a considerable sum of money was obtained by this means.

great difficulty receive its benefits—long before the days of stage coaches or railways—is evident from the following extract from Provost Macpherson's *Glimpses of Church and Social Life in the Highlands in Olden Times.* Of the people of Badenoch he writes :—

> Little as they could afford to spare at the time out of their scanty *sporrans*, collections in aid of that noble institution appear to have been periodically made in the Church of Kingussie. In a Minute of the Presbytery, of date 26th January, 1731, it is recorded that " Mr Wm. Blair did this day give in ten shillings sterling to the Moderator as the collection of Kingussie parish for the Infirmary at Edinburgh, to be transmitted." That similar collections were made in all the congregations within the bounds of the Presbytery appears from the following entry in the Presbytery records of date 27th April, 1731—" This day the collections for the Infirmary at Edinburgh were delivered to Mr Lewis Chapman to carry south, viz. : From Aberfeldy £7 : 4 : od. ; from Kingussie, £6 ; from Kirkmichael, £7 : 4 ; from Alvey, £6 ; from Cromdale, £13 : 16 ; and from Duthil, £18 ; and the said Mr Lewis Chapman was appointed by the Presbytery to deliver the said money to David Spence, secretary to the Bank of Scotland, and get his receipt therefor."

For many years the attendance of the medical and surgical staff was conducted on a system of rotation. The Fellows of the College of Physicians, on the eve of the opening of the hospital, " considering that the Infirmary is now in readiness of receiving patients, and that it will be necessary that they attend the same, doe therefore unanimously agree to attend the Infirmary in their turns for the space of a fortnight, until some settled method be agreed upon . . . "[1] So the Fellows and Licentiates visited in the order of their seniority on the Roll of the College, each physician attending for the period of a fortnight ; and, when the roster was exhausted, the same process was repeated. As the Roll, in 1729, contained the names of twenty-four Fellows—with a certain number of Licentiates in addition—and with fresh names added from time to time, it is obvious that the medical staff of the hospital assumed very considerable proportions. For the same reason also the intervals between the periods of service of each

[1] Minute of the Royal College of Physicians, 5th August 1729.

physician became longer. Such a system undoubtedly had its drawbacks and, failing to give entire satisfaction, the managers were compelled to forbid the Licentiates, on and after 1st January 1738, from continuing their visits on account of the inconvenience arising from the attendance of so many physicians.[1] The minute of 19th December 1737, is of sufficient importance to merit quotation :—

> The Managers of the Infirmary being sensible of the inconvenience of so many physicians attending the Infirmary do unanimously agree that the attendance be performed from and after the first day of January next by such physicians only as are Fellows of the Royal College, that the College be acquainted with this resolution at their first meeting, and the continuance of the attendance of the Fellows be humbly desired in the name of the Managers and thanks be returned to them for their attendance and their good offices to the Infirmary hitherto.

This enactment remains in force at the present day, the Fellowship of the Royal College being a necessary qualification for appointment to the honorary medical staff of the Royal Infirmary. Many years afterwards an unsuccessful attempt was made by the General Council of the University of Edinburgh to effect a change in the regulation governing the eligibility of physicians for appointments to the Royal Infirmary. The Council, in 1888,[2] petitioned the managers so to alter their rules that the degree of M.D. Edinburgh should be held as a sufficient qualification for election to the staff of the hospital. To this request the Board replied that "both by the original Charter of 1736 and by subsequent resolutions of the managers, the Board is absolutely bound to elect their physicians from the Royal College of Physicians of Edinburgh."[3] In the following April the General Council again wrote to the managers of the Infirmary, pointing out, first, that the Charter did not contain the need of this qualification and, secondly, that as the Board itself made the condition, it could equally

[1] An exception was made in the case of two Licentiates who had attended since the opening of the hospital. (Minute, Royal Infirmary, 14th January 1738.)

[2] Minute, General Council, 26th October 1888.

[3] Minute, Royal Infirmary, 26th November 1888.

well remove it.[1] In their reply the managers merely stated that the question had been amply considered, and the decision previously communicated to the Council was adhered to.[2] In the preamble to the Royal Charter of 1736 the following reference is made to the staffing of the Royal Infirmary: The interest of the fund collected " by agreement of the subscribers and donors is to be applied for erecting a house in Edinburgh, wherein poor sick . . . are to be entertained and taken care of by the royal college of physicians of Edinburgh, and some of the most skilful surgeons." The interpretation placed upon these words by the Board of Management restricts the election of physicians and surgeons to the Infirmary to those who are Fellows of the two Royal Colleges.

The first Fellow to attend as physician on 6th August 1729 was John Drummond, senior, a graduate of Aberdeen University, during whose presidency the Royal College had inaugurated the movement for the erection of a hospital. He became a member of the first group of managers of the Infirmary. He was followed during the second fortnight of August by Robert Lowis, a graduate of Leiden, and elected president of the Royal College in 1735.

In January 1729, some months before the hospital was opened, Alexander Monro offered to provide medicines at cost price for a period of one year, and " to attend the sick in Chyrurgical operations and other wayes as frequently as possible he can." The committee accepted his offer. But two months later the system of attendance by rotation was suggested by the surgeons of the Incorporation, each to act for a period of one month: " to furnish the sick and wounded in the Infirmary with medicines and operations in a Society way for two years gratis and agreed to the list of medicines; and in consequence ordained the Deacon and William Mitchell to attend in the terms aforesaid for the first month; the Treasurer and John Douglas the second month and, for the remainder of the two years, the eldest and youngest

[1] Minute, General Council, 16th April 1889.

[2] Minute, Royal Infirmary, 29th April 1889.

members of the Incorporation successively each month . . ." [1] —a suggested arrangement presented to the committee of the Infirmary on 3rd March 1729.

After giving careful consideration to this proposal the committee reached the decision that the surgeons individually could not be bound by their Corporation Act to perform a deed and service of charity such as was involved by attendance at the hospital, nor could the service of that institution be made dependent upon such a basis. Consequently the committee suggested to the Incorporation that the hospital should be served by such of its members as were willing to undertake the duties, stating in writing their proposals as to how the work should be conducted.[2] Acting on this decision Alexander Monro and five other surgeons presented the terms on which they were prepared to serve.[3] The year would be equally divided amongst them : they would dispense gratis from their own shops the medicines prescribed by the physicians and they would consult each other on all extraordinary surgical cases. Each would detail to his successor the condition of the patients who had been in his hands, and they would continue to give their services till the number of patients in the hospital exceeded ten, or as the committee were pleased to restrict them. These terms were accepted. Thus it came about that during the life of the Little House the surgical work was in the hands of six surgeons and was not undertaken by all the members of the Incorporation who then numbered between forty and fifty.

Robert Hope, Alexander Monro, John McGill, Francis Congalton, John Douglas and George Cunynghame became the first surgeons to the Infirmary. Hope, Monro and George Cunynghame were elected managers when the first Board was formed in February 1730. In those early days, therefore, both the medical and surgical staff were represented on the Board of the hospital. With the exception of John Douglas, the surgeons were men of considerable experience. Monro

[1] Minutes, Incorporation of Surgeons, 10th February and 2nd May 1729.
[2] Minute, Royal Infirmary, 7th April 1729.
[3] Minute, Royal Infirmary, 7th July 1729.

was professor of anatomy and surgery in the University and John McGill had been professor of anatomy at Surgeons' Hall prior to Monro's appointment there in 1720. McGill's term of office as surgeon was brief, as he died in 1735. The vacancy in the group of six was then filled, with the concurrence of the other five surgeons, by the selection of George Balderstone who had expressed his willingness to serve. He had specialised as a lithotomist and it was thought that his appointment would add to the reputation of the hospital.

In the Rules of the Infirmary published in 1730, the physician or surgeon on duty was required to seek the advice of his colleagues in all extraordinary cases, and an instance of this practice is related by John McGill in his description of a case of traumatic aneurism of the brachial artery.[1] As the diagnosis of the condition presented some difficulty, the physician in attendance and the other five surgeons met him in consultation at the bedside of the patient. Having unanimously agreed upon the nature of the condition it fell to the lot of John McGill to perform the operation. Before doing so he summoned his colleagues in order to determine the method of procedure and to receive their assistance. A successful operation was performed, the patient making a good recovery.

Thus at the beginning the managers had no voice in the selection of the medical and surgical staff of the hospital, the physicians attending on a system of rotation, while certain of the surgeons offered their services. The story, as it proceeds, will disclose that a period followed in which some of the members were appointed by the Board while others attended by rotation. Finally, the time arrived when attendance by rotation was abandoned and all the appointments to the staff were made by the Board of Management.

Following the foundation of the faculty of medicine and the opening of the hospital, systematic and clinical instruction in the theory and practice of medicine at Edinburgh underwent a profound change. This was not merely the result of the provision of better facilities for study, but was due also to the

[1] *Medical Essays and Observations*, vol. ii, p. 255. (Edinburgh, 1734.)

fact that in the young university school were teachers possessing a wider comprehension than formerly of the science that underlay the art of medicine, men who were, at the same time, capable of expounding it. Already a steady increase in the number of students was taking place and clinical instruction in the hospital was evidently proving a great attraction. Consequently the managers, in November 1730,[1] found it necessary to issue somewhat stringent regulations to meet a situation which was threatening to become unmanageable. The visiting staff were finding it increasingly difficult to examine the sick persons, and even to perform operations, owing to the overcrowding of the somewhat limited accommodation. The patients, too, expressed alarm at the great number of persons present in the consulting room during their examination.

Such a contingency had probably not been anticipated as no regulations had been drawn up relative to the conduct of clinical instruction in the hospital. To meet the emergency the following rules were issued and a copy affixed in the consulting room, so that no one could feign ignorance of them :—

1. That no person whatsoever presume to enter the consulting room while the physicians and surgeons are advising any case.

2. That no student of physic or surgeon's apprentice be admitted at any operation but such as have a ticket from his physician, then in waiting, or from any of the six gentlemen surgeons attending the hospital.

3. That neither the physician in waiting nor any of the six gentlemen surgeons, who attend the hospital, shall have power to give more than two tickets at one time, it being always understood that any member of the College of Physicians may be present at every operation if they please.

The ban thus placed upon attendance in the consulting room was a serious handicap to the student, but the managers very properly were anxious to safeguard the comfort and interests of the patients. Accommodation in the Little House was very limited and the students were increasing in numbers.

[1] Minute, 2nd November 1730.

Alexander Monro, who had been teaching anatomy for ten years, had in the autumn of 1730 eighty-three pupils enrolled in his class, a proportion of whom probably desired to see the practice of the hospital. The number of the visiting staff in consequence of the system of attendance then in vogue undoubtedly added to the difficulty, as their pupils and apprentices naturally expected to receive clinical instruction.

The rules issued by the managers governing the attendance of students at the hospital provided for a definite limitation of their number at any one time ; but, in the circumstances, the regulation forbidding entrance to the consulting room was probably not rigorously enforced. A fee of two guineas was exacted by the Board for the privilege of "walking the hospital," and the money thus received supplemented the annual income of the Infirmary.

Six months after the opening of the Infirmary the managers were elected. For more than a year all the preliminary arrangements had been in the hands of the representative committee of twenty-one appointed by the contributors on 16th December 1728. They had laboured to some purpose. The house in Robertson's Close had been obtained, adapted and furnished as a hospital : the services of the domestic staff had been engaged and provision made for the attendance of the physicians and surgeons, while rules for the election and re-election of managers and for the conduct of the hospital had been drawn up, criticised and adjusted. For six months the patients had been under treatment. It only remained for the committee to render an account of their stewardship.

For this object a General Meeting of Contributors was summoned to attend in the Burgh Room on the afternoon of 13th January 1730. The rules and regulations were twice read and each Article separately considered and finally approved. An adjournment was made till 26th January for the election of the managers, but on that date, "the meeting not being as frequent and numerous as was expected, for the first election of managers the same was adjourned to Monday, the second of February next at three in the afternoon." So reads the short minute.

The management at the adjourned meeting on 2nd February 1730 was intrusted to twenty persons, all donors to the hospital: they were selected from the following "classes or societies" in the city:—

> The Lord Provost of Edinburgh for the time and in his absence the Dean of Guild; the Deacon Convener of the Crafts of Edinburgh for the time; the President, and in his absence the Vice-President of the Royal College of Physicians at Edinburgh for the time, and four other members of the College, whereof two are of the Professors of Medicine in the University of Edinburgh, when such are at the time; the Professor of Anatomy in the University of Edinburgh at the time; and two of the Surgeons of Edinburgh, or three if there is no Professor of Anatomy; one of the Senators of the College of Justice; one of the Faculty of Advocates; one of the Society of Writers to the Signet; one of the Ministers of the Gospel in Edinburgh; and six others who have been donors to the Hospital; of which twenty, seven to be a quorum.

The twenty managers were to choose from amongst themselves twelve as Ordinary Managers, having a quorum of five, the remaining eight to be Extraordinary Managers. A statutory General Meeting of Managers was to be held twice annually, the Ordinary Managers meeting each quarter.

While the original Board of Management was elected by the donors to the Infirmary, the managers annually thereafter nominated and elected themselves in the month of January. The method of doing so is thus quaintly expressed in the rules printed in 1730:—

> They shall consider and agree who amongst them ought to be eased and disburden'd of the Trouble of Management and elect and assume others in their Place out of the same Classes or Societies to which the Persons dismissed do belong, the Number to be altered at one Time, not exceeding Six, or less than Four, and in the case of Decease of any during the Currency of a Year, that the first General Meeting of Managers thereafter, elect and assume one in his Place out of the Society to which he belonged, to serve the Remainder of the Year.

No specified limit was attached to the period of service of any individual member of the Board, and George Drummond and Alexander Monro, two of the original members, continued to serve the Institution for many years. Drummond sat on the Board for probably more years than any other member has done. In 1762-63, as Lord Provost of the City for the sixth time, he was again officiating as chairman. In his Diary, 13th October 1738, he writes: "Forwarding the building of the Royal Infirmary is the only amusement (*sic*) I have allowed myself in of a great while." For 140 years there was no change in the above procedure of election until the Edinburgh Royal Infirmary Act, 1870, introduced radical alterations in the principle underlying the system of nomination and election to the Board. In 1841, however, at the instigation of the managers themselves, one small change was introduced in connection with the nomination of the six donors or contributors, to which reference will again be made (p. 74).

The contributors to the Infirmary, however, had their interest maintained in the internal administration of the Institution, as under Article XXVII of the first Rules: "Every Donor to the Hospital shall have free access to the Books and Records of the Hospital, that they may offer their Advice to the Managers, if anything occurs to them, for the Benefit and Advantage thereof." In this early rule lies the germ of the future Committee of Contributors annually elected, after the Royal Charter had been granted, to revise the proceedings of the managers and the Treasurer's accounts, a committee which was appointed for the first time in 1738 (p. 72).

The inclusion of the Dean of Guild of the City, *ex officio*, to sit in the absence of the Lord Provost was again provided for in the Charter of 1736 and in the Royal Infirmary Act, 1870. It is interesting to note at this point that on 4th January 1742 the Dean of Guild, Thomas Crocket (Crokat), presided at two meetings of the Board and at the General Court of Contributors in the absence of the Lord Provost. Two professors of medicine amongst the five managers selected from the Royal College of Physicians indirectly gave the Senatus Academicus of the University of Edinburgh representation on the Board, the occupant of the chair of anatomy being also a member of the Senatus. His selection as a manager was undoubtedly made in recognition of the valuable part taken by Alexander Monro in the promotion of the Infirmary. The professor of anatomy retained a seat on the Board till the Edinburgh Royal Infirmary Act, 1870, altered the constitution. Monro *primus*, *secundus* and *tertius*—the three Monros—were repeatedly ordinary managers and actively engaged in the business of the Board, but their two successors in the chair prior to 1870, John Goodsir and William—Sir William—Turner, as extraordinary members, took a lesser part in its affairs.

At the first General Meeting of the Managers on 9th February 1730, the twelve Ordinary Managers for the year were selected, and the Treasurer, the Clerk to the Incorporation and the Housekeeper were appointed. David Spence, secretary to the Bank of Scotland, who had already given so much of his time to the work of the committee, accepted the office of Treasurer, continuing to give his services gratuitously: Henry Balcanquhal, Writer, was appointed Clerk to the Incorporation at a salary of £10 Sterling, and Mrs Nisbett previously chosen by the committee was re-elected Mistress or Housekeeper. Later, the name of a fourth official appears from time to time in the minutes of the Infirmary, described as the "officer," and various small sums are voted to him as salary. He appears to have been an employé of the College of Physicians, in more than one instance the gardener at Fountain Close, his duty at the Infirmary apparently being to issue to the managers the notices summoning them to the meetings.

The duties of the ordinary managers were many and diverse. They had the power, subject to the review and correction of the General Meeting of Managers, of investing the Stock of the hospital: they examined and controlled at each quarterly meeting the accounts of the Treasurer: they selected and paid the servants, provided the furniture, ordered the repairs: they established the rules for the conduct and behaviour of servants and patients, and enquired into such diseases and circumstances of persons who ought not to be admitted to the hospital: they regulated the daily attendance of the physicians and surgeons. An important part of their duties was the monthly visitation of the hospital by two of their number. That these visits were regularly made is shown in the several minutes of the Board which record that the managers reported the result of their inspection of the hospital. Sir Henry Burdett in his *Hospitals of the World* has expressed the opinion that the efficiency in the administration of the voluntary hospitals in this country was undoubtedly increased through the system of visitation. A Minute of the Board of 7th November 1814 records that "those managers who fail to make their statutory visit be fined five shillings!"

The method of staffing the Infirmary in Robertson's Close by six surgeons and the reason assigned for this arrangement have already been recorded. But no account of the early Infirmary would be complete without brief reference to the Surgeons' Hospital which, for two years, was a rival charity. The members of the Incorporation of Surgeons in all probability had a feeling of disappointment that their offer of service, made before the Little House was opened, had not been accepted; and, when a proposal to erect a second hospital was made by some of their number at a meeting of the Incorporation in February 1736, it received the unanimous approval of that body.[1]

Impressed by the fact that many necessitous poor were unable to receive treatment at the Infirmary, twelve surgeons, as private individuals, proceeded to collect subscriptions, themselves contributed to the scheme, and offered their services and medicines gratis to the new hospital. Although they had no reason to suppose that their design would clash with the Infirmary or prove prejudicial or hurtful to it, they brought their scheme to the notice of the managers in a letter, dated 5th March 1736, at the same time proposing a coalition between the two charities. In their communication the

[1] Minutes, Incorporation of Surgeons, 13th February 1736.

surgeons also expressed the view that not only would more sick persons thus receive hospital treatment but greater facilities would be provided for students to see the practice of physic and surgery, both these objects having been in the minds of the original contributors to the scheme of a hospital in 1725. In proposing a coalition the surgeons undertook to give their attendance for six years, along with the six surgeons who had hitherto served the Infirmary, and to furnish at their own charge the necessary medicines ; undertaking, further, to become donors to the Infirmary and to persuade the contributors to their scheme to allow their subscriptions to be transferred to the Stock of the Infirmary, so that all might work with the same single purpose in view.

As the managers were not quite clear whether the surgeons really intended to erect a hospital, as signified in the first part of their letter, or only desired to introduce themselves into the Infirmary, as proposed in the second part of the letter, a meeting between the two bodies was arranged. But even then as there was still some doubt as to what was meant by a coalition, the surgeons were asked to put their proposals in writing. While reiterating the suggestions made in their former letter, they amplified the statement concerning the supply of medicines and, further, made the promise that after their admission to the Infirmary they would as donors hand over to that Institution the sum of 2000 Merks Scots.[1]

In their memorial,[2] based on these proposals, the managers of the Infirmary stated that the number of surgeons would thus become greater than in any similar hospital at home or abroad and, as all their apprentices would claim their privileges, it would be necessary to readjust the number and attendance of students at the infirmary ; the offer concerning the supply of medicines, certainly a benefit to the Infirmary, would require to be carefully considered ; and, while the promise to contribute 2000 Merks was very generous, it would be satisfactory to learn what sum had been raised by the surgeons in subscriptions and donations towards their new

[1] In Scotland the Merk was of the value of 13s. 4d.

[2] Minute, Royal Infirmary, 7th June 1736.

hospital. The managers fully recognised the advantages that the students would have of increased facilities for study: nothing was nearer their own hearts, but, as soon as a larger house was procurable, they hoped to remove the inconvenience due to the small size of their present house. They felt, however, that the erection of a rival hospital would retard the charity and, at the same time, increase the expenses necessarily arising from the support of two houses. They hoped, therefore, that the twelve founders of the new hospital, who were so charitably disposed, would transfer their subscriptions to the Infirmary, thus avoiding the risk of the censure and criticism of those citizens who were indifferent to works of charity, adverse criticism which might interfere with future contributions.

No further discussion took place at that time on the question of coalition and, in July 1736, the Surgeons' Hospital was opened in College Wynd, a narrow alley lying to the west of Robertson's Close and leading up from the Cowgate to the College Buildings on Kirk-o'-Field.

Two years elapsed before a second proposal for coalition was renewed on the part of the surgeons who again desired to serve the Infirmary and to have their apprentices and students attend the hospital without distinction or partiality, provided that sufficient security was given to the Incorporation that all their members would be admitted to the service of the Infirmary. After considerable deliberation between both parties the agreement, finally concluded between them in July 1738, was drawn up in the following terms: (1) As soon as the first part of the new building under construction is completed, all the Masters of the Incorporation resident in the city and suburbs and engaged in their profession, *who expressed their willingness to act*, will be admitted as surgeons to the Infirmary on the same footing as the six surgeons already in attendance, their service and practice to be regulated by the managers from time to time; (2) the same privileges will be extended to all future members of the Incorporation on signing a paper expressing their desire to serve; (3) all those studying physic and surgery in Edinburgh, whether as appren-

and you may know likewise what small progress we made in it, the soumes subscribed not amounting to above 2000 libs. However small this fund the Infirmary has been sett on foot. You may remember likewise that we thought it impracticable to carry it much further without publick encouragement, which was scarcely to be expected for reasons not very proper to be mentioned. The enclosed memorial will I hope convince you that it may be done without disobliging any body, except some privat Harpyes who I hear are to apply for it or have done it allready. You could not certainly do a more charitable thing than to put us on a way or method to obtain the premisses and use your interest for that purpose. One thing attending it is the looseness of our Society, which consists of a numerous list of voluntary subscribers, who in a late generall Meeting gave the management of the hospital to a committee, who pass under the name of managers (to shun that of directors) to be chosen annually. The Crown has been in use to incorporate such charitable societies by Charter gratis, as particularly Q. Ann did the Society for propagation of Christian Knowledge. These two favours if they could be done, would establish the most charitable work that was ever projected in this Country.—Adieu.[1] J. C.

More than five years elapsed, however, before the Charter received the Royal signature at the Court at Kensington on the 25th day of August 1736.

Now, know ye, That we having taken into consideration the charitable intention of the petitioners, and being desirous to promote so good and laudable a charity, by virtue of our prerogative royal, and out of our special grace, certain knowledge and mere motion, have Erected, Created and Incorporated, and by these presents, for us, our heirs and successors, do Erect, Create and Incorporate, all and every the said contributors, who have already contributed to the said charitable design, and all such persons as shall hereafter contribute thereto, into one body-corporate and politic, by the name of the Royal Infirmary of Edinburgh. . . .

Translated into Latin by Thomas Ruddiman, then Keeper of the Advocates' Library and, with the Great Seal appended, the Charter was read at the General Meeting of the Managers on 4th November following, and the oath *de fideli administratione* was administered to the members present by the Lord Provost

[1] *More Culloden Papers. V. From 1725 to 1737.* Edited by Duncan Warrand, M.A. vol. iii, 1725-1745, pp. 37 and 38. (Robert Carruthers & Sons, Inverness, 1927.)

in the chair. A fee of £94, 4s. 2d. was paid by the Treasurer of the Royal Infirmary to the Lord Advocate's clerk for the expenses connected with obtaining the Charter; and the managers further authorised the payment of a special fee to him of £15, 15s. od. "for his own pains during the three years the matter was in dependance, with the managers' thanks for his care and diligence."

Having created the body-corporate the Charter then proceeded to place the direction of its affairs in the hands of twenty managers,

> whereof the Lord Provost of our city of Edinburgh for the time being, shall be always one, and in the case of his absence, the Dean of Guild shall be always one, and the President of our Royal College of Physicians of Edinburgh, and in case of his absence, the Vice-President, shall be always one other, and the Deacon Conveener of the Crafts of our said city for the time being shall be always one other:

the remaining seventeen to be annually elected from the following Classes,

> four out of our said Royal College of Physicians, whereof two shall be of the Professors of Medicine in the University of Edinburgh, if there are any such at the time, the Professor of Anatomy, of the said University, if there be any such at that time, and two out of the Incorporation of Surgeons of our said city, or three out of the said Incorporation of Surgeons, if there is no Professor of Anatomy at the time, one out of the Senators of the College of Justice, one out of the Faculty of Advocates, one out of the Society of the Clerks to our Signet, one out of the Ministers of the Gospel in Edinburgh, and six more to be elected out of the number of the contributors to the said charity, residing in or near the said city, if such can be found to undertake the office.

Seven of the twenty managers constituted a quorum.

Having named the first twenty managers to hold office the Charter then proceeded in the following terms:—

> And the said managers shall, on the said first Monday of January, assemble between the hours of two and four in the afternoon, in the borough-room of our said city of Edinburgh; and they, or any seven of them, shall there and then, by a majority of voices, elect and nominate out of the several classes, and in the proportions before described, so many fit persons, as, with the Lord Provost of Edinburgh,

or, in his absence, the Dean of Guild, the President of the Royal College of Physicians, the Deacon Conveener of the said city, and the Professor of Anatomy of the said University, when there is such professor there, will compose the full number of twenty managers for directing and governing the affairs of the said Corporation for the year ensuing.

Although the actual method of procedure at each annual election was not laid down in the Charter, nevertheless " the easing and disburdening of the trouble of management of not more than six or less than four of their number at one time " —as originally carried out prior to the Charter—was continued as the annual practice, regularised in the By-Laws and Rules framed by the managers appointed in 1737, and subsequently approved by the General Court of Contributors. No time limit was laid down in the Charter defining the period of service, and those relieved by their colleagues for a year or more were eligible for re-election on future occasions. In the event of any of the managers refusing to accept office or to take the oath *De Fideli*, or, if any happened to die within a year after their election, then a quorum or more of the managers were authorised to name another manager in place of the person deceased.

At the first meeting in each year they elected twelve of their number as Ordinary Managers, with five as a quorum, to hold quarterly meetings and call to their assistance the eight Extraordinary Managers, as often as they deemed necessary. Upon the ordinary managers devolved the conduct of the hospital in all particulars : they chose annually the Treasurer to the Corporation and the Clerk thereto, to whom they administered the oath, and selected such other persons as they deemed necessary, affixing their salaries with the consent of the extraordinary managers and removing or discharging these officials, if they saw reason to do so. The Treasurer, under the direction of the ordinary managers, had the custody of the Corporation's monies. It was, however, expressly laid down in the Charter that in no circumstances and on no pretext whatsoever was it permissible for the managers to break in upon the Capital Stock of the Corporation, but only to apply the annual interest or revenue as they should judge fit and necessary for the aims and uses of the Infirmary. In several respects, therefore, the terms of the Charter of 1736 closely followed the enactments of the managers elected in 1730.

In the preceding Chapter (p. 62) reference was made to Article XXVII of the First Rules of Management of the Infirmary, printed and circulated in 1730, whereby the contributors were given access to the books and records so that they might offer their advice to the managers, if anything occurred to them that would prove of advantage to the hospital. The Charter considerably extended this privilege by giving a measure of authority to the contributors in the management and government of the Corporation. It established a General Court of Contributors, making it

> lawful to, and for all and every the members of the said corporation or body-politic who shall have contributed five pounds Sterling each, or more, towards the said Infirmary, to assemble and meet together on the first Monday of January next . . . and for ever thereafter yearlie.

Full power and authority were given to this Court

> to make and constitute such by-laws, ordinances, and regulations for the management and government of the affairs of the said corporation, as to them shall seem meet, so that such by-laws, ordinances, and regulations be not contrary to the true intent and meaning hereof, nor repugnant to the laws of our realm.

It was furthermore ordained that at the second and every succeeding General Court the managers shall give an account of their stewardship during their time of office, present a statement of the Capital Stock of the Infirmary in lands, money and other effects, with a report upon all the patients treated in the hospital during the preceding year.

When the General Court met for the second time, on 2nd January 1738, and the managers, in pursuance of the Charter, presented the record of their proceedings during the previous year, a step was taken which was not defined in the Charter. On the suggestion of the chairman, Charles Erskine of Barjarg, then Lord Advocate and one of the managers, a committee were appointed to revise the records submitted and to report their opinion at an adjourned meeting of the Court on the first Monday of March. Seven of the members present were thereupon elected, of whom five, or a majority of the committee, were managers of the Infirmary. The Court further recommended that the ordinary managers at their early convenience should summon a meeting of this committee: at the same time the Court resolved that this method of naming a committee should be observed yearly in time coming as one of the By-Laws of the Corporation.

In the course of time the composition of this committee changed both as regards numbers and personnel. Perusal of the minutes of the Board of Management over a number of years shows that there was a considerable variation in its numbers from time to time, from the original seven to as many as nineteen, and that a quorum of five of the committee became accepted for the transaction of its business. The number of managers appointed to it gradually became fewer and, in 1775, their representation had apparently ceased, without any reason being assigned.[1] The appointment of a committee to revise the annual report of the managers was not provided for in the Charter but came as a suggestion from the contributors. The Committee of the Court annually discharge these duties. The members give purely voluntary service: many retain their membership for a number of years and, in their report to the Court at its adjourned meeting, sometimes make useful suggestions for the consideration of the Board of Management.

During the long period of one hundred and thirty-four years the terms of the Charter of 1736 governed the number of managers appointed, the procedure followed at their election and re-election out of certain "classes," the unrestricted period of their service, and their subdivision into ordinary and extraordinary members: the qualification necessary for membership of the General Court of Contributors also remained

[1] As the volume of Minutes, 1776-1788 inclusive, is missing, no further information on this point is obtainable. In the subsequent volume, commencing in 1789, there were again no managers on the committee of that year.

unchanged during that time. When the Edinburgh Royal Infirmary Act, 1870, was placed on the Statute Book definite alterations were made in the constitution of the Board of Management, in the method of electing its members, and in the qualification necessary for membership of the General Court.

Prior to the Act of 1870, however, one important although limited modification was introduced into the method of electing one group of managers. In the hope of increasing the interest of the public in the work of the Infirmary the managers, in 1840, resolved to consult the wishes of the Court of Contributors in regard to the choice of their representatives upon the Board. Accordingly they adopted the following resolution :—

> To request of the Contributors, assembled at the General Meeting held on the first Monday of January yearly, that they should be pleased to furnish a list of six persons, qualified as contributors, in terms of the Charter, and willing to serve the office of Manager ; to the effect that such six persons may be chosen Managers in the manner specified in the Charter, and that one-half of them may be named Ordinary Managers. And seeing that much benefit may result from the same individuals being continued in the management for more than one year, the Managers are of opinion that it should form no ground of exclusion from the foresaid list, that the names proposed to be inserted in it have been included in that of the preceding year.

Encouraged by this action of the managers in conferring upon the contributors the privilege of suggesting the names of those willing to sit on the Board, the Fellows of the College of Surgeons addressed a similar request to the managers, that the same arrangement might be adopted not only on their behalf but also in favour of the other bodies mentioned in the Charter.[1] But the managers, although admitting that the alteration had proved generally satisfactory to the public, regarded it as inexpedient to make any further changes in the old accepted procedure. It was not till 1870 that the Infirmary Act established the general principle whereby

[1] Minutes, Royal Infirmary, 22nd February, and 27th October 1841.

representatives were sent by the several " classes or societies " to sit on the Board of Management.

While the formalities were proceeding in connection with the application for the Charter the question of erecting a new hospital came under the consideration of the managers. The Capital Stock of the Infirmary was surely, if slowly, increasing and in 1733 the sum of £3620 had accumulated. The number of occupied beds in the " Little House " had also increased from six to eight. At the Meeting of the Board on 7th June of that year David Spence, the Treasurer, reported that a large area of ground was for sale at the head of the College Wynd. The property, on which stood " some thatched houses and one slated house," belonged to Patrick Crawfurd, merchant, who was willing to dispose of it. As 3000 Merks Scots was the price asked, a sum equivalent to £2000 sterling, it was obviously more than the managers were prepared to consider. This site is not again referred to in the minutes.

In November 1736, however, after the Charter had been granted, it was intimated to the Board of Management that the trustees of George Watson's Hospital were prepared to negotiate for the sale of an area of ground known as Thomson's Yards in close proximity to Robertson's Close. In 1724, the trustees had purchased the Yards or Gardens of John Thomson, writer in Edinburgh, as the prospective site for their " hospital " or school, but building operations had never been commenced. The conduct of the school had been placed by the trustees in the hands of a body of governors and the two parties were at variance on the question of sites. The governors preferred a larger site in Lauriston on Heriot's Croft just outside the Flodden Wall, while the trustees, on the other hand, objected to this alternative position on the ground of its unnecessarily large size and of its remoteness from the centre of the city. Finally, yielding to persuasion, the trustees acquired the ground at Lauriston from the Heriot Trust for the sum of £420, and they sold Thomson's Yards to the managers of the Royal Infirmary for a similar sum. The suitability of the

Yards as a site for the new Infirmary was approved in January 1737 at the annual meeting of the General Court of Contributors who authorised the settlement of the transaction with all possible speed. This was accomplished in the month of November following.

When the managers thus successfully completed their negotiations with George Watson's trustees in 1737, no one would have ventured to predict that history would repeat itself on three future occasions—in 1869, 1891-92, and in 1924—and that negotiations would again be opened between these two parties, when the question of expansion and extension of the Infirmary came under consideration. But history has a habit of repeating itself and the records of the Infirmary will disclose, as this narrative proceeds, how the Infirmary came to make fresh contacts with George Watson's College for Boys, as the Hospital was afterwards designated.

The site thus acquired for the Royal Infirmary was the western part of the area of land, formerly the property of the Dominican Order of the Black Friars to whom it had been granted, in 1230, by Alexander II of Scotland and enjoyed by them for more than three centuries. Upon this site the Friars built their monastery, church and school, their guest house and infirmary; and they cultivated their gardens or yards on its southern and western aspects, while along the northern fringe of the estate they feued small plots for building purposes. The whole area was from six to seven acres in extent. The historic interest attaching to this property and the uses to which it was put, subsequent to the demolition of the conventual buildings of the Friars at the time of the Reformation, are so closely linked with the story of the development and progress of the Infirmary and of the Edinburgh School of Medicine that its topography and further history are deserving of more than cursory mention.

The Black Friars occupied the eastermost of the three ecclesiastical properties lying on the slope of the rising ground to the south of the old Burgh. Adjacent to the Black Friars on the west side was St Mary-in-the-Fields or the Kirk-o'-Field, while further west and separated from the latter by some open croft land were the grounds and buildings belonging to the Grey Friars. The whole of this extensive area was originally outside the city wall but, after the defeat of the Scots on Flodden field in 1513, the town wall was extended southwards for defensive purposes as far as the summit of the rise, so as to include these Church lands within its protection.

After 1513 the property of the Black Friars was defined on the north by the Cowgate, on the south and east by the Flodden Wall,[1] while on the west it marched with the Kirk-o'-Field. Immediately beyond the eastern boundary wall a winding roadway ran southwards from the city to the suburb of St Leonards; it was subsequently called the Pleasance, the name being derived from the Convent of Sancta Maria of Placentia, a religious house of the Franciscan Order of Nuns, which once stood on the west side of the roadway a short distance from its origin at the Cowgate Port. Today the boundaries of the old Black Friars' property can still be defined, but in somewhat altered terms. The Flodden Wall has almost entirely disappeared. The Cowgate and Pleasance are on the north and east and on the south is Drummond Street. At the angle where the Pleasance and Drummond Street meet, there still stands a corner tower, the only remnant of that part of the ancient wall. On the west of the old property the boundary line corresponds to the backs of the houses on the South Bridge opposite the façade of the University and is thence prolonged northwards to the Cowgate across Infirmary Street by the line of Robertson's Close.

In order to give the Friars access to the High Street, a narrow transe or lane, subdividing the northern portion of the area, descended to the Cowgate to open opposite the foot of Black Friars Wynd, up the steep ascent of which the High Street was reached. From the upper or south end of this transe a footpath led in a south-westerly direction to the

[1] At some period in the fifteenth century the Friars received a gift of three acres of croft land to the south of the line afterwards defined by the Flodden Wall (W. Moir Bryce, *Book of the Old Edinburgh Club*, vol. ii., 1909).

Kirk-o'-Field. In the course of years the transe became the High School Wynd and the much widened footpath was named Infirmary Street,[1] when the new Infirmary was built.

After the demolition of the ecclesiastical buildings in 1559, the object of the Reformers was to secure a fund to enable them to meet their new obligations—the support of the ministry, the care of the sick poor of the city and the maintenance of education. Therefore the Town Council, in 1561, adopted a resolution in the following terms :—

> It is thocht gude that the renttis annuellis and utheris emolimentis quhilikis of before war payit furth of landis and tenementis within this burgh to papistis preistis freris monkis nonis and utheris of that wilkit sort for manteinying of idolatrie and vane superstitioun seing it hes plesit the Almychti to oppin the eis of all pepill and to gyf thame the knawledge of sic vane abussis thairfoir that the saidis renttis and emolimentis be applyit to mair proffitable and godlie ussis sic as for sustenying of the trew ministeris of Goddis word, founding and biging of hospitalis for the pure and collegis for leirnyng and upbring of the youth and sic other godlie warkis.

Having been granted in 1562 the lands of the Grey Friars and Black Friars by Charter of Queen Mary, the Town Council considered the erection on the latter property of a hospital for the relief of the poor. No hospital, however, was built there, the site of the Trinity Hospital in Leith Wynd being utilised a few years later for that purpose.[2]

In default of the hospital, however, the resolution of the Town Council found practical expression during the ensuing years in other "proffitable and godlie ussis," philanthropic, educational and scientific. Prior to the acquisition of Thomson's Yards in 1737 by the Infirmary Corporation, certain portions of the property had been feued to various individuals for the erection of private residences, the central area to the Earl of Cromartie, the south-east corner to Sir John Skene, afterwards Lord Curriehill, and the westermost

[1] In Ainslie's map of Edinburgh published in 1780, Infirmary Street is named Jamaica Street.

[2] Chapter II, p. 16.

of the old gardens passed through various hands into those of John Thomson. The larger portion of the property, however, had been allocated to other purposes. The High School for boys, previously administered by the Abbey of Holyrood, and which had passed into the control of the Town Council, required rebuilding. Accordingly they erected, in 1578, a school at the head of the old transe and on its east side, almost in the position previously occupied by the monastery. It was pulled down in 1777 and the second High School was erected with its yards or gardens: this building still stands today. In 1647, the first Lady Yester's church was built on the north-west corner of the Friary ground in the angle formed by the transe and the footpath. Converted into a parish church it was supported in part from the rents and properties which had formerly maintained the priests and monks. The second Lady Yester's church, providing more accommodation, was built in 1803 on the present site a little to the west of that of the original church. Finally, the Incorporation of Surgeons, in 1656, purchased from the Town Council the south-east corner of the property along with the dilapidated mansion of the Curriehills. There the surgeons, in 1697, erected their Hall and Anatomical Theatre which, as already related, became the cradle of the Edinburgh School of Anatomy.[1]

With the purchase of Thomson's Yards and the erection of the Infirmary thereon, a hospital for the care of the sick poor had at last been placed on the ground of the former property of the Black Friars, thus fulfilling the resolution of the Town Council of 1561 that a portion of the land should be applied "for the founding and biging of hospitalis for the pure." It was raised, however, by voluntary subscription and not as an act of the Local Authority.

While projecting a building that would eventually accommodate two hundred and twenty-eight patients, the managers recognised the necessity of constructing in the first instance only a part of the hospital, as much indeed as could

[1] Chapter IV, p. 34.

be maintained on the income derived from the Capital Stock. With part of the house completed and occupied, they had no doubt that charitable persons would be well disposed towards a hospital which made provision for a considerable number of patients and which was maintained on economic lines. They felt that, in these circumstances, contributions would increase and eventually permit of the extension and final completion of the building. George Drummond, continually solicitous for the well-being of the Infirmary, made this entry in his Diary on 17th March 1738 :—

> Royal Infirmary : I have given a great deal of my time to it this winter. We have got a plan for our house ; it is to hold about 200 patients. We propose to build at present so much of it as will accommodate 66, and 5 cells for lunatics, and being restricted by our charter from encroaching on our capital we have no other fund for building (and would cost a private man £1600) but charitable contributions, in getting of which we go on with good success. I look to the Lord about it, to make it a blessing to the place and Nation.

In the month of April 1738, the ordinary managers prepared a memorandum in which the financial position of the hospital was carefully set out, and the opinion expressed as to the prospect of maintaining about one hundred patients in the part of the hospital first constructed. " The building " they said in the preamble to the report " ought to be solid and erected of the most durable material, not slovenly, and yet that very little or no expense should be paid out in useless ornament. . . . In order to form the plan in the best manner, they applied to William Adam,[1] architect, who has generously assisted them with a plan of the whole work which, when finished, will conveniently accommodate 200 patients allowing each patient a bed."

In order to defray the expense of maintaining about one hundred patients the managers submitted prospective sources

[1] William Adam of Maryburgh, Fife, was a well-known Scottish architect and the father of two distinguished sons, Robert and James, the former, amongst other important works, designing the plan of the present University in South Bridge, the foundation stone of which was laid in 1789.

of revenue, along with a calculation as to the annual income which might thus be realised :—

Interest on Present Capital of about £5000 . . .	£250
Interest from the King's Scots' Invalid Fund of £6000 .	300
Hospital tickets of 100 students and apprentices at £2, 2s. od. per annum	210
From the Ladies of the Dancing Assembly, the Assembly of the Church of Scotland, and Episcopal congregations in the city from one Sabbath collection annually .	240
	£1000

They further computed that £10 would be a reasonable allowance for the annual entertainment of each patient; consequently, the income thus raised would permit of the provision of the hundred beds suggested.

Wise, cautious and prudent, however, in their new venture they were " unwilling to act too forwardly in this matter " and therefore proposed " to build no more at present than what will accommodate 66 patients," of whom only 40 would be a regular charge on the hospital. They proposed that 26 beds would be set aside for domestic servants, their masters paying the charge of their maintenance. At the same time as there was no institution in Scotland for the care of insane persons, " five cells " were to be provided for these patients in the part of the hospital first erected. The architect estimated the expenditure on this section at £1573, 16s. 2d. sterling: as its completion was not anticipated, at the earliest, before the end of 1740 there was ample time to secure the building funds necessary to meet this outlay. The Treasurer already had in hand £279, 15s. 11d. subscribed for the purpose by the Parish Churches throughout Scotland, by the Episcopal congregations in Edinburgh and by certain charitable individuals. During the progress of construction it was believed that an additional sum of £1140 would be obtained from further Church collections, from the Faculty of Advocates and the Writers to the Signet, and from a tax which the Freemasons had imposed upon themselves in order to assist the hospital; and lastly, from the accumulation of the annual unexpended income on the maintenance of the Little House in Robertson's Close during the next three years. A total sum of £1419, 15s. 11d. would thus be available to meet the estimated contract.

There was every reason to hope, however, that William Adam's estimate would be considerably reduced and that a sum of £428, 16s. 10d. would be saved by obtaining certain quarry privileges for stone, gifts of slates, the use of lath and lime in place of deal, and through the generous proposal of the masons to give some of their services gratis. With the estimated cost of the building thus reduced to £1144, 19s. 4d., and the sum of £1419, 15s. 11d. in hand to meet the outlay, there was a comfortable balance in the event of unexpected contingencies.

With these figures before them the managers unanimously approved of the architect's plans for the whole Infirmary and agreed that the construction of the limited portion should be forthwith undertaken with all diligence, and that the necessary funds should be collected. George Drummond, Alexander Monro, professor of anatomy, Andrew St Clair, physician, and George Cunynghame, surgeon, were appointed members of the Building Committee of the Board ; and, at the meeting of the General Court of Contributors in January 1739, the managers were able to report that the work on the new hospital had commenced and was already well advanced.

In its general design the Royal Infirmary was of the simplest character. Facing the north and overlooking the Cowgate valley, with the high ridge of the city beyond, it was planned with the object of accommodating 228 patients. It comprised a body, 210 feet in length, with east and west wings, each 70 feet long, directed to the north from either extremity and embracing the fore-court. The central portion of the body was in relief, projecting 12 feet beyond the rest, the exterior of this part being made more decorative by the addition of a pillared façade, surmounted by a specially designed attic and cupola.

The building was of four floors, the top or fourth floor being designated as the " attick story " : in the roof were garrets.

The ground or first floor, which contained the administrative departments, was also fitted with " 12 cells " for the accommodation of insane persons. The wards were placed on the three upper floors, those in the body of the house, six in number, containing 24 beds in each, and thus capable of accommodating 144 patients. A similar number of wards of smaller design, in the two wings, each containing 12 beds, made provision for 72 patients, the whole, including the 12 cells, completing the proposed 228 beds. The wards on the second and third floors of the body and wings were assigned to the medical cases, 144 in number :[1] while the 72 beds on the fourth or attic floor were allocated to surgical cases, partly on account of their proximity to the operating theatre and, being situated in the higher part of the building, there was less noise and a greater supply of fresh air. The east half of the hospital was to accommodate the male patients, the women were to occupy the west half.

The central or principal staircase leading to the several floors was spacious and of easy ascent permitting the transport of patients without great difficulty. Two smaller staircases were added, each being placed at the junction of the body with the wings. The accommodation for nurses was very limited, a small room on each landing, where the body and wings joined, providing for both the large and small wards. Heating was obtained by fires, lighting by oil lamps and candles. The water supply was at first carried to the hospital in buckets. This having proved laborious and expensive, a supply pipe was connected in 1743 with the main pipe of the city.

The central part of the fourth floor of the hospital was elevated in the form of a domed projection within which was placed the operating theatre, capable of accommodating two hundred students, and " the same serving as a chapel." From the centre of the dome rose a turret or cupola " having windows to different parts of the hemisphere, which may occasionally be used as an astronomical laboratory." This elevation, decorated with a balustrade and vases, along with the pillared façade beneath, relieved the otherwise plain, drab appearance

[1] Fever cases were then treated in the general medical wards.

of the stonework of the building and provided a little ornamentation. In an alcove between the two central pillars and above the main entrance there was afterwards placed a life-size statue of George II in Roman dress.[1] When the present Infirmary was opened in Lauriston Place in 1879, this statue, standing on a stone pedestal, was erected on the right side of the flight of steps giving access to the main hall of the hospital. In William Adam's engraving of the north elevation of the old Infirmary there is depicted, between the two windows of the operating theatre, a large stone on which were carved four figures illustrating a patient in the hands of a surgeon and his attendants, and above the figure the text : "I was sick and ye visited me." It is probable that this design was never actually executed on stone as, in Sandby's engraving and in the photograph of the building taken shortly before its demolition in 1884, a third, central window occupies this position. But two scriptural texts were inscribed on tablets between the pillars, "I was a stranger and ye took Me in," "I was sick and ye visited Me." When the building was demolished the ornamental façade of the theatre came into the possession of Mr Robert Andrew Macfie of Dreghorn who incorporated it in the walls of the stable in the grounds of Redford House. Here it may still be seen by the traveller as he passes the gate of the avenue on his pilgrimage to Swanston Cottage, the country home of Robert Louis Stevenson in his boyhood's days. The stable has now become a garage.

For many years the Infirmary was exposed to "a' the airts the wind can blaw," and benefited too from the available maximum of sunshine, till in the closing years of the eighteenth century the tenements of the South Bridge, the high eastern face of the University Buildings and the houses in Drummond Street rose as barriers to air and light. Originally the College Garden provided an open space on the west side, and within the hospital enclosure were gravel walks for the outdoor recreation of the convalescent patients. In the boundary wall

[1] The King's statue was brought from London and erected when the Infirmary obtained the benefits derived from the King's Invalid Fund in 1755.

separating the fore-court of the Infirmary from the public thoroughfare, Infirmary Street, stood a handsome, ornamental, iron gate flanked on each side by a stone balustrade. The gate was approached from the roadway by a semi-circular flight of stone steps which precluded its use as a carriage entrance. History records that the gate always remained closed and was never used either by patients or by the hospital staff, access to the grounds being obtained through a doorway placed further west in the boundary wall. When the original Infirmary building was pulled down in 1884, the gate, balustrade and stone steps were removed and placed in the railings on the north side of Drummond Street. There the gate gave access for many years to the City Fever Hospital and, subsequently, to the Natural Philosophy Department of the University, a function it continues to perform today.

Constructive work was commenced on the east portion of the body of the hospital, the Foundation Stone being laid on 2nd August 1738, with considerable ceremony, in the presence of a large gathering of prominent citizens. The Lord Provost, Magistrates and Council attended officially, walking in procession from the Council Chamber down the High Street and Black Friars' Wynd, and thence across the Cowgate and up the High School Wynd to the scene of operations. Behind them walked the Free and Accepted Masons with all the paraphernalia of their Order. The President and Fellows of the Royal College of Physicians marched from their Hall in Fountain Close, the Surgeons from their Hall in the immediate vicinity of Thomson's Yards: there were also in attendance the managers of the Royal Infirmary, Senators of the College of Justice, many members of the Faculty of Advocates, of the Writers to the Signet, and of the Presbytery of Edinburgh, along with a number of the Incorporations of the city. "The Grand Master, the Earl of Cromartie, Master Mason of the Work, and the Preses of the Managers of the Royal Infirmary, George Drummond, coming to the East Corner of the Foundation, where the Stone was to be laid, placed the same in its bed: the Right Hon. the Lord Provost, Archibald Macaulay, having first laid a Medal under it, each in their turns giving

3 strokes upon the Stone with an Iron-Mallet, which was succeeded by 3 Clarines of the Trumpet, 3 Huzzas and 3 Claps of Hands."[1] After the ceremony the Lord Provost and Magistrates along with a number of the company met in the Council Chamber, when the Health of His Majesty and the other members of the Royal Family was drunk and prosperity to the Royal Infirmary was toasted. The occasion was utilised for making a collection for the Building Fund and, at a meeting of the managers in the following month, it was intimated that £132, 19s. 2d. had then been obtained. Of this sum the physicians contributed £39, 18s., the friends of the erectors of the Surgeons' Hospital £34, 3s. 2d., and the Incorporation of Surgeons £20. The skinners, candlemakers and goldsmiths also gave donations.

Notwithstanding the decision, previously reached on financial grounds, to proceed with the building of the hospital in stages, the whole fabric, as originally designed, was actually in course of construction before the first patients were admitted in December 1741 to the beds in the east part of the hospital. This had undoubtedly been made possible by the vigorous action taken in raising funds and by the ready and wide response to the appeal. There could be no question that the completion of building operations at as early a date as possible would add to the comfort of the inmates and to the amenity of the surroundings.

All who were interested in the hospital were greatly indebted to the devotion and untiring energy of George Drummond who presided at almost every meeting of the ordinary managers and, with forethought and shrewdness, directed the appeal for funds. In an appeal dated 1st August 1739, he wrote :—

> The restriction on us by the Charter, to employ no part of the Capital to the Building, lays us under a Necessity to address ourselves to every Person or Society from whom we can hope for it, for their charitable Assistance to foreward this Great and Good Work ; in itself, the most necessary and most beneficial to the publick of any one Undertaking of this Nature which has been at any time set on Foot.

[1] *The Caledonian Mercury*, 3rd August 1738.

APPEAL BY GEORGE DRUMMOND, 1739

The Honourable State of Burrows met in Convention in July last, having recommended a Collection for it to all their Members, by their Act inclosed, we humbly pray it may be complied with as soon as possible, and the Collection remitted to Mr David Spence, Secretary to the Bank of Scotland, our Treasurer.

Two of your Number, viz. the Burrows of Perth and Stirling, have set a very laudable Example to their neighbours in this Matter. Upon an Application from us to them last Winter; they, by an Act of their Council, divided their Town into so many Quarters, and, after Intimation made thereof from the Pulpits, ordered a Magistrate, a Town Counsellor and a Deacon to go from House to House in the Quarter allotted to them, to receive from the several Inhabitants what they were pleased to give. The Collections were handsome. They did Honour to these Burrows, and stand recorded in our Books with Gratitude. We humbly presume to mention this, that if you please you may follow their good Example in making your Collection in the same Manner; since we find by Experience that those made at Kirk-doors turn to very little Account.

We do not know a more useful, a more general Charity than this we are humbly recommending; and the Belief we have, that we are addressing ourselves to Christians, who consider the Import of that Text I John III 17. "But whoso hath this World's Good, and seeth his Brother hath need, and shutteth up his Bowels of Compassion from him, how dwelleth the Love of God in him?" Makes it that we'll add no more than to assure you there is Danger of the Good Work's stopping, if we are not assisted. We are with greatest respect,

Gentlemen,

Your most faithful and most obedient humble Servants,
Signed in Name and by Order of the Managers, by

(Signed) GEORGE DRUMMOND, 1739.

After his death in 1766, to commemorate his good work, his bust, executed in marble by Joseph Nollekens, was placed in the entrance hall of the Infirmary and inscribed "To George Drummond, to whom this country is indebted for all the benefit which it derives from the Royal Infirmary." This and an admirable portrait, painted in 1752 by J. Alexander, are preserved in the Infirmary today as valued mementoes of a great benefactor.

The appeal for subscriptions was not confined to the city, nor indeed to Scotland : how widely the net was spread over these islands, over the continent of Europe and the plantations of the New World is revealed by a study of the minutes. Scotsmen and others not only resident near home but in distant lands gave practical proof of their sympathy. Subscription lists were opened in London and in the county of Kent. George Drummond made a special overture to the Mayor and Aldermen of the City of Canterbury, to the Dean and Chapter of the Cathedral, and to the Ministers, Elders and people of the Presbyterian and Anabaptist congregations.

One of the most active bodies in the community was the Society of Friends, and in the person of Miss May Drummond, the Quaker sister of George Drummond, the Infirmary possessed a zealous and diligent helper. Travelling through the English provinces she pleaded its cause before the Corporations of Newcastle, Durham, York, Leeds, Nottingham and Exeter, and her applications were endorsed by letters from the managers to the Mayors of these cities ; she also addressed the Quakers in Dorset and Somerset. The interest of the Friends in the South of Ireland was stimulated by one of their number who had brought his son from Cork to study medicine in the Edinburgh school. It is recorded on the mural tablets of the Infirmary that the sum of £379, 8s. 8d. was raised in 1739 by the members of the Society of Friends resident in towns in the north of England. In acknowledgment of the services thus rendered

> the Managers taking into serious consideration the liberal donations they have already received from the charitable and well disposed people called Quakers, both in Great Britain and Ireland, towards carrying on and perfecting the building of the Infirmary, wherein they still continue to show a readiness to contribute more and more until the good work is finished, think they should be wanting both to themselves and the charitable design, if such a large and extensive charity, the peculiar characteristic of these friendly people, were not acknowledged with the highest mark of gratitude and esteem and duly recorded in the minutes of their proceedings, as a notable example of their universal charity so natural to these good and friendly people.

The Prince and Princess of Wales, each sent £100 sterling.

Scotsmen engaged in business in Stockholm and Gothenburg, in Rotterdam and other cities of Holland, and in the Hanseatic city of Danzig agreed to collect from their exiled fellow countrymen: in France and as far south as Lisbon similar collections were made. The assistance of the Governor of New England was solicited: Scotsmen too in Pennsylvania and Maryland answered to the call of the homeland. In the West Indies considerable sums were raised, the island of Jamaica alone contributing over £1000, and from the islands of the Windward group, Antigua, Barbados and Montserrat varying sums were received.

One further source of supply is worthy of mention. Mr Thomas Topham offered to perform his feats of strength for the benefit of the building, an offer which the managers gratefully accepted and agreed to attend at the door of the house to collect the money! There is no record as to whether they fulfilled their promise.[1]

The material required in the construction of the hospital was not entirely the product of the soil of Scotland. Timber was imported from foreign soil, and when the ship, from the Baltic port of Stralsund, carrying the massive beams necessary for the support of the floor of the operating theatre, failed to arrive at Leith, great consternation ensued. To remedy this defect George Drummond ordered from London four joists of red-wood, each thirty feet in length and fourteen inches square. Lime was brought from England, and hundreds of carts were procured for its transport; 7000 unglazed paving tiles, each eleven inches square, were imported from Holland. Interest and enthusiasm were aroused in all classes of the community. A large hospital was a novel undertaking and appealed to the imagination. Gratuitous gifts and service were forthcoming. Thus, six thousand planks of wood were sent by the tenants of the Duke of Argyll and timber by the merchants in Leith: the farmers lent their carts for haulage and the masons and labourers gave gratis one day's work in the month.

[1] Minutes, Royal Infirmary, 3rd July 1739.

In March 1740 the Building Fund had reached the very considerable sum of £2447 and there was every prospect of more to follow. Thus encouraged the managers decided to proceed with the construction of the west half of the body of the house and, on 14th May, a second foundation stone was laid. The ceremony was not quite on the same grand scale as in 1738. James, Earl of Morton, as Grand Master Mason officiated, proceeding with the dignitaries of the Order from St Mary's Chapel in Niddry Wynd to the Infirmary.

Nothing now remained to complete the hospital but the erection of the two wings. This was made possible, in 1741, through the generosity of members of his Majesty's Revenue of Excise who, learning that only lack of money hindered their construction, solicited subscriptions for the purpose from the Officers of Excise throughout Scotland, sufficient to defray the wages of the masons working on both wings. In the same year the Building Fund amounted to £4795.

Thus the whole fabric was in process of construction prior to the transference of the patients from Robertson's Close and their admission to the east section of the new hospital in December 1741. In February 1743 the managers resolved to give up their lease of the "Little House" and "prayed its discharge from the Town Council." It was not till 1748 that the Royal Infirmary was completed and the whole building was ready for the reception of patients. Ten years had been spent on its construction, but many more were to elapse before full advantage could be taken of all the accommodation it provided.

CHAPTER VII

THE ROYAL INFIRMARY IN THE EIGHTEENTH CENTURY

THE ADMISSION OF PATIENTS—A SYSTEM OF MAINTENANCE BY SPECIAL PAYMENTS—THE MATERNITY WARD—EARLY LEGACIES—LEASING ROOMS IN THE HOSPITAL AND ADJACENT BUILDINGS—THE BAGNIO OR PUBLIC BATH HOUSE—MEMBERS OF THE HOSPITAL FAMILY—THE MATRON—THE CLERK OF THE HOUSE—THE PHYSICIANS' AND SURGEONS' CLERKS—THE PORTER—THE APOTHECARY—THE COOK—THE NURSES—THE CHAPLAIN.

On 1st December 1741, "the Family" was transferred from the Infirmary in Robertson's Close across the old footpath trodden daily by the Friars two centuries earlier, and was accommodated in the east section of the new building. No formal ceremony marked this important event. The first and second floors of this part had been furnished as wards, the central portion of the body of the hospital being adapted for administrative purposes. At first, only thirty-four beds were in daily use as the interest from the Capital Stock was insufficient to maintain the full complement of sixty-six, the number previously suggested.

Some amplification of the rules governing the admission of patients became necessary. The managers had profited by their experience in conducting the early hospital. It was made quite clear in the first of the new regulations that patients of all countries or nations were to be admitted : power was also given to the physicians and surgeons to place no restriction upon the admission of cases of an acute nature and those suffering from serious accidents. In the event of those not so afflicted it was necessary for some responsible person to come under an obligation to remove the patient when he or she was deemed fit to return home ; or, if such obligation was not forthcoming, the patient was required to deposit ten shillings sterling in the hands of the matron to indemnify the hospital

" from any charge that might arise from burying or removing them." " Patients suffering from incurable or very tedious diseases " were not to be admitted, nor were those with venereal disease, till special wards were prepared for them. Women with young children could not be accepted unless arrangements were first made elsewhere for the proper care of the latter.

Reference may be made at this point to the employment of " subscribers' letters " as a method of recommending patients for admission to the voluntary hospitals. For many years the system was in use at the Royal Infirmary. The managers, when preparing the new statutes for the conduct of the Royal Infirmary following upon the Charter, made a rule that those " who had given or shall give £50 sterling or pay £5 sterling annually to the Infirmary, may, during life, have one patient (not excluded by the rules), constantly entertained and taken care of as a patient in the Infirmary upon their recommendation ; and double, triple, etc., those sums shall entitle them to a proportional number of such patients." Thus, the system of subscribers' letters was introduced. The patients bearing this recommendation were to be given preference over others, when all applying could not be entertained without exceeding the number allowed by the managers, and when the cases were nearly equally urgent. If those, thus recommended, could not be immediately admitted they were treated as out-patients, receiving advice and medicine gratis. This system of recommendation by letters was finally abandoned.[1]

Every possible source of income was explored in order that the Infirmary might give the maximum service and make use of all the beds provided. But it is obvious from the minutes of that period that this could not be accomplished without departing from the principle of purely voluntary support which formed the basis of the hospital movement in the eighteenth century. At least three groups of in-patients came under treatment : those on the ordinary establishment, supported by the annual revenue from invested capital ; those

[1] The actual date has not been ascertained. It is possible that the missing Minute Book, vol. v, November 1775 to December 1788, inclusive, contained the reference.

maintained by special funds raised for certain definite purposes; and lastly, those who were frankly "paying patients" financially responsible for their own care and treatment while in hospital.

In 1742, the Infirmary was greatly indebted to the beneficence of the second Earl of Hopetoun who not only helped to maintain the limited number on the ordinary establishment but provided a special fund for the maintenance of incurable patients. Holding at that time His Majesty's Commission as one of the Lords of Police in Scotland, he intimated to the Board of Management that, so long as he retained the office, he would hand over annually to the Infirmary £400 sterling from his salary.[1] He desired that this sum should be allocated in the following manner: £100 annually towards augmenting Capital; £150 for the maintenance of sick persons in the hospital; £100 towards furnishing the part of the house already built, on reparations, or for building purposes, or, at the discretion of the managers, to be used as ordinary annual income; and £50 annually for the continued care of five poor patients who were deemed incurable after a period of treatment in the wards. Lord Hopetoun's "Incurable Fund" proved of great value, for a number of years maintaining annually four or five patients of this class. In 1743, he was elected an extraordinary manager, and his portrait, painted and presented by Allan Ramsay, occupies today a prominent position in the Board Room of the Royal Infirmary.[2]

Another source of revenue which served the double purpose of maintaining the ordinary establishment and of providing beds for sick soldiers was obtained through the King's Invalid Fund, raised in Scotland prior to the Union in 1707. It will be recalled that in the memorandum prepared by the managers in 1738, when calculating the sources of income for maintenance in the new hospital, a sum sufficient to provide £300 annually was anticipated from this fund (p. 81). It was not, however, till early in 1755 that the Lords of the Treasury agreed to give the Invalid Fund to the Town

[1] Minute, Royal Infirmary, 21st April 1742. [2] *Ibid.*, 7th November 1748.

Council of Edinburgh on the condition that they granted Bonds for the payment of annual interest to the Infirmary at the rate of 3½ per cent. But a further condition was attached by the Treasury to this transaction, namely, that the managers should prepare and fit up sixty beds for the reception of as many soldiers certified as suitable by the Commander-in-Chief of the Forces in Scotland. The Infirmary was to receive fourpence per day for each soldier treated and dieted, this sum, however, to be deducted from the soldier's pay! This stipulation was agreed to. The total amount of the Invalid Fund was £8723, 17s. 3d. and, in 1756, the special beds were ready for occupation.

The question of the accommodation of soldiers in the Royal Infirmary had been brought to the notice of the authorities a number of years before the acceptance of the Invalid Fund had made the managers responsible for the provision of military beds. In August 1744, Sir John Cope, then Commander-in-Chief of the Forces in Scotland, submitted certain proposals for the care of the sick and wounded in the garrison. These entailed the preparation of a ward of twenty-four beds of which the surgeon of the regiment, supplying the medicines, dressings and bandages, was to be in charge: the physicians to the Infirmary, however, were to have the privilege of visiting the patients, accompanied by their pupils who would receive clinical instruction. The hospital was to provide meals similar to those prepared for the civilian patients, and two shillings and sixpence per week for each soldier was to be handed over by the paymaster to the Treasurer of the Infirmary. With the acceptance of these terms the ward on the second floor of the west section of the body of the building was prepared for their reception.

During the Rising of the '45 the Infirmary assumed very largely the character of a military hospital. The young Prince Charles Edward Stuart having landed on the beach at Arisaig in July 1745, reached the capital with his Highlanders on the eve of the battle of Prestonpans. On the following day, the 21st September, he defeated the King's troops under Sir John Cope. From that date, till the termination of the Rebellion on Culloden Moor in April 1746, soldiers formed the majority of the patients in the hospital, the number of civilians being reduced to very small proportions: indeed, at the end of December 1745 only ten ordinary patients were returned on the books of the Infirmary. Fresh demands, however, were made upon its resources in January 1746, the Physician-General to the Hospital of the Army requesting the accommodation of the whole available part of the Infirmary, with the exception of the two wards originally assigned to the ordinary patients. Application was also made for "the use of all the dishes and utensils and all the beds so far unemployed," and, after their distribution, the Government would provide what might still be necessary. "Coals, candles, nurses, servants, clerks and loaves of bread" would also be supplied and paid for by the Army, the managers binding themselves to prepare a special bill of fare for the soldiers. The sum of 4½d. sterling per day was at first paid for each soldier, but with the rise in the cost of provisions this was later raised to 5d.; and for those on a full diet a charge of 7½d. per day was made.

For many years after the Rebellion soldiers were regularly treated in the hospital in pursuance of the terms on which the Invalid Fund had been accepted: they constituted a considerable proportion of the patients entertained in the house. In 1761 as many as 301 were admitted, the civilian patients during the same year numbering 447. At the termination of the Seven Years' War, with the Peace of Paris in 1763, many soldiers were disbanded from the army and those falling sick near Edinburgh, while on their journey home, applied for admission. Although under no obligation to receive or to maintain disbanded soldiers, the managers, in testimony of their regard for the men who had fought in the late war, resolved "that all sick soldiers of disbanded regiments applying for admission should be received without fee or reward so as to be cured of their several diseases, while those who were still in the Infirmary should remain until they were cured and able to return to their respective homes." [1] Ten years later,

[1] Minute, Royal Infirmary, May 1763.

in the annual return of the patients under treatment in the hospital, 447 soldiers passed through the wards, forming nearly one-third of the total number of admissions.

The personnel of the Royal Navy also received attention. In the event of applications being made for their maintenance, it was calculated that 6d. per day per head would indemnify the hospital, as there was no desire to make profit from this source. When, however, the Board of Excise in 1774 proposed that the sailors from His Majesty's Excise Yacht should be admitted, it was decided to receive them on the basis of ordinary patients.

Another section of the community to receive particular consideration and for which a special fund was raised for maintenance were the domestic servants in the employment of the "well-disposed families in town." The physicians attending the Infirmary had reported that, owing to lack of suitable accommodation in many of the houses in the city, servants suffering from an acute illness frequently succumbed. To remedy this state of affairs the managers had proposed, in their memorandum of April 1738,[1] to set aside twenty-six of the sixty-six beds in the east half of the hospital, when available, for the reception of these cases, on the express condition that the masters and mistresses should pay the cost of maintenance. No action, however, was taken at that time, and it was not till 1755 that the matter was again considered. The proposal was then made that beds should be reserved for the above purpose and that the occupants should be maintained, not by their employers as originally suggested, but from a special fund. Accordingly a petition was presented to the Town Council and to the Presbytery of Edinburgh in favour of a collection at the doors of the Churches in the city and suburbs. Two wards, each capable of accommodating ten beds, were prepared—one for men and one for women—and the arrangement was made known through an advertisement in the public Press.[2] The first special collection yielded £194, 15s. and similar petitions for the same object were renewed from time to time. A Mr James Hunter bequeathed a sum of

[1] Chapter VI, p. 81.

[2] Minute, Royal Infirmary, 5th April 1756.

£200 for the same purpose. The number of domestic servants entertained during successive years varied considerably, doubtless due to the changing incidence of the infectious fevers. Forty were returned in 1756, but the number reached 193 in 1774, the last year during which data are available. Many years afterwards, in 1842, the managers, with the approval of the Court of Contributors, " admitted no person to the privilege and seclusion of the female servants' ward, except the servants of those who contributed £1 annually to the Infirmary. This may help to increase the funds, and it will not prevent any individual from resorting to the Infirmary as a patient in the ordinary wards."

There still remain for consideration the patients paying for their maintenance. Among these, persons mentally afflicted formed an important group. Arrangements for the care of the insane were contemplated when William Adam prepared his plans of the Royal Infirmary, there being at that time no " Asylum " in Scotland for their treatment. A small number of " cells " was therefore fitted up in the part of the hospital first constructed. Establishments for the treatment of the insane then resembled prisons rather than hospitals and they constituted a link with medieval times. But towards the end of the eighteenth century legislation provided special institutions for the care of this class of patient, and the Royal Scottish Asylum at Montrose, founded in 1779, was the first hospital in Scotland to arrange accommodation for the mentally afflicted. Largely through the influence of Andrew Duncan, senior, physician to the Royal Infirmary, the Royal Edinburgh Asylum received its Charter in 1807, and a few years later it opened its doors for the reception of patients.

Members of all classes of the community without distinction of social status, when considered insane, were eligible for admission to the Infirmary. Before admission, however, an obligation was signed by the relatives accepting responsibility for the payment of board and treatment. This was made payable quarterly and in advance and, in the event of the death of the patient, the expenses of the funeral were also to be a charge upon the relatives and friends.[1] At first a sum of £5 sterling per quarter was exacted, but in response to complaints of its excessive character it was afterwards reduced to £3. The patients were placed under the care of the visiting physicians and surgeons.

It is appropriate at this stage to refer to the payment of fees by patients admitted into the Lock wards of the hospital, although there is no reference to such payments till the early part of the nineteenth century. Persons suffering from venereal disease were originally excluded from the Royal Infirmary by the early regulations of the managers[2] but, in 1750, a ward containing twelve beds for female patients was opened on the fourth floor.[3] In 1811, the Board of Management minuted a resolution that these patients should pay a fee of £3, 3s., it being left, however, to the discretion of the physicians to dispense with payment, in whole or in part, as they might judge proper. Some years later 10s. 6d. was exacted from the women on admission.[4] The income received from this source was returned in the annual statement of revenue, but after 1863, when the new Lock Hospital was established in the building formerly used by John Bell as a lecture room, no further payments appear to have been made.

With the provision of a Lying-in Ward in the hospital in 1755, a limited number of maternity patients was admitted on a free basis, but a small sum was requisitioned for the maintenance of those above that number. As the Infirmary has once again accepted responsibility for the treatment of maternity patients and for the instruction of students in midwifery, brief reference may suitably be made to the early history of the movement. When the faculty of medicine was created in February 1726, the Town Council of Edinburgh, on the recommendation of the Incorporation of Surgeons, appointed Joseph Gibson, a member of that body and a practitioner in the town of Leith, as "City Professor of Midwifery."

[1] Minute, Royal Infirmary, 19th January 1742.
[2] In the Infirmary in Robertson's Close a "salivating" room was established.
[3] Minute, Royal Infirmary, 5th November 1750.
[4] Minutes, Royal Infirmary, 15th January 1811 and 28th March 1831.

His rôle as a teacher, however, was confined to the instruction of midwives in whose hands the practice of midwifery was mainly conducted. Shortly before his election the Magistrates had insisted upon the production of certificates from a qualified physician or surgeon testifying that these women had received instruction prior to practising their profession. There is no evidence that Gibson lectured to students in the University. But his successor, Robert Smith, whose commission made him "Professor of Midwifery in the City's College," and who was recognised as a member of the Senatus Academicus, possibly gave some tuition to students as well as to midwives.

With the appointment of Thomas Young, then Deacon of the Surgeons and a graduate of the University, as professor of midwifery, a systematic course of lectures was given for the first time to students of medicine; and in order that clinical instruction might be provided he applied to the managers for permission to use the maternity ward in the Infirmary.[1] The following arrangements were made:

that Dr Young should fit up a ward at his own expense on the attic floor of the east wing of the hospital and be responsible for the repairs from time to time: for six months in the year he should have four maternity cases maintained in the Infirmary and, in addition to these, four other cases as he might think proper, for which he should pay at the rate of sixpence per day for each patient. The House would be responsible for all the charges connected with the maternity nurses in his ward—their board and lodging—but he would pay their salaries. It was further agreed that those students who formerly had a ticket for attendance at the hospital for two years, and students actually attending the hospital, should be allowed admission to the lying-in ward.

In this way yet another group of patients was accommodated in the Infirmary, outside the ordinary establishment of the hospital, payment for their care and treatment being made by a member of the medical staff! For several years these

[1] The Minutes of the Royal Infirmary, dated July and October 1755, state that Thomas Young, professor of midwifery, applied to the managers for a maternity ward and that students should have liberty to attend for instruction. In *Edinburgh University Calendar* the year 1756 is given as the date of his appointment to the chair of midwifery.

arrangements remained unchanged but, in 1760, the number of maternity beds chargeable on the funds of the hospital was increased from four to six. Two years later, in response to an urgent appeal by those students who had not had opportunities of receiving clinical instruction in midwifery, permission was given to the professor to conduct a summer course, the ward being kept open for two months longer than had been originally arranged.

In 1780, Alexander Hamilton, who became joint-professor with Young, and his successor three years later, continued the practice of obstetrics in the Infirmary, "restricting his clinical tuition among outdoor patients to students who under the designation 'annual pupils' paid a fee of ten guineas." That arrangement, however, proving inadequate for the training of students and nurses, proposals for a Lying-in Hospital were discussed and steps were taken to establish the same. In 1793, Park House—close to the site now occupied by the University Union—was fitted as a private hospital and named the Edinburgh General Lying-in Hospital, from which eventually arose the Royal Maternity and Simpson Memorial Hospital. The maternity ward in the Infirmary was therefore closed in August of that year and used as a fever ward for female patients.

Thus for thirty-eight years, during the eighteenth century, the Royal Infirmary made provision for the care of the parturient woman and for instruction in practical midwifery. After the long interval of nearly 140 years the Infirmary has again assumed a similar responsibility, upon a greatly extended scale, by accepting the transfer and management of the Maternity Hospital with the object of providing obstetrical wards in the new Simpson Memorial Maternity Pavilion, when that building should be completed.

Very early in the history of the Infirmary the grim spectre of the "waiting list" made its appearance. While cases of acute illness or of persons who had met with serious accidents were, in all circumstances, given first consideration, there were numerous occasions when applications for the admission of those suffering from minor disabilities exceeded the available accommodation, and arrangements had to be made to cope with this difficulty. In the Statutes of the Infirmary, revised after the Charter had been granted, it was expressly stated that a sick person might be admitted as a "supernumerary" patient on the payment of sixpence per day till a bed on the ordinary establishment became vacant, this sum being considered sufficient for maintenance. As security one guinea had to be deposited with the Clerk of the House and when "the *Depositum* is consumed a new one is to be made; and, if there is any Remainder of any of them, it shall be returned at such Patients' going out." In some instances the supernumerary patients were cured so that their transference later to the wards occupied by the ordinary patients was unnecessary. In 1767, the managers accepted a proposal of the Earl of Galloway to lodge £5 sterling with the Clerk for the same purpose. When this sum became exhausted he promised to pay sixpence per day for any supernumerary patients who, in the opinion of the physicians, ought to be admitted to the house till vacant beds were available in the wards.

For a number of years a special return of this group of in-patients was made in the annual reports. In one year as many as eighty-seven were stated to have been under treatment. In 1771, the managers required that a monthly report should be made along with a statement of the names of those recommending their admission and of the number who had paid. On one occasion fifty-three supernumeraries were returned of whom only five had paid! This request for monthly returns suggested that some doubt had arisen as to the regularity with which payments were being made. An arrangement existed, however, which gave the physicians discretionary power to admit supernumerary patients without payment, up to the number of ten, "who, from the nature of their ailment and poverty together, could not be rejected without doing violence to the laws of humanity."

In 1749, on the suggestion of the managers, John Clerk, one of their colleagues and a Fellow of the Royal College of Physicians, designed the Crest of the Royal Infirmary from which a Seal was cut on steel and used as a stamp on the official documents. An error having been detected in the original armorial bearings, the late Sir James Balfour Paul, Lord Lyon King of Arms, was asked in 1914 to make the necessary correction. His description in heraldic terms reads :—

> Argent on a mount in base proper, a Castle triple towered Sable, masoned of the first, windows, portcullis and vanes Gules, between two Æsculapian rods in the flanks proper : above the shield is placed a helmet befitting their degree with a Mantling Gules dubbed Argent, and on a wreath of their liveries is set for Crest, a pelican in her piety proper, and in an escrol over the same this Motto, " Ad sanitatem gentium " and in another below the shield this Motto, " Patet Omnibus." [1]

Although the hospital was " open to all," it is perfectly clear from the foregoing account that the managers of those days were not prepared to admit and maintain gratuitously all and sundry.

Proof of the increasing interest taken in the Royal Infirmary, at a time when financial help was so much desired to place the whole of the new hospital at the service of the sick, has been exemplified in the Earl of Hopetoun's Annual Fund for the maintenance of incurable persons, and in the legacy of Mr James Hunter for the care of domestic servants. The practice of bequeathing legacies, thus originated, has grown from year to year and they now constitute the greater proportion of the Extraordinary Annual Income of the Infirmary. Another legacy was unexpectedly obtained from the Jamaican estate of Dr Archibald Ker who died in 1750 while on the voyage to England. His property on the island was valued at a figure yielding in the currency of Jamaica £306 annually, and when converted to sterling, the sum of £218, 11s. 5d. Some years later Mr John Henderson of Kingston, Jamaica, bequeathed £500 to the hospital, a further testimony of the keen interest maintained in the institutions of their native land by Scotsmen resident overseas. Numerous other legacies varying from £10 to £500 were received during the ensuing years, thus materially assisting the funds of the hospital.

[1] In heraldry, the Pelican in her piety represents the old belief that she fed her young with her blood and she thus became the emblem of charity.

An interesting sidelight is thrown upon the methods adopted at this time to raise additional revenue by leasing to townsmen parts of the unoccupied building as business premises. Thus Scott & Laurie, druggists, rented for two years a room in the west wing of the hospital at £7, 10s. per annum, afterwards raised to £10. Hamilton & Co., printers, were given a ward on the third floor of the same wing, along with a small room at the top of the stair as a printing room and warehouse at the same rent. Some cellars in the basement were occupied as dwellings, but as the tenants of these persisted in coming in at all hours of the night, it was found necessary to get rid of them.

Another and by no means negligible source of annual income was derived from the disposal of hospital tickets to students attending for clinical instruction, a subject which will be more appropriately dealt with when teaching in the medical school comes under consideration. But an interesting and unique eighteenth-century relic is preserved in the Board Room of the Infirmary, a playing card, the ten of clubs which has been used as a hospital ticket. Dated 1st November 1768, signed by Alexander Hunter, the preses of the Board on the day of its issue and countersigned by Gilbert Laurie, the Treasurer, it admits John Goodsir, student of medicine, for one year, the fee charged being £3, 5s. 6d. What became of the other fifty-one cards of the pack? Were the managers of that period of a more than usually economical frame of mind? John Goodsir, whose hospital ticket is thus preserved, became a practitioner in Largo, Fife, and was the grandfather of John Goodsir, the professor of anatomy at Edinburgh, 1846 to 1867.[1]

As the possibility of future expansion of the Infirmary was not lost sight of, the managers availed themselves of every opportunity of acquiring property in its immediate neighbourhood. By this means they not only increased the value of their Capital Stock but, by leasing the purchased buildings on favourable terms, added to their annual revenue. The Flodden Wall to the south and the University buildings and

[1] The card was presented to the managers by Professor John Chiene.

garden on the west side of the hospital precluded any extension in these directions ; but on the east side the area was less circumscribed. Standing between the Infirmary and the High School and opposite the head of the High School Wynd was the house of Mr Archibald Stewart, formerly belonging to the Earls of Cromartie. Although in a very dilapidated condition, the house was bought for £400 sterling, on the advice of William Adam, the architect, as he considered that, if rebuilt, the rent would in course of time more than repay the initial expenditure. The Countess of Haddington became tenant of the new house and grounds, paying £50 annually ; but she proved to be a very troublesome occupant, repeatedly demanding repairs and improvements. As she lived till the age of ninety she was for a long time a thorn in the flesh of the Treasurer of the Infirmary. Many years later the resident house physicians occupied a building on this site.

Other houses were purchased, from time to time, for which tenants were obtained : particular mention may be made of Roehead's Brewery on the east side of Robertson's Close and behind Lady Yester's Church. Bought for £1050, it was leased to Lady Seton for twenty years at the annual rent of fifty guineas.

It was not always as a business transaction, based on the ulterior motive of increasing the annual income of the hospital, that vacant accommodation was temporarily disposed of by the managers. On more than one occasion friendly assistance was extended to their near neighbours, the surgeons and physicians, and to the members of the Royal Medical Society. In the days of adversity the Incorporation of Surgeons was sometimes compelled to lease to tenants the Hall and adjoining dwelling-house. It was then necessary that they should find a suitable place in which to deposit their collection of books and the " curiosities " in their possession. Accommodation was obtained in the Infirmary, the surgeons retaining the liberty of borrowing the books, on giving the necessary security to return them.[1] In 1763, the books were withdrawn and transferred to the University library as the surgeons desired

[1] Minute, Royal Infirmary, 27th July 1761.

to encourage the scheme, then projected, of making the latter more complete and useful. Three years later the Royal College of Physicians, finding the accommodation in the Hall in Fountain Close insufficient for the storage of their books, sought " an empty ward in the Infirmary if such could be spared for the College Library."[1] The request was granted, and for fifteen years the hospital provided a temporary asylum.

The establishment of a Bagnio or Public Bath House proved another source of revenue. In William Adam's original plan of the Royal Infirmary, accommodation was reserved on the ground floor of the east wing for hot and cold baths for the use of the patients in the hospital, but these had not been introduced when the building was finally completed. As the supply of water had been improved in 1743 by laying down a special pipe to connect with the main conduit to the city, Alexander Monro in September 1748 proposed that a Bagnio or bath house along with a wash house should be built, the bath to serve for the use of the public. After a considerable interval it was decided to raise subscriptions for this purpose and Mr James Adam, architect, was invited to prepare plans.

The institution of a public bath house in connection with a large establishment like the Infirmary was not unknown in those days when private dwellings lacked the necessary bathing arrangements. The surgeons, near neighbours of the Infirmary, had experimented and failed to make a profitable concern of a bath house in connection with their Hall. The surgeons' Bagnio, handsomely and expensively paved with white marble tiles purchased in Holland, had been opened in 1704, but, as the years passed, it failed to maintain its earlier success. The prices charged for admission had to be reduced and, finally in 1740, the baths were closed and the ornamentation disposed of to the best advantage.[2] A similar unsuccessful attempt had been made by the physicians in the ground adjoining their Hall in Fountain Close by converting some dilapidated

[1] Minute, Royal Infirmary, 9th June 1766.

[2] *Royal College of Surgeons of Edinburgh, 1505-1905*, by C. H. Creswell (Edinburgh, 1926), p. 52.

buildings adjacent to the Cowgate into a pavilion for cold-water baths. For the use of the bath a charge of 12 shillings Scots (1 shilling sterling) was made, with one penny to the attendant, while those who subscribed one guinea had the privilege of using the baths when they pleased. The physicians, having found it inconvenient to superintend the establishment, leased the building in 1714, but the speculation did not prove satisfactory as frequent requests were made to reduce the rents, and demands for repairs interfered with the profits.[1]

Undeterred by the example of these failures, the managers of the Infirmary proceeded with the construction of their public Bagnio in the west wing of the building to which the citizens were to have entrance through a separate door. Equipped with marble bathing troughs and "finished in the neatest manner in all the other parts of its furniture," the bath house was opened in July 1756. The subscriptions collected for its erection had been received from several sources: from the ladies of "the Assembly," £69, 3s. 1d.; from Mr John Jardine, Minister in the city, 100 Merks Scots, while further subscriptions amounting to a sum of £27, 6s. included £21 from the Duke of Hamilton. The hours of admission were from 9 A.M. to 7 P.M. Both sweating and massage treatment were provided. Those contributing ten guineas or upwards had the right to use the baths during life, those giving one guinea to the building fund were entitled to use them for one year. For sweating, a fee of four shillings was exacted, for a warm bath two shillings and for a cold bath one shilling; and on no account might a rubber or other attendant accept a gratuity under pain of dismissal.

The venture met with more success than those previously attempted by the surgeons and physicians, as in 1823—sixty-seven years after the baths were opened—the appointment of a new keeper of the baths is recorded in the minutes of the hospital. There is possibly truth in the story that when George IV visited Edinburgh in 1822 he used the Bagnio. This may or may not be the case, but the minute of 26th

[1] *Historical Sketch and Laws of the Royal College of Physicians* (Edinburgh, 1925), p. 40.

August of that year records with gratification His Majesty's donation of two hundred guineas to the Royal Infirmary. In 1836-37 the baths yielded a sum of £65, 6s. 4d. and in the following year £96, 6s., but no further reference is made to the public baths in the accounts. Close to the site of the old bath house now stand the City Corporation Baths erected by the Town Council for the use of the public, after the demolition in 1884 of the old Infirmary building.

After the granting of the Charter new Statutes were drawn up by the managers which received the approval of the General Court of Contributors at their annual meeting in 1743. The duties of the various officials engaged in the internal administration of the hospital were clearly defined and, while no radical changes were introduced in the conduct of its affairs, some increase in the number of the staff became necessary in the larger establishment in Infirmary Street.

The posts of Treasurer and of Clerk to the Corporation continued to be separate and held by two individuals: these offices remained, as before, in the hands of David Spence and Henry Balcanquhal, respectively. But in the spring of 1744, David Spence who, from the inception of the hospital movement in 1725, had given his services gratuitously, tendered his resignation as Treasurer on the ground of age and ill-health. On his retirement in the month of August the managers minuted "their grateful thanks and approbation for the faithfulness and accuracy with which he had discharged his trust as Treasurer and for his charitable diligence so long voluntarily bestowed in the service of the hospital without fee or reward." Mr Gavin Hamilton, late bailie, a bookseller in Edinburgh, was elected his successor and received a small annual salary. At the same time an Accountant was appointed, Mr Alexander Chalmers, whose duties were to prepare a full statement of the affairs of the Infirmary from the books of the Treasurer and the minutes of the managers and, from these, to present an abstract for the consideration of the committee of the General Court of Contributors. His salary was £36. This is apparently the first mention of the appointment of an auditor. The " strong box " in which were deposited all the vouchers of the funds of the hospital was very carefully protected, being provided with two locks, with different works and keys : one key was kept by the Treasurer and the other by a manager, selected yearly. No paper could be removed from it by the Treasurer or by any other person without a previous order of the ordinary managers or of the General Court of Managers, or Court of Contributors, the order specifying the papers to be taken out, the occasion for doing so, and the person to whom they were to be delivered. The duties of the Clerk to the Corporation consisted in attendance at all the meetings of the Board and of the Courts, in summoning the managers to the same, in the keeping of the minutes and of those receipts not coming within the sphere of the Treasurer.

The Matron or Governess—her alternative title—continued in office, with control over the nurses and servants and with the charge of the inventory of all the household furniture which was inspected and checked with the articles themselves once yearly by a committee of the managers. She was required to make a ward visit daily, to purchase the provisions and to keep an exact register of all donations in kind, coals, meal, blankets, etc.

The Clerk of the House was another new official with considerable responsibilities. In those days there was no superintendent, an office which was not established till the latter half of the nineteenth century. The Clerk was a man educated in medicine and unmarried : he was required to live in the house and to give all his time to his duties, discharging the functions of medical registrar and house physician and surgeon. He kept a record of all the patients on the waiting list, wrote their histories on admission, to which he added in his ledgers the notes of their further progress dictated to him by the physicians and surgeons. He visited the wards morning and evening. He had to acquaint the matron with the form of diet prescribed for each patient and to send the apothecary a copy of each prescription for the purpose of dispensing. He was responsible to the Clerk to the Corporation for the preparation of the annual return of all the patients under treatment.

His duties also entailed inspection of the students' tickets before they could be admitted to the operating theatre. On Saturday afternoons he dictated the case-notes to such students as attended and, when desired, transcribed copies of these notes for which he was allowed to charge the students threepence per page, a sum afterwards reduced to twopence. All the instruments, dressings and printed books belonging to the Infirmary, with the price of each article attached, were in his charge: any of these might be borrowed by the visiting staff, the borrower requiring to deposit the price annexed in the inventory, "along with a twelfth part more, the price being returned when the book or instrument is given back in good condition; but the twelfth is to be retained, for the use of the book or instrument: whereas if any book or instrument is damaged or injured, the price is also to be retained, the borrower keeping the book or instrument." The professor of anatomy and surgery appears to have been a specially privileged person as "he may, upon depositing the price, borrow from the Clerk the instruments for his course of lectures without paying any premium for the use of them, on condition that he shall once a year demonstrate to the licensed students the mechanism and manner of using all the instruments." The Clerk might also sell any instruments or dressings at the prices marked in the inventory, but he was required to replace them by others. He had to render an account of all these transactions to a committee of the managers.

The important post of Clerk of the House was given to Robert McKinley, at first without a salary, but on consideration of his manifold duties the managers decided, in 1745, to pay him £10 per annum, this allowance to be calculated from the date of his original appointment. The clerk and the matron were frequently in disagreement. He accused her of various misdemeanours—she spoke harshly to the patients, she watered the milk, her rice puddings were deficient both in eggs and milk and she constantly entertained her friends to tea. On enquiry the managers satisfied themselves that, although she had occasionally spoken roughly to the patients, the other complaints were untrue and malicious. The matron was reprimanded for the former offence and the clerk was admonished and warned not to interfere with matters that did not belong to his department. But the clerk was a troublesome fellow, and a year or two later attacked the Treasurer, accusing him of substituting for the physicians' prescriptions the drops of a certain Dr Maximilian, a " German practitioner." Mr McKinley apologised for his groundless calumny and was permitted to remain ; but becoming lazy and in arrears with his report, in 1747 his services were finally dispensed with. Mrs Waldie, the matron, who had succeeded Mrs Nisbett, the first matron, remained in her post for fourteen years, finally resigning on the grounds of age and infirmity.

After the dismissal of McKinley, Mr Petrie and Mr Sutherland assumed the twofold duties of Clerk and Apothecary, serving alternately in these posts, each with an annual salary of £10. They resided in the hospital and both could not be absent at the same time. For several years the managers had been considering the introduction of an Apothecary's Shop so that the patients might be more readily provided with medicines. When the original hospital was opened the surgeon-apothecaries had supplied the drugs at their own cost, but with the increase in the number of patients in the new Infirmary and in order to free the surgeons from this increasing expense, it was decided to open in 1747 a " shop " or dispensary within the building and to apply the sum of £10 for that purpose. Petrie having resigned in 1750, Sutherland became apothecary, and very careful instructions were prepared as to how he should conduct the dispensary. In 1754 the number of out-patients, many of whom received medicines, had reached one thousand. The managers then advised the discontinuance of the supply of medicines to out-patients, a proposal which received the approval of the Court of Contributors. When the annual expenditure on drugs amounted to the sum of £15 and continued to increase, the managers appealed to the Town Council for the lease of a portion of the adjacent College Garden, where they might grow herbs and roots for the service of the " shop." This was granted free of rent with certain conditions and reservations.

After Petrie's resignation, Physicians' and Surgeons' Clerks were appointed. The clerks were students of medicine : they lived in the hospital and were allowed to attend classes in the University, provided the hours did not interfere with their duties in the Infirmary. An annual salary of £10 was paid to each, an allowance which was eventually discontinued.[1] Eligibility for these posts was later restricted to those students who had completed two sessions at the University and at least one year of attendance in the Infirmary, the appointment being then limited to a period of two years.[2]

The duties of the physicians' clerks were somewhat similar to those previously discharged by the Clerk of the House and do not require to be restated. The clerks, however, were responsible for keeping an account of, and receiving, the monies from the patients from whom payment was exacted, the soldiers and sailors, the domestic servants and supernumeraries. The duties of the surgeons' clerks included the notification of operations, the summoning of the surgeons to consultations, the care of the instruments and the direction of the dressers with instruction in bandaging. They had permission also to perform minor surgical operations, such as cupping, bleeding and the introduction of setons. It came to the knowledge of the managers that some of the clerks were in the habit of conducting private practice while engaged in their hospital duties, and intimation was at once made that this practice must cease.[3]

Gratuities were sometimes given to the physicians' clerks for the important work they did in collecting the money from those patients who paid for their treatment. Thus, when a certain Mr William Butter resigned on taking his doctor's degree, after ten years of service as clerk, he was given £10, 10s. in recognition of his long and faithful services ; similarly

[1] Minutes, Royal Infirmary, August and September 1791.
[2] Minute, Royal Infirmary, April 1695. [3] *Ibid.*, August 1775.

Mr Alexander Monro Drummond, in 1765, received a gratuity of £21 "for his extraordinary trouble in collecting the money on behalf of the supernumerary patients and the soldiers"; he was also allowed ten shillings per quarter for his laundry. On his resignation in 1770 he received another gratuity of 20 guineas. On this occasion the managers considered the expediency of discontinuing this form of remuneration; nevertheless, in the following year, they gave Mr Huggan five guineas for faithful service. It is difficult to understand why the collecting of such fees was not placed from the first in the hands of the Treasurer to the hospital. In 1773, Wilkinson Manuel, one of the physicians' clerks, applied to have his personal laundry done in the Infirmary, or alternatively, to be granted an allowance for that purpose. Two years later the managers authorised the payment of £2 sterling for laundry to each of the resident clerks for a period of one year till the whole matter was given fuller consideration. But it was not till 1st October 1909 that an allowance for laundry was finally granted to the resident physicians and surgeons, the sum given to each being £4 per quarter.[1] After 1800, new regulations were adopted and the managers approved of a resolution that the clerks should pay £20 yearly "as a consideration for their entertainment of bed and board in the Infirmary."[2] In a subsequent minute that sum was apparently raised to 30 guineas.[3] The tables had indeed been turned! On 27th February 1854, the resident clerks were named Resident House Physicians and House Surgeons: they were then qualified medical practitioners.

The ledgers, in which the case histories and notes of the patients while in hospital were recorded by the clerks, belonged at first to the Infirmary; and, from time to time, the minutes contain references to requests from members of the visiting staff for permission to publish cases in the medical press, a request invariably granted by the managers. A rule was

[1] No salary is attached to the post of house physician and house surgeon.

[2] Minute, Royal Infirmary, January 1803.

[3] Minute, Royal Infirmary, 31st March 1818. In 1839-40 the accounts show that the receipts obtained from the board of resident clerks totalled £442, 10s. A sum of £1663 was received for students' hospital tickets in the same year.

established that the signature of "the chief" should be attached to the ledgers kept by the clerks as a guarantee that the records they contained were authentic accounts of the character and nature of the disease of each patient admitted to the Infirmary. In 1844, this regulation led to an unfortunate dispute between the managers and the Senatus Academicus, when James Syme, professor of clinical surgery, refused to docquet the reports of his cases made by his clerk. The managers threatened to dispense with Syme's services to the hospital if he persisted in his refusal. The matter was finally settled by his compliance, on the advice of the Senatus on grounds of expediency, although his colleagues in the Senatus did not approve of the regulation.[1] Syme's letter to the Board, dated 13th January 1845, was ordered to be engrossed in the minutes :—

Gentlemen, when you intimated to the Senatus Academicus that my connection with the Infirmary depended upon docqueting the cases, I at once declared my resolution to be guided by the opinion of my Colleagues.

The Senatus, while not approving of the Regulation in question, having on grounds of expediency advised me to comply with it, I now acquaint you with my intention of doing so for the future. At the same time I take the liberty of expressing my deep regret for being forced to perform a duty which will every week prevent me from forgetting how little respect for my opinion as to the professional details of the Hospital is entertained by the Managers—and how lightly they value my connection with the Infirmary. I have the honour to be,

Gentlemen,

Your most obedt. servant,

(Signed) James Syme.

Syme very reasonably held the view that the clerks, who were not nominated by him, were not sufficiently qualified to write accurate accounts of the cases.

A Porter was also appointed to the new hospital : he too resided in the house and could not absent himself unless on the service of the Infirmary or with permission of the matron.

[1] Minutes, Royal Infirmary, 28th October 1844 and 13th January 1845.

John Forbes, the first to occupy the position, had a very brief tenure of office, as notwithstanding repeated instructions to the contrary he accepted monetary gifts from visitors to the hospital " to the great prejudice of the Charity Box," and he accepted " tips " from curiously-minded persons whom he admitted to the theatre to see operations. A successor was appointed at a salary of £6 sterling yearly, " who on no pretext whatsoever shall accept or receive for his own use or benefit any money or gratification whatsoever from any persons who shall happen to come and see the Infirmary."

The regulations controlling the duties of the Cook to the hospital found a place in the printed statutes. Every morning she required to wait upon the matron to receive from her the bill of fare and the daily provisions, and to submit to her a sample of each kind of food prepared for the patients before sending it to the wards. Three kinds of diet were prescribed by order of the physicians and surgeons, low, middle and full diets. The low diet consisted mainly of bread and milk with oaten or barley meal porridge, also of rice and milk ; the middle diet contained, in addition to the above, broths prepared with beef or mutton with a small allowance of ale ; in full diet, boiled beef or mutton, broth and a larger allowance of small beer were supplied. Various fruits in their respective seasons were included in the dietary. In the weekly Bill of Fare, it is stated that for breakfast each patient received, in the form of porridge, four ounces of meal with three gills of milk, or, alternatively, a bap, weighing six ounces, and one mutchkin of milk.[1]

The nursing establishment comprised " Ordinary " and " Supernumerary " Nurses. Each ward was in charge of an ordinary nurse whose duties were to clean the ward before nine o'clock in the morning, make the beds, attend generally to the patients and carry the medicine bottles to and from the apothecary's shop. The salary of the ordinary nurse varied from £3, 10s. to £5 per annum. Supernumerary nurses were engaged for those who required constant attention by day and night. They received a special fee of fourpence or even

[1] A mutchkin measures about three-quarters of an imperial pint.

sixpence per night: they were forbidden on any pretext whatsoever to accept gratuities. There did not appear to be any ordinary nurse on night duty. On one occasion the female patients complained that the nurses distributed the porridge first to the male patients. The complaint was rectified by the managers giving instructions that the women were not to be given cold porridge!

At the request of the managers, the ministers of the city and suburbs agreed to visit the sick in the Infirmary in rotation, at first for the period of a fortnight and later by weekly attendance. In 1755, the proposal was made to appoint a Chaplain at a small salary, and the suggestion was remitted to the Court of Contributors for their consideration. In the following year Mr Willis, Minister of the Gospel, was elected first Chaplain to the house at a yearly salary of £12. He agreed to preach once each Sunday and, in addition, to visit the wards twice weekly and to attend any call made on behalf of a dying patient. It became part of his duty also to open with prayer each meeting of the Board of Management.

CHAPTER VIII

THE ROYAL INFIRMARY IN THE EIGHTEENTH CENTURY—*Continued*

PHYSICIANS-IN-ORDINARY FIRST APPOINTED BY THE BOARD OF MANAGEMENT—SURGEONS-IN-ORDINARY APPOINTED BY THE BOARD —END OF THE SYSTEM OF ATTENDANCE BY ROTATION.

IN the previous chapter a brief account has been given of the duties of the officials responsible for the conduct of the business of the Infirmary—the Treasurer, the Clerk to the Corporation and the Accountant—and of the members of the domestic staff resident in the hospital, and sometimes referred to as " the Family," a term now long in disuse but happily expressive of the little household of bygone days. The procedure adopted in appointing the physicians and surgeons, although referred to in an earlier chapter, requires fuller explanation as, during the long life of the Infirmary, it has undergone more than one important change.

It may be recalled that when the original hospital was opened in Robertson's Close in 1729, the physicians gave their services gratuitously, attending the patients for short periods of time on a system of rotation. Originally all the Fellows and Licentiates on the roll of the Royal College of Physicians served the Institution along with six members of the Incorporation of Surgeons. A few years later, however, the managers found it necessary to limit the medical staff to the Fellows of the Royal College, as the attendance of so many physicians caused considerable inconvenience. The surgical staff, on the other hand, at first six in number, became augmented later in consequence of the agreement concluded in 1738 between the managers and the " erectors " of the Surgeons' Hospital, whereby all those members of the Incorporation, who expressed their willingness to act, were admitted as surgeons to the Infirmary on the same terms as the six originally appointed.[1]

The system of attendance by rotation was still in operation when the new building was occupied in December 1741. The unsatisfactory nature of this arrangement, however, became more and more apparent with the steady increase in the number of those joining the two Incorporations who, during their residence in the city and suburbs, were eligible to act as members of the staff of the Infirmary. The system presented many disadvantages. The managers were denied any voice or participation in the selection of those placed in charge of the sick persons for whose proper care and treatment they were ultimately responsible. They had no option but to accept the physicians and surgeons on the roll of their respective Incorporations—the old and the young, the experienced and the inexperienced, the able and the inefficient—without any opportunity of estimating their worthiness for their duties. The visiting staff, on the other hand, were handicapped by too brief periods on duty and by longer intervals between their terms of service, as the new Fellows and members claimed their privileges. The staff were thus deprived of the opportunity of acquiring the experience derived from constant attendance on the sick, denied continuity of time for the observation and study of disease, and compelled to interrupt their service at the hospital for months at a time. It was becoming evident also that certain of the senior members of the Incorporations, conscious of the weakness of the system, were withdrawing themselves from hospital attendance. Furthermore, the frequent changes in the personnel were undoubtedly detrimental to the interests of the patients, placed as they might be in the care of young and inexperienced men, some of whom had probably just received their licence to practise. Attempts to minimise the risks attending this unsatisfactory state of affairs are seen in the somewhat elaborate regulations made by the managers for consultations between several members of the staff in difficult cases, especially when the question of the performance of a serious operation arose.

[1] Chapter v, pp. 66, 67.

Nor did the system tend to enhance the reputation of the school of medicine in which an ever increasing number of students was seeking education. It was essential that clinical teaching and the professional practice of the hospital should be maintained, as far as possible, on a uniformly high level and not subjected to periods during which an inferior quality of instruction and a poor standard of professional skill were exhibited. Weakness in both these respects was readily detected by discerning and critical students and did not redound to the credit of the school.

It is not surprising, therefore, to find the managers in January 1751—twenty-two years after the first hospital had been opened—resolving to make a definite change in a system, of the evils of which they had so long been conscious. They decided, as a commencement, to lay before the Court of Contributors a plan designed to alter the procedure regulating the attendance of the physicians. The minute of 7th January of that year reads as follows :—

> It having pleased God in his providence to dispose the hearts of many well inclined persons to become contributors to the charitable purpose intended by the establishment of the Royal Infirmary, whereby the number of patients taken in has been of late very much increased, and it appearing by the present state of the funds that the well-grounded prospect they have of considerable future benefactions that there will be room to take in a still greater number of distressed, by which the trouble and attendance of the physicians who have hitherto very generously given their assistance and advice gratis is likely to be much increased, unless some remedy is found for their relief at least in part of that burden, therefore humbly moved that the following proposal be laid before the General Court of Contributors for their consideration ; namely, that two fixed physicians may be appointed for the constant and daily attendance on the patients, under the title of Physicians-in-Ordinary to the Infirmary, and that the ordinary managers be authorised to elect and nominate such physicians as they shall think proper, and to make them such allowance for their trouble as they shall judge reasonable, due regard being had to the condition of the Infirmary's funds at the time ; this to take place on 24th June next, and that the Royal College of Physicians be entrusted to give their advice and confidence in these matters.

The Court of Contributors meeting on the same day approved of, and agreed to, this proposal. At the same time the thanks of the Corporation were conveyed to the Royal College of Physicians for the attendance which the Fellows had hitherto given to the sick poor. The Court further begged them to continue their good offices by appointing some of their number to attend monthly by rotation, or in whatever way they thought proper, to visit the house once or twice weekly to give their advice and assistance to the two physicians-in-ordinary, when the latter considered it necessary. To this request the President of the Royal College replied that " they did most cheerfully agree to what is thereby desired, namely, to continue their good offices to the Infirmary by appointing some of their number monthly by rotation, or in what other way they think proper, to visit the house once or twice a week." Thus the physicians accepted without demur the new arrangement of attendance at the Infirmary notwithstanding the curtailment of the privileges to which they had hitherto been entitled. The two ordinary physicians attended the hospital daily, examining the patients under their care. Those selected by the College of Physicians—called extraordinary physicians—attended for one month in rotation, once or twice weekly, their duties being mainly those of consulting physicians, one for in-patients and one for out-patients, giving their advice to the ordinary physicians in cases of importance.

By the appointment of two physicians, with no time limit attached to their tenure of office, the managers provided for continuous and uninterrupted attendance, thus removing one of the objectionable features of the old system. For the first time too in the history of the Infirmary, the Board of Management was responsible for the selection of members of the visiting staff. At the same time there was introduced a system of payment for services rendered to the hospital by members of the medical staff. Hence in two important particulars, in the payment for treatment by certain classes of patients, as previously related, and in salaries to members of the visiting staff, a practice was established contrary to the principle on which the conduct of the voluntary hospital was based.

The managers, with the powers given to them by the Court of Contributors, elected as physicians-in-ordinary to the Infirmary, David Clerk and Colin Drummond with instructions to commence their duties on 24th June 1751: they also granted them " an annual allowance or salary of £30 sterling to be paid to each out of the annual revenue of the House during the time that they so officiate." They accepted office and appeared before the Board to take the oath *De Fideli*. Both men were young physicians, graduates of the University of Edinburgh and Fellows of the Royal College of Physicians. Clerk had been qualified for five years and had taken a post-graduate course at Leiden, but Drummond, the younger man, had taken his degree only in the previous year. David Clerk served the hospital for seventeen years till his death in 1768; Colin Drummond resigned in 1773 after giving twenty-two years of service. A time limit was not imposed till 1824 when a physician-in-ordinary was appointed for a period of seven years. David Clerk's successor in office was John Hope, professor of botany in the University: John Steedman succeeded Colin Drummond in 1773. The first two physicians were members of the Board of Management at the time of their election to the staff; and it is interesting to note that they then voluntarily resigned their position as managers, but again took the oath *De Fideli* on their appointment to the staff of the hospital. The custom of administering the oath to members of the medical and surgical staff, when first appointed, remained for one hundred and nineteen years, the last reference to this appearing in the minutes in 1870. It is perhaps regrettable that this old time formality, which afforded an opportunity of introducing the members of the staff to the Board of Management, should have been discontinued.

John Hope, a son of Robert Hope one of the original six surgeons on the staff of the Infirmary in Robertson's Close, was an eminent botanist, occupying the chair from 1761 to 1786. A disciple of Linnæus, he introduced into Scotland the Linnæan system of the classification of plants and was responsible for the transference of the old Physic

Garden from its damp and somewhat sunless area at Trinity Hospital to a more favourable position on the west side of Leith Walk in the vicinity of Gayfield Square. For a brief period in 1774 Joseph Black, the discoverer of carbonic acid gas and of the principle of latent heat, and the successor of William Cullen in the chair of chemistry in 1766, was one of the physicians-in-ordinary to the Infirmary, acting conjointly with John Steedman. His tenure of office was brief, however, as he resigned at the end of one month.

If the faults and inconveniences of a system of attendance by rotation demanded the change adopted in 1751 in the case of the physicians, some similar drastic measure was even more necessary in the case of the surgeons. The defects already detailed, were aggravated in their case by the very irregular manner in which some of the surgeons attended the hospital, sending substitutes in their place who, in turn, often failed to put in an appearance. Arrangements for the necessary consultations and for obtaining decisions regarding the incurability of certain diseases were thus difficult to adjust, while the maintenance of discipline amongst the surgeons' clerks and dressers was becoming more impracticable. Irregular attendance on the part of the surgeons was not a recent phase. As far back as 1748 it had been found necessary to stiffen the regulations as to attendance, so that when a surgeon was negligent of his duties on a second occasion and failed to provide a deputy, the Clerk of the House was given authority to remove his name from the list of those to be summoned in rotation.

At their meeting on 7th July 1766, the managers took action :—

they being fully sensible of the inconveniences attending the practice of surgery in the hospital on the present plan, and desirous of establishing regulations to prevent them in the future, do hereby statute and ordain that all the members of the Incorporation of Surgeons shall attend monthly by turns as at present, each surgeon during his one month of attendance to perform the operations which shall occur and advise the surgical cases in the Infirmary, but shall not have the power of substituting any other in his place either for advising or operating.

In order to effect a regular attendance of surgeons in the House agreeably to the plan pursued so successfully with respect to the physicians, they hereby nominate and appoint four surgeons, all members of the Incorporation . . . and declare them, Surgeons-in-Ordinary to the Royal Infirmary, ordaining them, in addition, to attend during the month which shall fall to them by rotation, together with the surgeon whose turn it shall be to wait on the Infirmary, and, in his absence, to advise the surgical cases and perform the operations and to attend all consultations, to commit to their care the direction of dressers and dressings, the records of cases and the inspection and management of the Apothecary's shop. . . .

At the same time the managers authorised the Treasurer to pay annually to each of the four surgeons the sum of £10 Sterling as salary, their office as Surgeons-in-Ordinary to commence on 1st August 1766.

The four surgeons selected by the managers were James Rae, Peter Adie, John Balfour and Alexander Wood, men occupying a senior position on the roll of the Incorporation. James Rae, then fifty years of age, had been Deacon of the Surgeons in 1764-65 ; he was a surgeon of repute and a skilful dentist. He delivered at Surgeons' Hall a course of lectures on surgery along with practical teaching on important cases in the Infirmary, and was the founder of instruction in clinical surgery in Edinburgh. Peter Adie had been a member of the Incorporation of Surgeons since 1751, and John Balfour a member for fifteen years, and Deacon in 1760. Alexander Wood, the junior member of the quartet, was forty-one years of age ; he had joined the Incorporation in 1756 and had been Deacon in 1762. Affectionately spoken of as " lang Sandy Wood," he was a well-known figure in the city : he is depicted in *Kay's Portraits* crossing the North Bridge wearing a periwig, cocked hat and knee breeches with an umbrella under his arm. He is said to have been the first man in Edinburgh to use that serviceable article. Alexander Wood " enjoyed the confidence of the public and the esteem of all good men " and added to the reputation of the surgical department of the Infirmary. He died in 1807 at the ripe age of eighty-two years.

The plan of attendance at the Infirmary and the subdivision of the work submitted by the four surgeons-in-ordinary were approved of by the Board. Commencing with the senior member of the group, each surgeon was to visit the hospital daily for a period of two months, the next in order always acting as his assistant and taking his place in the event of his unavoidable absence, thus forecasting the office of assistant surgeon to the Infirmary. Further, all were from time to time to attend the hospital together, when consultations or operations demanded such collaboration. In this way a more regular attendance was ensured and provision was also made for the constant service of surgeons of experience. At the same time the somewhat haphazard procedure previously in force, by which the surgeon attending in rotation could ask any member of the Incorporation to take his place, was terminated, as any one of the four surgeons-in-ordinary was, in these circumstances, to act as the substitute.

The new arrangement, however, was not accepted by the Incorporation of Surgeons in the same cheerful spirit as was displayed by the Royal College of Physicians on the appointment, in 1751, of two physicians-in-ordinary. On the contrary, the appointment of surgeons-in-ordinary was regarded as invidious and in distinct contravention of the agreement entered into, in 1738, between the managers and the Incorporation.[1] Although sensible of the defects of the existing system and acknowledging that they had accepted it subject to any alterations that the managers might in future deem necessary, the surgeons nevertheless felt that, when handing over to the managers of the Infirmary the Surgeons' Hospital and their funds, they had acquired for all their members in time coming security of the privilege of acting as surgeons to the Infirmary.

A somewhat protracted discussion ensued between the members of the two bodies, and Counsel's opinion was sought by the surgeons. Many months elapsed before a final settlement was reached, the surgeons maintaining the position that all their members should be free to act on the staff of the hospital; the managers, on the other hand, remaining unanimously of the opinion that the Incorporation of Surgeons had no power to appoint substitutes to officiate in place of the

[1] Pp. 66, 67.

absent surgeons. In order to reach an amicable understanding, a compromise was suggested by the managers in the form of certain alterations and amendments to their resolution of 7th July 1766, the chief proposal being that one of the four surgeons-in-ordinary should be changed each year, another member of the Incorporation being elected in his place.

On this basis, agreement was reached on 3rd April 1769—so long drawn out had been the consideration of the position. The managers then minuted the following resolutions :—1. They will change one of their four ordinary surgeons annually and will elect another of the Incorporation in his place ; 2. They will make this annual change and election according to seniority on the list of those surgeons willing to act ; and 3. This shall continue until altered by the managers. The list presented by the Incorporation contained the names of only sixteen members willing to attend the hospital monthly in rotation, eight of whom were also prepared to act as surgeons-in-ordinary or substitutes. As the complete resident membership of the Incorporation at that date was probably thirty-two, only half intimated their readiness to serve the Infirmary, while one fourth of the total number declared their willingness to accept the duties of surgeon-in-ordinary !

At this period surgery in Edinburgh was ably represented by the two families of Bell, the older, in the person of Benjamin Bell, " the father of the surgical school," the younger, by John Bell. Both men, before settling in practice in the city, had profited by years of study in European schools. Benjamin Bell, a native of Dumfries, joined the Incorporation of Surgeons in 1771 and, in the following year, applied to the Board of Management to be enrolled on the staff of the Infirmary as one of the surgeons in rotation,[1] serving the hospital in that capacity till the system of rotation was abandoned in 1800. His advice and surgical skill were in great demand : " he had an impressive mode of expressing himself, giving great assurance and confidence to the sick, and in all the excitement of a surgical operation he displayed the greatest composure." In his clinical teaching Bell emphasised the danger that might

[1] Minute, Royal Infirmary, 3rd August 1772.

follow the entrance of the atmospheric air into a large abscess when opened freely with the knife and, to obviate that risk, he recommended drainage of the pus by the introduction of a seton; he recognised too that the cancerous tumour was in the first instance a local condition and that early removal was essential if a cure was to be expected. His *System of Surgery* passed through seven editions and for many years remained a standard work: it was translated into French and German.[1] John Bell, born in Edinburgh, was not only an anatomist and surgeon, but an accomplished scholar, a musician and draughtsman. He earned the reputation of being one of the most skilful members of the surgical staff, but, conservative in his outlook, he was unwilling to regard operations as the be-all and end-all of surgery. John Bell died in Rome in 1820. His burial place is marked by a Celtic Cross erected by the Royal College of Surgeons of Edinburgh in 1891, and by its side is the nameless grave of John Keats, the English poet.[2]

For the moment matters had been amicably adjusted between the Infirmary and the Incorporation of Surgeons. The missing Minute Book, 1775-88 inclusive, interrupts the story; but it is significant to find that in December 1793 a committee was appointed to enquire once again into the attendance of the surgeons. One of the defects attendant upon the service by rotation had clearly not been removed and indeed had become aggravated, as the younger and more recently qualified surgeons were placing their names on the list for service, while the older and more experienced members of the Incorporation were declining to do so. As the result of the committee's enquiry the following resolution was minuted by the Board on 3rd February 1794, "That no future Intrant Member of the College of Surgeons shall be admitted to practise as an Attendant Surgeon in the Infirmary till after the lapse of five years from the time of his being admitted a

[1] Benjamin Bell's great grandson was Joseph Bell, surgeon to the Royal Infirmary, and the prototype of Sir Conan Doyle's "Sherlock Holmes."

[2] *The Edinburgh School of Surgery before Lister*, by Alexander Miles, M.D. (A. & C. Black, Ltd., London, 1918, p. 75.) Minutes, Royal College of Surgeons of Edinburgh, 3rd February and 16th May 1891.

member of the Incorporation of Surgeons."[1] Obviously the system of attendance by rotation still left something to be desired.

The arrangements recently completed remained in operation till 1800 when the whole question of surgical attendance was again opened up in a very acute form, in consequence of the printed Memorial[2] prepared and presented to the managers by James Gregory, one of their number, and the professor of practice of physic. This Memorial brought matters to a crisis. It strongly condemned the whole system of rotation and was the spark which ignited a conflagration that persisted when its original and admirable purpose was achieved, for it led to bitter personal controversies between members of the medical profession in Edinburgh, and found expression in numerous abusive pamphlets.

Conscious of the fact that the surgical department of the hospital was not being conducted either to the best advantage of the Institution, or in accordance with the interests of a public charity, the managers were again stirred to take prompt action. But before proceeding to consider new regulations they desired to ascertain the opinion of the Royal College of Surgeons.[3] The surgeons, thus given the opportunity, submitted to the Board a plan in which the old, vexed question of service by rotation for short periods still formed an important consideration. Two surgeons-in-ordinary were to attend according to seniority for six months, and the two surgeons next in rotation were to be present for at least one month before coming into office as ordinary surgeons. The proviso, however, was made that these surgeons should have been Fellows of the College for at least three years. They suggested also that three consulting surgeons should be appointed by the managers to attend when required and to assume duty should any sudden emergency arise. Thus, in the election of consulting surgeons the managers were to retain some responsibility in the choice of members of the staff, but in the attendance

[1] By a new Charter of 1778 the College was incorporated as the Royal College of Surgeons of Edinburgh.

[2] Minute, Royal Infirmary, 4th August 1800. [3] *Ibid.*, 1st September 1800.

of the surgeons-in-ordinary the system of rotation was to be perpetuated. Two clauses in the proposals submitted must have raised considerable criticism : the consultations were not to be confined to the two ordinary and three consulting surgeons but " any gentleman who may accidentally happen to be present shall be called upon to give his opinion and that, in particular cases, the ordinary surgeons shall have it in their power to call any and whatever number of the members of the College they shall think proper." *Quot homines, tot sententiæ!* Moreover, the ordinary surgeons were to have the power of selecting any of the Fellows of the College to assist them at their operations.[1]

Although the managers acknowledged that the new proposals submitted were in some respects an improvement upon the existing system of attendance, they could not see their way to perpetuate the indiscriminate method of rotation, however qualified, and which failed at the same time to place the election of the surgeons in the hands of the Board.[2] Their objection was still further strengthened by the knowledge that the proposals made by the Fellows had been carried in the College by the narrow majority of one vote, fifteen having voted in favour, and fourteen against, the minority also entering a protest against the measure.

Accordingly the managers proceeded to draw up a new system of attendance: this was, in brief, that six surgeons, Fellows of the College of at least three years standing, resident and practising in Edinburgh, were to be appointed by the Board, the two first on the list to act as surgeons-in-ordinary for two years, " when they shall resign and be succeeded by the two next on the list, they in like manner resigning at the end of the next two years to be succeeded by the remaining two of the first election." At the end of every second year two other surgeons having similar qualifications to the above were to be elected and placed at the foot of the list. No surgeon after acting as ordinary surgeon for two years was to be again eligible for appointment till the expiry of four years after his

[1] Minute, Royal Infirmary, 17th November 1800.
[2] *Ibid.*, 1st December 1800.

previous period of attendance. In the absence of one or both of the two surgeons acting as ordinary surgeons, the others listed would officiate for them in the order of their nomination by the managers. The two surgeons next in succession were to attend the hospital regularly for one month prior to assuming office as surgeons-in-ordinary so as to become acquainted with the patients in the wards.[1] All the members of the Royal College were invited to be present at the operations in the theatre and "that the first bench next the pit shall be allocated for their accommodation exclusively."

This scheme was then presented to the College along with the intimation that the Fellows desirous of acting on the staff should send their names to the Treasurer of the Royal Infirmary. But as the surgeons disapproved of the principle and re-affirmed the right of the members of the College to attend the hospital in rotation, according to the terms of the agreement of 1738, they declined to consider it. A further attempt on the part of the managers to adjust the differences between the two parties having failed in its object they adhered to their deliverance. Thus a definite break was made with the past, the old system of rotation was abrogated and the election of all the members of the surgical staff passed into the hands of the Board. A Bill of Suspension was applied for by the Royal College, but the Court of Session, by a considerable majority, found that the managers were entitled to enforce their former regulations and that the agreement of 1738 was no bar to any reasonable change made in the interest of the patients.[2]

On 23rd December 1800, James Russell, Andrew Wardrop, James Law, Andrew Inglis, William Brown, senior, and John Thomson, Fellows of the Royal College, were elected surgeons in charge of the department in terms of the regulations above prescribed; and, on the following day at an extraordinary meeting of the managers at which they attended, they took the oath, *De Fideli*, on accepting office.

[1] Minute, Royal Infirmary, 1st December 1800.

[2] *Morrison's Dictionary of Decisions*, vol. xiv., Article Privilege, Appendix, Part I.

It was unfortunate, however, that the new arrangement deprived the Infirmary of the services of more than one surgeon of exceptional promise. John Bell, with his younger brother Charles—afterwards Sir Charles Bell—having voted at the College against the new scheme of the managers was consequently not in a position to offer himself as a candidate for election by the Board.[1] His retiral was a distinct loss to the hospital. His younger and more brilliant brother Charles, having become a Fellow of the College in 1799, would soon have been eligible to take his place as one of the surgeons to the Infirmary. This restriction of his opportunities probably greatly influenced his decision to leave Edinburgh and commence his distinguished career in London.

It is perhaps difficult at the present day, when unacquainted with all the contemporary circumstances, to understand why the managers hesitated so long in enforcing a change which would undoubtedly have been of material benefit to the hospital. At any rate in 1800 they had the satisfaction of knowing that the step which they finally took received general approbation. The marked division of opinion in the College of Surgeons when the vote was taken, the gradual withdrawal of the more senior Fellows from participation in a service which they no longer favoured, and a growing tendency on the part of the younger Fellows to be careless as regards regular attendance at the hospital, all pointed to an increasing disbelief in the merits of the system of rotation so long in vogue.

[1] Minute, Royal College of Surgeons, 1st November 1800.

CHAPTER IX

CLINICAL TEACHING IN THE ROYAL INFIRMARY IN THE EIGHTEENTH CENTURY

THE PROFESSORS OF MEDICINE IN THE EARLY AND LATER YEARS OF THE CENTURY—LECTURES IN CLINICAL SURGERY—FOUNDATION OF THE CHAIR OF CLINICAL SURGERY IN 1803—MEDICAL STUDENTS IN THE INFIRMARY AND THE SCHOOL OF MEDICINE—THE INFLUENCE OF EDINBURGH ON MEDICAL EDUCATION IN THE NEW WORLD.

HAVING sketched the main steps taken to effect a better service from the physicians and surgeons it is now necessary to trace the gradual development of the methods adopted for imparting clinical instruction in the hospital. With the opening of the new building of the Royal Infirmary, in December 1741, accommodation was obtained for an increased number of patients along with improved facilities for clinical teaching. The school of medicine had been in existence since 1726: St Clair, Rutherford, Plummer, Innes and Monro were still teaching respectively the theory and practice of physic, chemistry, anatomy and surgery in the University, while botany was being taught in the Physic Garden by Charles Alston. Since the opening of the Little House in 1729, clinical instruction had been given by the physicians and surgeons attending in rotation for short periods. Although the school in 1741 was still comparatively young, it was acquiring a growing reputation and was attracting students in increasing numbers from beyond the confines of Scotland.

The students of medicine while attending the hospital in Robertson's Close had received from the members of the visiting staff practical instruction in the small wards and operating theatre, and for this privilege the Board of Management exacted a fee of two guineas from each pupil, the money thus raised being applied to the ordinary annual revenue of the house. When the new building was opened this sum was reduced to one guinea in the case of the surgeons' apprentices.[1] Later, in 1756, a system of issuing "perpetual" hospital tickets was introduced for which the apprentices paid five guineas and other students seven and a half, these tickets admitting the holders to the practice of the hospital "in all time coming." [2]

In February 1748, however, after the completion of the new building, a further method of clinical teaching was introduced for which no additional fee was at first charged.[3] John Rutherford proposed to give a course of clinical lectures in the hospital to illustrate in a practical way the principles of medicine taught in his systematic class in the University. For some time he had encouraged his pupils to bring patients to him on Saturday morning, when he enquired into the nature of their diseases and prescribed for them in the presence of the class.[4] Learning, however, that some of his students who were desirous of attending the new course did not possess hospital tickets, and being unwilling for that reason to admit them into the Infirmary, he wished to postpone his lectures till the following winter session commencing in October 1748, making it a condition that all should then have the necessary hospital tickets. But "the managers, having considered the proposal, were of the opinion that, as the year of attendance in the Infirmary is far spent, it would not be reasonable to insist with the students who want tickets to take them now, and, as these lectures may be of very great service to the students and likewise an advantage to the house, they recommend to Dr Rutherford to begin his lectures immediately and agree to give him the use of a room in the Infirmary for that purpose, and that all who desire to attend them shall be admitted." [5]

[1] Minute, Royal Infirmary, 30th November 1741.

[2] Minute, Royal Infirmary, December 1756. The "Perpetual" ticket was afterwards made £10, 10s. and, in 1805, £12, for all students, the latter sum being the cost of the ticket at the present time, if taken in one payment, but, if in instalments, £12, 12s.

[3] Later in the century the University charged a fee of £3, 3s. for attendance on a qualifying course of lectures in Clinical Medicine.

[4] *Chambers's Biographical Dictionary*, vol. xxvi. : John Rutherford.

[5] Minute, Royal Infirmary, 1st February 1748.

Accordingly, Rutherford commenced his clinical lectures in February of that year. The course, at first, was given only during the period of his attendance at the Infirmary as physician-in-rotation, and suitable patients were selected from the several wards of the hospital. Alexander Bower, in *The History of the University of Edinburgh*,[1] states on the authority of a writer in the *Scots Magazine* that the first course was given in the winter session of 1746-47.[2] But the records of the Royal Infirmary do not confirm this date, the minute of 1st February 1748, above quoted, being the first reference to the subject. It is also interesting in this connection to quote an extract from the letter of a contemporary student of medicine, the first of the young colonial students from the American continent to take the doctor's degree at Edinburgh.[3] Writing to his father in Charleston, South Carolina, on 2nd February of the winter session, 1747-48, he says :—

> We are very busy just now in ye Colledges (courses of instruction), and Dr Whytt, our new Professor, who succeeded Dr St Clair as Professor of Institutes, fills ye Chair and gives satisfaction to all his hearers. We have a new Class set on footing here this winter by our Professor of ye Practice of Physic, which is to lecture on the Cases of ye Patients in the Infirmary, in which he gives the Diagnosis, Prognosis and Method of Cure, which Lectures are reckon'd very valuable and serviceable. I shall not attend him this Session as I have enough to do already, but shall ye next.

There was thus introduced a system of clinical instruction, at first confined to the teaching of medicine but afterwards extended to surgery, which has survived in the school to the present day and which, in the years that followed its inception, was adopted far and wide in other centres of medical training. Sir William Osler, when addressing the members of the Royal Medical Society of Edinburgh on 7th February 1907, alluded to Rutherford's lectures in the following terms, " they are of great value as a record of the initiation of clinical teaching in the English-speaking schools, and what has been called

[1] Vol. ii, p. 213. Edinburgh, 1817.
[2] *Scots Magazine*, 1750, vol. xii, p. 52.
[3] *University of Edinburgh Journal*, 1930-31, vol. iv, p. 274.

the 'Edinburgh Method' dates from the introduction by Rutherford of practical classes in the Royal Infirmary." [1]

Rutherford owed his inspiration as a teacher to his great master, Boerhaave of Leiden, and in his clinical lectures he systematised bedside instruction as he had seen it conducted in the old Convent Hospital of that city. Manuscript notes of Rutherford's lectures written by his students have been preserved, a few copies of which are still extant.[2] In his introduction to the course he explains the purpose he has in view :—

> As health is the greatest blessing we enjoy in this life, and gives a relish to all other enjoyments, so the Art, which restores it when lost, must be of great service to mankind . . . the physician is acquainted with the fundamentals of his Art, he understands the animal economy, he knows when Nature makes an effort, he supports her in all her operations, varies his practice as the symptoms change and in all things acts according to reason. . . .
>
> I shall examine every patient appearing before you that no circumstances may escape you : I shall give you the history of the disease, enquire into the cause of it, give you my opinion as to how it will terminate, lay down the indications of cure which will arise or, if any new symptoms happen, acquaint you of them that you may see how I vary my prescriptions : If at any time you find me deceived in giving my judgment, you will be so good as to excuse me, for neither do I pretend to be, nor is the Art of Physic, infallible. . . .

Thus Rutherford propounded the Hippocratic teaching that experience must be the chief rule of practice, reasoning must be based on observation and experience, and that hypotheses not founded on facts must be condemned. His clinical lectures were from the first a success, not only as a valuable form of tuition, but in augmenting the revenue of the hospital through the disposal of a larger number of students' tickets. Although the managers at that period were not infrequently presenting tickets gratis to a certain number of students, the receipts from those sold during 1747-48—

[1] *Scottish Medical and Surgical Journal.* Edinburgh, March 1907.

[2] The writer possesses a MS. volume written by a student at Edinburgh in 1758. Early notes of Rutherford's clinical lectures are also preserved in the Library of the Royal College of Physicians of Edinburgh.

sixty-eight in number—amounted to £95, 11s. But in the following year, 1st October 1748 to 30th September 1749, one hundred and twelve tickets were disposed of, the hospital receiving as revenue therefrom £172, 4s.; the additional £76, 13s. from this source were attributed "in good measure" to the success of Rutherford's course of instruction.

Although the early courses of lectures on clinical medicine were delivered by Rutherford, a similar privilege had been granted at the same time to all the "Professors of Medicine" in the University. The Statutes and Rules prepared by the managers in 1748, and approved by the Court of Contributors on 23rd January 1749, contain the following regulation: "The Professors of Medicine in the University may during their attendance give clinical lectures to the Licensed students on the cases of the patients in the Infirmary at any hour excepting the ordinary time of visiting and may have the perusal of the Ledger."[1] Further extensions of the facilities for this system of instruction were soon provided, and a clinical ward was opened in 1750 for the accommodation of the patients who were to illustrate Rutherford's lectures.[2] These beds, which at first were not to exceed ten in number, were placed on the ordinary establishment of the hospital, and there was every expectation that the students' fees would provide for their maintenance. Again, by a statute approved and adopted by the Court of Contributors on 7th January 1751, the limitation, previously restricting the delivery of the lectures to a specified time, was withdrawn and the professors were authorised to teach at any period "they shall find most beneficial for the students without limiting them to the time of the professors' attendance as physicians." With the increasing number of young men attracted by this form of instruction, it soon became necessary to provide additional clinical beds, the number being at first raised to fifteen in 1751 and to twenty in 1752.

Another step in the evolution of clinical instruction was introduced at the beginning of 1757 when the professors of

[1] *History and Statutes of the Royal Infirmary of Edinburgh, 1749.*

[2] Minute, Royal Infirmary, January 1750.

medicine proposed to give a conjoint course of lectures, a suggestion which at once met with the approval of the Board of Management.[1] Alexander Monro, *primus*, William Cullen, professor of chemistry, and Robert Whytt, then in the chair of institutes of medicine, joined forces with John Rutherford and proceeded to deliver a course extending over a period of five months, each of the lecturers teaching in turn during the space of five weeks. At the same time clinical wards were fitted up both for male and female patients, the number of beds being increased to twenty-nine. Alexander Monro, *primus*, professor of anatomy, hitherto an active member of the Incorporation of Surgeons and one of the original members of the surgical staff of the Infirmary, had been elected a Fellow of the Royal College of Physicians of Edinburgh in March 1756 and was thus qualified to act as a physician to the hospital.[2] His son, Alexander, *secundus*, recently appointed to assist his father in the work of the chair, liberated the latter for his new duties in the Infirmary. Monro, *primus*, having resigned his chair in 1758, continued to cooperate with his colleagues in the conjoint course of clinical medicine.

An explanation of the collective term " Professors of Medicine " is desirable at this point. To the managers of the Infirmary it was not unfamiliar through its employment in the Charter of 1736 and, many years prior to that date, the term was used in Acts of the Town Council, when, as patrons of the University, they appointed the early professors in the faculty of medicine.[3] As new subjects were added to the curriculum and their study made compulsory to qualify for the degree in medicine—materia medica, forensic medicine and general pathology—the occupants of these chairs also became professors of medicine ; and, provided they were Fellows of the Royal College of Physicians and practising as physicians, they were privileged if they so desired, on obtaining

[1] Minutes, Royal Infirmary, 27th November and 6th December 1756.

[2] On 1st January 1756, the University of Edinburgh conferred the degree of doctor of medicine on Alexander Monro, *primus*.

[3] Acts of Town Council of Edinburgh, 9th September 1685, 9th February 1726, and 31st March 1738.

the consent of the managers, to take part in the teaching of clinical medicine in the Royal Infirmary.[1]

As the years passed and the scientific subjects in the medical curriculum grew in importance and absorbed more and more of the time and attention of the occupants of the chairs, it eventually became difficult for them to combine satisfactorily the duties of the scientific chair with those of physician to the hospital. Consequently today the term professors of medicine has a more restricted application than it had in the eighteenth and early part of the nineteenth century.

What manner of men were these early professors of medicine who taught in the Royal Infirmary? John Rutherford, as the pioneer, is deserving of special mention. A Lowland Scot, born in 1695 in the Manse of Yarrow, he spent his childhood's days in the Border countryside, the history and scenery of which his grandson, Sir Walter Scott, delighted to chronicle in prose and verse. As a boy, Rutherford attended the Grammar School at Selkirk and in his daily journeyings to and from the Manse,

> He pass'd where Newark's stately tower
> Looks out from Yarrow's birchen bower.[2]

From the school at Selkirk he entered the faculty of arts in the University of Edinburgh and, after a period of apprenticeship with a surgeon in the city, he proceeded to London and eventually to Leiden where he completed his medical studies. After graduating at Rheims in 1719, he returned to Edinburgh to assist in the foundation of the medical school in which he became the first professor of medicine, delivering his lectures in Latin, a language in which he was highly proficient.[3] He

[1] The privilege was not exercised by every professor on his appointment to a chair in the medical faculty: neither John Hope (botany) nor Joseph Black (chemistry) gave clinical lectures. When the chairs of forensic medicine and midwifery were created, the subjects were not at first compulsory for medical students, consequently their occupants were not entitled to teach clinical medicine in the Infirmary. In 1833 these subjects became obligatory.

[2] *The Lay of the Last Minstrel.*

[3] As a clinical teacher John Rutherford imparted his instruction in his native tongue.

resigned the chair in 1765. Through the marriage of his daughter, Anne, to Walter Scott, Writer to the Signet in Edinburgh, Rutherford became grandfather to Sir Walter, "that eminent ornament of Scottish literature," who has described his forbear as one "To whom the school of medicine in our northern metropolis owes its rise, and a man distinguished for professional talent, for lively wit and for literary acquirements."

Robert Whytt, who succeeded to the chair of institutes of medicine in 1747, was conspicuous as a leader in medical science in the middle of the eighteenth century. Born in 1714, the second son of Robert Whytt of Bennochie, Fife, a member of the Scots Bar, the younger Robert graduated M.A. St Andrews at the age of sixteen. On the conclusion of his medical studies at Edinburgh, London and Paris he graduated M.D. Rheims in 1736 and returned to Scotland to practise in the capital. His reputation at home and on the continent of Europe added greatly to the contemporary fame of the Edinburgh School. Whytt's experimental investigations upon the nervous system embodied the subject of reflex movements and the localisation of reflex action in the spinal cord. He was the first to give a clear clinical account of tuberculous meningitis, under the title of "Observations on the Dropsy in the Brain," and although he did not recognise the specific nature of the disease the accuracy of the clinical syndrome is remarkable. He died in 1766 at the comparatively early age of fifty-one.[1] The family assumed the name of Whyte-Melville a name familiar to later generations through the writings of George Whyte-Melville, the sporting novelist, a grandson of the distinguished physician of the eighteenth century.

William Cullen, translated from the chair of chemistry in Glasgow to occupy a similar position in Edinburgh as one of the professors of medicine, commenced his long career as a clinical teacher in the Royal Infirmary in 1755. Prior to

[1] *Memoir of the Life and Writings of Robert Whytt, M.D.*, by William Seller. "An 18th Century Neurologist," by J. D. Comrie, M.D., *Edin. Med. Journ.*, November, 1925.

this he had been an active and vital force in founding the medical school in the western city. His reputation, like that of Boerhaave, rested mainly upon his gifts as a teacher, his clinical lectures illustrated by numerous examples of varieties of disease being characterised by clarity of thought and lucidity of exposition. Cullen's period as a university professor at Edinburgh covered thirty-four years, 1755 to 1789, during which time he occupied the chairs of chemistry, the institutes of medicine and the practice of physic: he was equally capable of giving instruction in botany and materia medica, and thus, like Boerhaave at Leiden, he was equipped to teach nearly all the subjects in the curriculum of medicine. He attracted to his classroom men from many parts, especially from the American colonies where his influence on his pupils materially affected the early development of medical education in the New World. Cullen may be said to have broken the Boerhaave tradition in the medical school: in his *Synopsis Nosologiæ Medicæ* he adopted a rigid classification of diseases based upon symptoms, a plan which simplified the study of medicine at that period, though its reputation as a text-book did not long survive its author.[1] Retiring in 1789, Cullen died in the following year: the preservation of his grave and monument in Kirknewton churchyard now rests in perpetuity in the reverent care of the Royal College of Physicians of Edinburgh.

While instruction in medicine at the bedside, as originally practised in the ordinary wards, continued to be conducted by the physicians attending in rotation, teaching by clinical lectures remained for many years entirely in the hands of the professors to whom the special clinical wards were assigned for that purpose. The explanation of this action on the part of the Board of Management is clearly expressed in the following quotation from *The History and Statutes of the Royal Infirmary of Edinburgh, 1778*:—

A School of Medicine having been for many years established in Edinburgh and having arisen, before the erection of this hospital,

[1] *The Life and Writings of William Cullen, M.D.*, by John Thomson. Edinburgh, 1859.

to a flourishing state, the Managers of the Infirmary resolved to spare no pains in cherishing it as far as the hospital could serve that purpose ; and foreseeing that its interests would soon be interwoven with that of the University, they resolved to adopt every measure that could tend to facilitate medical education, and to render it compleat . . . further, considering that the defect of clinical lectures in medical seminaries had often proved a ground of complaint gave liberty to the Professors of Medicine to lecture on such cases of the patients as they should find most conducive to the instruction of the students . . . this was the only branch wanting in the medical course.

Hence, at a very early period in the history of the Infirmary, the University was not only granted the sole privilege of giving courses of clinical instruction in medicine but also the use of special wards for that purpose. The extension of a similar privilege to the physicians-in-ordinary, first appointed in 1751, came at a much later date. In 1790, forty years after the delivery of John Rutherford's inaugural course, Henry Cullen, one of the two physicians-in-ordinary, was authorised to give a summer course of clinical lectures upon the patients in his own care ;[1] but his death in the autumn of the same year terminated the arrangement for the time being. With the appointment of Daniel Rutherford, professor of botany from 1786 to 1819, to fill the vacancy as physician-in-ordinary in 1790, clinical lectures were delivered by him and, after his resignation as physician in 1802, he lectured at the request of his professorial colleagues as one of the professors of medicine.[2] Eventually in 1829, when four physicians-in-ordinary, previously appointed for a period of seven years, sought permission to give clinical lectures, no opposition was raised by the professors of medicine and the request was granted by the managers.[3]

Thus, as a system of staffing and teaching evolved, two groups of physicians gradually became differentiated, superseding those who had formerly served by rotation. One comprised the professors of medicine in the University—sometimes styled in the minutes the clinical physicians—

[1] Minute, Royal Infirmary, 1st March 1790. [2] *Ibid.*, April 1791.
[3] Minutes, Royal Infirmary, 25th May and 1st June 1829.

to whom were assigned the duties of clinical lecturers with wards allocated to them for that purpose, their period of attendance coinciding later with the period of tenure of their chairs. The second group—the physicians-in-ordinary to the hospital—was appointed in charge of wards, primarily for the purpose of conducting the daily service of the Infirmary; and, in more than one instance, the occupant of a chair in the medical faculty was chosen to fill one of these posts.[1] To the ordinary physicians, but at a much later date, was extended the privilege of giving clinical lectures. Hence were established within the Royal Infirmary two groups of physicians, those representative of the University or academical school and those belonging to the extra-academical body of teachers who in the early years of the nineteenth century were in considerable numbers. The latter, although at first teaching as individuals without any cohesion as an organised school and subject to no disciplinary authority, later constituted themselves an association of lecturers making their own arrangements. It was not till near the end of the nineteenth century, in 1895, that the association sought a closer connection with the two Colleges in Edinburgh, established a Governing Board of the Fellows and formed a definite Extra-academical School of Medicine of the Royal Colleges.[2]

Among the professors of medicine in the second half of the eighteenth century were Daniel Rutherford, Francis Home, the Gregorys, John and James, and Andrew Duncan, senior. Daniel Rutherford, the son of John Rutherford and the uncle of Sir Walter Scott, made his reputation in the scientific world while still a young man as, in his graduation thesis in 1772, he announced as the result of experiment his discovery of nitrogen gas. He became a member of the Board of Management in 1806. "A little, sluggish-looking man, with a large placid face, who, through the inroads of frequent

[1] Professors John Hope, Joseph Black, Daniel Rutherford and others were at various dates elected Physicians-in-Ordinary.

[2] Minute, Royal College of Physicians, 5th August 1895. Constitution of the School of Medicine was adopted.

gout, moved slowly . . . his accents and manner, unless he happened to be cross, were mild, kindly and dreamy."[1] His portrait was painted by Sir Henry Raeburn. Francis Home, appointed the first professor of materia medica in the University, in 1768, occupied the chair for thirty years : in 1769 he was given permission to deliver a course of clinical lectures in medicine. A man of exceptional ability he was the first to describe " the croup " as a distinct disease and, in his *Principia Medicinæ* written in correct and elegant Latin, he enhanced his reputation on the continent of Europe. Outside the immediate province of his chair he contributed valuable observations on bleaching and wrote on the Principles of Agriculture. He died in 1813 at the advanced age of ninety-four.

The Gregorys, John and James, father and son, were members of a Scottish family distinguished in mathematics and medicine. John Gregory was a son of the " mediciner " at King's College, Aberdeen, but Edinburgh claimed his services in 1766 as professor of practice of physic and, along with William Cullen, he taught clinical medicine in the wards of the Royal Infirmary. A man of culture and of great personal charm, on intimate terms with Edinburgh's literary circle, he brought more than mere technical knowledge to the study of medicine. His career was unfortunately terminated in 1773, at the comparatively early age of forty-nine, when he succumbed to gout, a disease from which he had always dreaded an early death. His son James, elected to the vacant chair of institutes of medicine in 1776 at the age of twenty-three, became successor to William Cullen in the chair of the practice of physic, thus establishing a link between eighteenth century and nineteenth century medicine, as he occupied the latter office till his death in 1821. More virile than his father, " he was a man having authority impressed on every feature, radiant with affection for his friends, intolerant of enemies, asking his own way and getting his own way, loving, hating, thinking, speaking, feeling, always

[1] *Life of Sir Robert Christison, Bart.*, vol. i, p. 55. William Blackwood & Sons. Edinburgh, 1885.

with intensest ardour: a man whom none of his associates could regard dispassionately; they either loved him as a friend or hated him as an enemy."[1] He wasted much of his ability in controversial feuds with his professional brethren. Commencing clinical instruction in the hospital in 1777, his remarkable gifts as a teacher proved a source of attraction. "The Gregorian physic was free blood-letting, the cold affusion, brisk purging, frequent blistering and the nauseating action of tartar emetic" and, one might add, in the exhibition of the famous mixture which still bears his name.[2] Andrew Duncan, senior, became professor of the institutes of medicine in 1789, but his first connection with the Infirmary was in the winter session of 1774-75 when he temporarily discharged the duties of the chair and was granted permission to give clinical lectures. A man of genial disposition, generous and hospitable and untiring in his devotion to the interests of the medical profession in Edinburgh, his name has come down through the years as the founder of the Æsculapian Club and the Harveian Society, and as one who did much to secure Charters for the Royal Medical Society, the Royal Public Dispensary and the Royal Edinburgh Asylum.[3] He retained his vigour to a ripe old age, invariably climbing Arthur's Seat on May-day morning, a feat he accomplished for the last time in the year prior to his death. He died, in 1828, aged eighty-three years.

Practical teaching in surgery by means of clinical lectures, on lines similar to those already adopted in medicine, was introduced twenty years after John Rutherford gave his first course in the hospital.[4] Moreover, when in 1769 these lectures became part of the system of surgical instruction, they were delivered by the surgeons-in-ordinary to the Infirmary and not by professors in the University. The explanation of

[1] *The Academic Gregories*, by Agnes Grainger Stewart. Famous Scots Series, 1901.

[2] *The Life of Sir Robert Christison, Bart.*, vol. i. William Blackwood & Sons, Edinburgh and London.

[3] The Royal Edinburgh Hospital (Morningside Asylum) for Mental and Nervous Disorders.

[4] Minute, Royal Infirmary, 2nd October 1769.

this is simple. When the faculty of medicine was created in 1726, surgery was given no separate academic status, no chair in that subject being then founded. The instruction was a somewhat minor part of the duties of Monro, *primus*, the professor of anatomy ; consequently the University was not in a position to approach the managers, as had been done in the case of medicine, to ask for the establishment of a course of surgical lectures in the Infirmary.

The privilege of teaching surgery in the city was regarded by the Incorporation of Surgeons as their prerogative and, since the opening of the Infirmary, the surgeons attending in rotation had given bedside instruction in the wards. After the appointment of four surgeons-in-ordinary to the hospital in 1766, with the terms of their service, for the time being amicably adjusted,[1] a proposal to institute lectures in clinical surgery was made by the Incorporation of Surgeons.[2] The suggestion was submitted to the Board of Management by the surgeons, in response to more than one appeal by the students of surgery who recognised the advantages derived from a similar system of teaching in medicine. The surgeons, cognisant of contemporary progress in the science and practice of surgery both in London and on the Continent, and desirous of effecting some improvement in the methods of teaching in Edinburgh, asked permission to have the necessary accommodation in the hospital, a request which was at once granted. Thus the movement to institute surgical instruction by means of clinical lectures was of extra-academical origin.

The success attending the courses of instruction both in systematic and clinical surgery by the teachers outside the University encouraged them to take a further step in promoting the interests of the subject : in 1777, therefore, they memorialised the Crown with the view of founding a professorship of systematic surgery in the University. But the opposition of Alexander Monro, *secundus*, supported by his colleagues in the Senatus Academicus, thwarted this early attempt to raise the status of surgery by instituting a university chair. Monro's

[1] Chapter VIII, p. 124.

[2] Minute, Royal Infirmary, 2nd October 1769.

selfish opposition to the project induced him to seek and to obtain from the Town Council of Edinburgh a new Commission "expressly authorising him to be professor of medicine and particularly of anatomy and surgery." In granting this request, however, the Town Council wisely reserved to themselves and their successors the power to separate the two offices at any time after the decease of Alexander Monro.[1] Although the teaching of systematic surgery by means of a separate chair was thus postponed for more than fifty years, clinical surgery received academic distinction in 1803.[2] In the previous year, James Russell, one of the six surgeons appointed by the managers in 1800, petitioned the Town Council to erect his lectureship at the Royal College of Surgeons into a professorship of clinical surgery in the University, a recommendation which was favourably received both by the Town Council and the Senatus Academicus. In order that the chair might be endowed, the Crown was approached and, in June 1803, a Commission was received from George III creating the regius chair of clinical surgery with an endowment of £50 per annum.[3]

In 1802, a letter from the Principal of the University had been presented to the managers of the Infirmary relative to James Russell's probable appointment to the chair.[4] The purport of this communication was to seek information concerning the accommodation which might be available in the hospital if the chair were founded : "and it will be extremely obliging if the managers state their opinion as to how far there is a probability or a certainty, if the chair shall be established, of that accommodation being rendered permanent in all time coming." In minuting their appreciation of the fact that the Senatus contemplated rewarding Mr Russell's past services in this way and anxious to give him every assistance in their power, the managers replied "that they could not consistently with the regulations of the hospital

[1] *The Story of the University of Edinburgh*, by Sir Alexander Grant, 1884, vol. i, p. 320.

[2] The chair of systematic surgery in the University was founded in 1831.

[3] Sir Alexander Grant, *op. cit.*

[4] Minute, Royal Infirmary, 14th May 1802.

bind themselves or their successors by any promise or agreement to render permanent such accommodation as they might be induced to give to the professor. They must reserve to themselves the power of determining both by whom and in what manner such lectures shall be given in the Royal Infirmary. They, however, beg to assure the Senatus that they would be most happy to give every accommodation in their power to Mr Russell and his successors in office in so far as the same may not interfere with the lectures which the attending surgeons of the hospital are entitled to give or with those delivered by the Professors of Medicine." [1]

The Senatus had to be content with this assurance. As James Russell, at the date of his appointment to the Chair in 1803, had recently terminated a period of two years as one of the two surgeons-in-ordinary and could not again take office till after an interval of four years, according to the regulations of 1800, he became dependent upon the goodwill of his colleagues for the patients illustrative of his course of lectures. After two further short periods as surgeon on the staff he declined to seek re-election in January 1815, intimating his desire to forgo election so as to relieve the managers from their embarrassment consequent upon the number of candidates seeking appointment.[2] He was then given the privilege of "delivering clinical lectures during all the days of his life" and was entitled to attend all consultations in the hospital and, if required by the surgeons, might give his opinion upon the patients. While Russell held the chair of clinical surgery attendance at his lectures was not obligatory upon the students proceeding to graduation. The explanation is probably to be found in the fact that no security had been given to the University by the managers that efficient means of teaching would be always at the disposal of the professor and, without such an understanding, the clinical course of lectures could not be made compulsory.[3]

Professor James Russell occupied the chair till 1833, when

[1] Minute, Royal Infirmary, 14th May 1802. [2] *Ibid*, 26th December 1814.
[3] See evidence given by Professor W. P. Alison before the Royal Commission of 1826.

he resigned at the age of eighty-one. A man universally respected, "he was singularly free from the jealousies and rivalries of his contemporaries." A tall, thin, elegant gentleman of the old school, with his red wig, white neckcloth, tail-coat, knee-breeches and silk stockings he was not a stimulating teacher. As a lecturer he has been described by a contemporary as somewhat "somnolent—a quality which was aggravated by an evening class hour, and betrayed by an inveterate habit the Professor had of yawning while he spoke, and continuing to speak while he yawned." [1]

The creation of the chair of systematic surgery, in 1831, and the succession of James Syme to the chair of clinical surgery in 1833, with their repercussions upon the arrangements in the Infirmary, may be left for consideration in their proper chronological sequence.

Up to this point a brief description has been given of the changes considered advisable for the improvement of the medical and surgical service of the hospital and for promoting the interests of clinical instruction. The dual purpose underlying the origin of the Infirmary had been at no time lost sight of and, so far as it was economically possible, provision had been made to increase the accommodation necessary for the care of the sick poor and to advance the cause of medical education. But to complete this chapter it is necessary to sketch the progress of the Edinburgh School of Medicine during the eighteenth century, with its growing reputation and with the steady increase in the number of students severely taxing the resources both of the University and of the Royal Infirmary.

The course of training for the degree of doctor of medicine —the single qualification then conferred by the University— covered a period of three years, although residence in Edinburgh was not necessary during the whole of that time. Evidence was required of attendance at lectures on anatomy and surgery —practical anatomy in the form of dissection was not then compulsory — on botany, chemistry, materia medica and

[1] *Edin. Med. and Surgic. Journal*, 1805.

pharmacy, on the institutes or theory and on the practice of physic, along with the clinical lectures in the hospital.[1] Only one examination for the degree, held at the termination of the curriculum, required to be passed. A thesis written in Latin was presented and *viva voce* examinations were conducted in the same tongue by the professors in the faculty. A written commentary on an aphorism of Hippocrates, and an expression of opinion upon one or more cases prepared by the examiners, completed the test.

The buildings on Kirk-o'-Field which constituted the old Town's College presented a very different appearance from those which now occupy the same site. Some of them were in a neglected and ruinous condition and ill-adapted for the purpose to which they were applied. The classrooms were, in general, " mean, straitened and inconvenient and, with the exception of the library and Monro's anatomical theatre, there was little to recommend them." After the completion of the South Bridge spanning the Cowgate and with the extension of the main thoroughfare southwards, the foundation stone of the new University was laid in 1789. Although the students in the University in that year numbered 1090, of whom 440 matriculated in medicine, yet more than forty years elapsed before the whole of the much-needed classrooms were provided and the Adam-Playfair building of today was completed.

The accommodation in the Royal Infirmary both for patients and pupils might also be described as " straitened " and the lack of sufficient annual income prevented the utilisation of all the available beds. Although the hospital in Infirmary Street was originally designed to contain 228 patients, that number had not hitherto been accommodated at one time. When in December 1741 the eastern part was opened, with beds from sixty to seventy in number, only thirty-four were in daily use; but as funds permitted, these were raised at intervals by increments of ten, so that, in 1799, as many as one hundred beds were on the ordinary establishment of the hospital, maintained by the annual revenue from Capital.

[1] In 1833, the period of study was extended to four years, and from time to time new subjects were added to the curriculum.

But the actual number of patients entertained exceeded the ordinary establishment, the additional maintenance being provided by special funds:[1] these patients, as previously stated, included the insane, the domestic servants, the soldiers, the supernumeraries paying sixpence per day and awaiting admission to the establishment, and the few supported on Lord Hopetoun's incurable fund. Further, many sick and injured were treated in the out-patient department of which no statistics have been preserved.

The accompanying Table, compiled from returns entered in the minutes of the hospital, shows the progressive increase in the number of patients in selected years along with, when possible, the relative proportion of the different classes of patients for whose treatment special payment was received.

TABULAR STATEMENT ILLUSTRATING INCREASE IN IN-PATIENTS, 1742-1800

A. *Prior to Introduction of Classes of Patients Maintained on Special Funds*

Year 1742

Number of In-Patients . .	155	34 beds occupied on ordinary establishment.

Year 1745

Number of In-Patients—		
On 1st January . . .	25	34 beds occupied on ordinary establishment
Admitted during the year .	121	
Total	146	

B. *After Introduction of Patients Maintained on Special Funds*

Year 1758

In Hospital on 1st January .	111	Patients on ordinary establishment	440
Admitted during the year . .	678	Soldiers	274
		Domestic servants . . .	75
Total	789	Total	789

Year 1768

In Hospital on 1st January .	119	Patients on ordinary establishment	721
Admitted during the year . .	975	Soldiers	234
		Domestic servants . . .	102
		Supernumeraries	37
Total	1094	Total	1094

[1] Chapter VII, p. 93 *et seq.*

Year 1789

In Hospital on 1st January .	147	
Admitted during the year . .	1830	No figures supplied.
Total	1977	

Year 1800

In Hospital on 1st January .	169	
Admitted during the year . .	1836	No figures supplied.
Total	2005	

Note.—The number of patients remaining in hospital on 1st January of each year indicates approximately the beds in occupation.

A summary of the figures compiled from the returns made during the years 1742-46—the first quinquennial period in the Royal Infirmary—will give a more comprehensive picture of the number of patients then in the care of the physicians and surgeons than can be obtained from the returns of the two years 1742 and 1745, recorded in the above Table. During the five-year period, 676 patients were treated in the wards but, unfortunately, no records are extant differentiating the medical and surgical cases, or the proportion of beds allotted to these two departments of the hospital. The surgical operations performed during the five years numbered 141 : of these, 31 were amputations, being nearly 22 per cent. of the total ; the operation of lithotomy was performed on 29 persons, *i.e.* on 20.5 per cent. ; the removal of malignant disease occupied the third place on the list. Throughout a period of one hundred and forty years or more in the history of the Infirmary, patients suffering from the infectious fevers, typhus, smallpox, scarlet fever, etc., were treated in the same building with the other cases, consequently the statistics invariably include patients who are today relegated to special hospitals.

To what extent, therefore, was the hospital, with its somewhat limited number of beds in daily use, able to provide the material necessary for the clinical instruction of the students of medicine ? Although various sources of information attest to the growing popularity of the Edinburgh School of Medicine at that time, it is difficult to arrive at an accurate estimate of the actual number of students attending the Infirmary year by year. The hospital tickets issued by the Treasurer, the class lists of the professors, the matriculation and graduation rolls of the University, and a few figures relative to the number of apprentices receiving the diploma of the College of Surgeons are available for the purpose. Much that is instructive can be learnt from their study, but the defects in the system of registration then employed make accurate deductions impossible, so that the number of those attending the hospital can only be estimated approximately. No subdivision was then made into first, second and third year students with a specified time in the curriculum of training assigned for clinical instruction : in all probability the hospital was visited by some during the greater part of the period of study, by others for only a limited time, while a number came to Edinburgh to sit in the classrooms of the professors of medicine, without seeking tuition in the Infirmary. Moreover, only a proportion of the students proceeded to graduation at Edinburgh, many afterwards qualifying elsewhere, while others who attended were already qualified.

The records of the Infirmary are unfortunately lacking in detail, nor do they cover the whole period under review. Further, it may be recalled that a uniform fee was not exacted by the managers from all the students attending the hospital, the sum chargeable to the apprentices of the surgeons being two guineas, to the other students, three guineas, and no indication is given in the minutes as to the proportion of tickets distributed to each group. In 1759, 79 tickets were disposed of, for which £225, 15s. were received, a sum suggesting that the greater proportion was sold at three guineas. During the triennial period 1760-63, 304 tickets—an approximate average of 100 per annum—yielded the sum of £852, 11s. In 1765-66 the income of the hospital from this source was £410, but no statement is made as to the number of tickets distributed ; in 1773 the sum of £356, 9s. was received. The missing minute book and the absence of figures during the closing decade of the century preclude further information from this source.

When the records of the University are explored the same difficulty is experienced. Prior to 1762, the matriculation roll makes no differentiation between the students of medicine and those entering the other faculties. In 1763, however, the names of the former are for the first time entered alphabetically and the subjects studied by each student are appended, but even these lists are incomplete, so that the following figures give only an approximate estimate of the actual number who enrolled.[1] In that year 223 matriculated in medicine, of whom 93 entered for clinical lectures and the study of obstetrics, two subjects necessitating attendance at the hospital. In 1773, the number of matriculates was 293, with 112 enrolling in the same two subjects ; and in 1783 matriculation had reached the maximum figure of 444, with 119 attending clinical lectures and obstetrical practice. In the closing year of the century the total was 417, with 150 enrolling in the two special clinical classes. At the two periods 1763 and 1773, when some comparison is possible between the figures furnished by the sale of Infirmary tickets and the attendance of those at the clinical and obstetric classes, there is approximate agreement (p. 150). The limited basis, however, on which the university calculation is made, is open to criticism, and students, other than those enrolling in the two specified classes, probably " walked " the hospital : to these the apprentices of the surgeons must be added.[2] In those days, therefore, notwithstanding the increasing number of patients, year by year, both physicians and surgeons must sometimes have experienced considerable difficulty in obtaining the necessary cases to meet the growing demand for clinical instruction.

For several years after the foundation of the school of medicine the majority of the students were Scotsmen, among whom were a few Englishmen. But, after the disturbances created by the Jacobite rising of the '45 had ceased and

[1] *University of Edinburgh Journal*, vol. viii, No. Two, 1936. "Dr Alexander Morgan on Matriculates in the Faculty of Medicine Prior to 1858."

[2] From 1790-94 inclusive, 113 diplomas were granted by the Royal College of Surgeons of Edinburgh, an average of 22 apprentices qualifying in each of these years.

Scotland was in a more settled condition, the cosmopolitan character of the school, which became one of its distinctive features, was soon firmly established. The combination of a university education along with clinical instruction in the hospital, modelled on the pattern of Leiden, offered an academic training in medicine not obtainable elsewhere in Britain at that period. At Glasgow and Aberdeen a similar development took place at a somewhat later date, but at Oxford and Cambridge no steps were then taken to adopt the scheme initiated at Edinburgh. In London the old apprenticeship system of training became supplemented by the introduction of the proprietary schools teaching anatomy, of which that carried on by the Hunters, William and John, in Great Windmill Street, was an example ; and, in the hospital schools of St Bartholomew's, St Thomas's and Guy's, anatomy and physiology were taught along with medicine and surgery in preparation for the examination for the diplomas licensing the recipients to practise.

Men flocked to Edinburgh in the eighteenth century for the same reason as their predecessors in the seventeenth had rallied to Leiden, and the Scottish capital became the new medical Mecca, gradually supplanting and finally eclipsing its nursing mother. The impressions left on the mind of a Danish physician who had spent some months in the city as a student in 1765, are thus recorded : " At the University of Edinburgh, Americans and West Indians, Portuguese and Italians, Frenchmen and Englishmen, Irishmen and Dutchmen, Germans and Swiss, Russians and Danes wandered together," a graphic description recalling similar scenes of former days at Leiden. While the matriculation lists, after 1762, record the majority of the names of students enrolling in medicine at the University they do not invariably state the country from which these men entered. The graduation roll, on the other hand, inscribes in every instance the latter fact, so that an approximate estimate may thus be made of the cosmopolitan character of the medical school. From 1726 to 1799 inclusive, 1143 men qualified in medicine and, of these, 237 graduated as Scotsmen, 254 as English, and 8 as Welsh, 280 as Irish, 195 from the

West Indies and the North American continent, 2 from South America (Brazil), 1 from the East Indies, and 26 from the nations on the continent of Europe. The total 1143 is completed by the addition of 140 graduates designated as British, with no distinction made as to whether they were Scottish, English or Welsh.[1]

The influence of the teaching of the Monros, *primus* and *secundus*, of John Rutherford, Whytt, Cullen, and Black, of John Gregory and John Bell, and the methods adopted in the Edinburgh School thus became widely diffused, and nowhere was this more markedly revealed than in the development and growth of the young schools of medicine on the North American continent. In the early colonial days medical education had received little consideration : the young men graduated in Arts in the first American Colleges, but the apprentices in medicine imbued with scientific enthusiasm, many of them of Scottish descent, had to turn to the old country to seek more adequate instruction than was then obtainable in the New World. They went, therefore, to Edinburgh and to London to study under the leaders in the profession. As early as 1744 the first colonial student, who came from the island of Antigua, took his degree at Edinburgh and, five years later, John Moultrie of Charleston, South Carolina, graduated. They were followed by others, some of whom, on returning to their own country, became founders of the early schools of medicine in America and pioneers in medical education. Even after the War of Independence, many, as citizens of the United States, sought further experience at Edinburgh.

The first medical school in America was created in 1765 in Philadelphia as a department of the young College of Pennsylvania, before it had received university status, and above the entrance to the medical buildings is still emblazoned the thistle, the emblem of its debt to the country of its parent institution. It was founded by the young Pennsylvanians, William Shippen and John Morgan, pupils of John Hunter and

[1] Prior to the creation of the Faculty of Medicine, in 1726, the degree of doctor of medicine was conferred upon 21 candidates, thus making the total number of graduates, 1164, during the eighteenth century.

students and graduates of Edinburgh, who on their return impressed upon the trustees of the College the necessity for a medical school. Shippen taught anatomy and Morgan the institutes and practice of physic ; they were soon joined by their compatriots, Benjamin Rush and Adam Kuhn also Edinburgh graduates. Both Rush and Kuhn signed at Philadelphia, in 1776, the Declaration of Independence. The Scottish influence was still further maintained, at a later date, by Caspar Wistar and Philip Syng Physic, graduates of Edinburgh, who became professors in the medical faculty of the University of Pennsylvania. The leader in the foundation of America's second school of medicine, King's College, New York, was Samuel Bard, a graduate of Edinburgh in 1765 : he was made the first professor of the theory and practice of physic and, like Benjamin Rush, was one of the most distinguished American physicians of that period.

It was not till the commencement of the nineteenth century that students from those parts of the North American continent that continued under the British flag enrolled from Canada, Nova Scotia, New Brunswick and Newfoundland. In Montreal, a school of medicine, which afterwards constituted the medical faculty of McGill University, founded in 1821, was created mainly through the zeal and labours of a small group of men who had received their training and taken their degree at Edinburgh. About the same time the first students of medicine arrived from New South Wales and from the Cape of Good Hope, and they were followed by increasing numbers from Australian territory, New Zealand and South Africa. Thus the Greek spirit in Medicine, revived at the Renaissance in Bologna and Padua and borne across the Alps to Leiden and Edinburgh, spread overseas to enrich the medical schools of the New World and the Edinburgh influence played its part in cementing the foundations of the Empire.

Notwithstanding the fact that fewer subjects were included in the curriculum of study in the eighteenth century than at the present day, and that instruction was mainly by means of the formal lecture—practical classes in the laboratory being unknown—the student, like his successors in the twentieth century, found his days fully occupied. Then as now there was a daily routine, though it differed considerably in matters of detail. A serious student "at the College" in the winter session of 1771-72 has left on record how he rose about 7 o'clock and read till 9, when he attended the lectures of William Cullen. He then breakfasted at 10 o'clock, after which he transcribed his notes. From 12 to 1 he "walked the wards" of the Infirmary and from 1 to 3 o'clock he was in the anatomical department with Monro, *secundus*. Having dined in his lodging between 3 and 4 he proceeded to Thomas Young's classroom to listen to his discourse on midwifery and from 5 to 6 he recast his notes taken at the lectures of Monro and Young. His working hours were not yet at an end as the hour 6 to 7 found him at the anatomical demonstrations of Dr Innis, Alexander Monro's "Dissector." He supped at 9 o'clock and then worked in his lodgings till midnight. In addition to the above, he attended, on two days in the week at the Infirmary, the clinical lectures of William Cullen and John Gregory. The cost of his tuition during the winter session was £17, 18s. 6d., a sum which included 9s. 6d. in the payment of "tips" to the janitors and the porter at the Infirmary! The cost of living varied with the type of lodging selected. "I have everything found but washing" he wrote to his father, "and I pay £10 per Quarter, which is the lowest one can get boarded in a genteel manner, and there is as high as £12 per Quarter."[1]

[1] *University of Edinburgh Journal*, vol. viii, No. One, p. 57.

CHAPTER X

THE ROYAL INFIRMARY IN THE NINETEENTH CENTURY, 1800-1870

THE FEVER EPIDEMICS, 1817 TO 1848—CHOLERA IN 1832 AND 1848—THE PHYSICIANS AND CLINICAL TEACHING—PROPOSED CHAIR OF CLINICAL MEDICINE—APPOINTMENT OF PATHOLOGISTS TO THE INFIRMARY, 1839 — EARLY SPECIALISATION — THE CONVALESCENT HOUSE AT CORSTORPHINE, 1867—THE FINANCIAL PROBLEM.

With the advent of the nineteenth century progressive developments both in town and country were of such a nature as to have an important influence on the immediate future of the hospital. The perennial burden associated with finance and the constant difficulty of making both ends meet—the balancing of the annual budget—were increased rather than diminished. The New Town was rapidly extending in all directions—north, south, east and west. The people, no longer confined within the old walled town, numbered in 1800 along with Leith, 100,000 souls. The lofty tenements of the Old Town, now vacated by the wealthier classes, became even more congested than formerly with the families of the poor and all that that implied. Better intercommunication with the country districts, as the result of improvement in the roads and accelerated means of transport, widened the area from which patients, attracted by the reputation of the Infirmary, sought advice and treatment from its medical and surgical staff. In the medical school, also, the progress of which has been detailed in the previous chapter, there was a steady increase in the number of students : in 1805-06 the matriculation roll in medicine contained 703 names and, five years later, as many as 934, an exceptional figure. All these circumstances naturally had their repercussion on such facilities as the Infirmary could provide.

In the meantime, to aggravate the situation, the managers

were obliged to face the grave responsibility of coping with a series of epidemics of relapsing and typhus fevers which broke out amongst the poor of the city. The first of these commenced in 1817 and recurrences took place at intervals till 1846-48.[1] The soil had been favourably prepared for the development of typhus fever in the years immediately preceding the first of these outbreaks. The Napoleonic campaigns, in which Britain was involved, had interfered with the prosperity of the country. There was increasing unemployment, a rise in the price of foodstuffs with consequent ill-nourishment and a lowering of the vitality of those least able to bear the strain. In addition, the bad harvest in Scotland in 1816 increased the impoverishment of the people and, over and above, was the overcrowding in the badly ventilated, ill-lit and insanitary dwellings of the poor, conditions which favoured the spread of typhus fever.

As no " Fever Hospital " existed in the city in those days, the onus of treatment of infectious fevers fell upon the Infirmary which in normal times provided at least two wards for that purpose. It is a matter of interest to note that even during an epidemic of fever it was observed that, with the segregation of these patients in separate wards, infection was not carried to the other patients living under the same roof. With the outbreak of the epidemic in 1817 three additional wards were opened, yet these were insufficient to deal with the emergency. Accordingly the Lord Provost and a number of influential citizens approached the Government with a view to utilising Queensberry House Barracks, then unoccupied.[2] This old and somewhat gloomy mansion, standing near the foot of the Canongate and on the south side of the thoroughfare, shortly after its erection in 1681 had passed into the hands of the Dukes of Queensberry who used it as their town residence. It was eventually sold in 1801, by "Old Q," William Douglas, Duke of Queensberry, and purchased by the Government as barracks. Permission for its use having been granted to the managers of the Infirmary they undertook the administration

[1] Epidemics of 1817-20; 1826-29; 1837; 1842-43 and 1846-48.

[2] Minute, Royal Infirmary, 17th January 1818.

of the house as a fever hospital, trusting that the public would respond in such a way as to provide the necessary increased expenditure. The unused wooden beds which it contained were exchanged for iron bedsteads and bedding transferred from Greenlaw Barracks—the Glencorse Barracks of today—and wards were opened capable of accommodating from sixty to eighty patients. A matron, an apothecary and a nursing staff were appointed and Benjamin Welsh, a graduate of medicine in 1818, became superintendent at a salary of £40 per annum.[1] James Hamilton, senior, and Thomas Spens, physicians-in-ordinary to the Royal Infirmary, acted as visiting physicians to Queensberry House and two physicians'-clerks were selected as residents. One of these, Robert Christison—later Sir Robert—who suffered from more than one attack of relapsing fever, has recorded in his autobiography a graphic account of his symptoms. Permission was given by the Magistrates of the City to make a collection at the doors of the churches, and the County Conveners were asked to stimulate interest in procuring contributions for the upkeep of the hospital.

The epidemic of typhus of 1817 was not of a virulent character and few deaths occurred: the patients admitted into Queensberry House during the twelve months, 1st March 1818 to 28th February 1819, numbered 1676, of whom 1605 recovered and 71 died, a low mortality rate of slightly more than 4 per cent. The expenditure incurred during the year 1818 in maintaining the Infirmary and the Annexe was £8376, a sum considerably in excess of any previous annual outlay which the managers had required to meet.

Although the first epidemic abated in 1820-21, Queensberry House continued to be used for fever patients till the autumn of 1823. When in 1825 the Government desired to sell the buildings, the managers as a precautionary measure leased the premises for ten years at a rent of £80 per annum. It was fortunate that they had made such provision, as a second epidemic, on an even larger scale than the previous one,

[1] Benjamin Welsh, brother of Dr John Welsh of Haddington, was the uncle of Mrs Thomas Carlyle; after succeeding his brother in the practice at Haddington he died a comparatively young man.

prevailed during 1826-29. Consequently the Barracks were again opened and 150 beds were kept constantly occupied to supplement those used in the Infirmary for a similar purpose.

With the outbreak of the third epidemic in 1837, the Infirmary was again called upon to make provision to deal with it. The lease of Queensberry House having then expired the necessary accommodation was obtained in the Infirmary, nine wards being appropriated for the purpose, containing approximately 140 beds. This arrangement had been made feasible through the transference of the surgical patients, in 1832, to the old High School building purchased in 1829. In addition to these wards the house, previously used as the Lock Hospital and containing thirty beds, was temporarily handed over to the Fever Board of the city which provided the necessary funds for its maintenance. The patients under treatment with typhus fever from 1st October 1837 to 30th September 1838 numbered 2244 and between the latter date and the end of December a further 527 patients were treated.[1]

It is unnecessary to enter into the details of the two subsequent epidemics of 1842-43 and 1846-48 : it is sufficient to state that they were on a larger scale than the previous outbreaks and that the resources of the Infirmary, both as regards the provision of accommodation and the funds required to meet the increased expenditure, were taxed to the utmost limit. In addition to the buildings previously fitted up for the reception of these cases, tents were borrowed from the Ordnance Store at Edinburgh Castle and from the Archers' Hall and were pitched in the vicinity of the Infirmary : even the chapel was requisitioned for a similar purpose, " the force of the objections which might otherwise have existed to this step being materially diminished by the inability of the great proportion of the patients to attend Divine Service." [2] During the years 1841 to 1848, inclusive, no fewer than 17,542 patients suffering from infectious fevers were under treatment in the Royal Infirmary. A striking feature in connection with the two last epidemics was the great proportion of Irish among

[1] Minute, Royal Infirmary, January 1839.

[2] Report of Managers, 3rd January 1848 and 1st January 1849.

the sufferers. The disease apparently first broke out among "the wandering Irish"; and, in the report of the Committee of the Court of Contributors appointed in January 1849, the opinion was expressed that more stringent measures ought to be adopted to prevent the exposure of the community to the injurious effects following the importation of the numerous paupers and vagrants from Ireland.

When in the autumn of 1831 grave apprehension was felt in Edinburgh regarding a probable visitation of cholera early in the following year, a Board of Health was set up by authority of the Privy Council [1] upon which three members of the Board of the Infirmary were invited to sit.[2] By the end of June 1832, six hundred deaths from cholera had occurred in the city. Every precaution was taken by the physicians to prevent the admission of suspicious cases into the Infirmary and, when such presented themselves, they were at once transferred to one of the district hospitals opened for that purpose by the Board of Health. One of these was Queensberry House and, another, a house situated at Fountainbridge.[3] Application was also made by the same Board for the use of old Surgeons' Hall, recently vacated by the Surgeons; and in a minute of the Town Council of 4th January 1832, the following statement occurs:—"The College of Surgeons at the earnest solicitation of the Board of Health granted to that body the use of the old building and, conditionally, that of another house of which they are proprietors for the important purpose of providing accommodation for cholera patients, if such accommodation should be required." The Hall was opened temporarily as the Drummond Street Cholera Hospital. When a second epidemic of Asiatic cholera visited the city in 1848, the managers, having resolved that these cases should not be admitted into the Infirmary, placed at the disposal of the Board of Health the old Surgeons' Hall which they had in the interval bought and used as a Fever Hospital,

[1] *Edinburgh, 1329-1929*, p. 15. Oliver & Boyd, Edinburgh, 1929.
[2] Minute, Royal Infirmary, 31st October 1831.
[3] Since 1853 Queensberry House has been used as a House of Refuge for the Destitute.

on the express understanding, however, that, although supplying the beds and bedding and providing the nurses, the funds of the Royal Infirmary were not to be made liable for any of the expense incurred in maintaining patients suffering from cholera.

It is evident, therefore, that the Infirmary was used as a fever hospital to an extent greatly beyond the original intention. Although in certain large cities—London, Manchester, Dublin—separate hospitals were maintained for that specific purpose, neither in Edinburgh nor in Leith had any similar provision been made. The Infirmary had found it increasingly difficult to provide the funds for the accommodation of the ordinary medical and surgical cases during the periods when serious epidemics prevailed, consequently the opinion was expressed that a separate fever hospital ought to be established and that the community, benefiting by such a safeguard, should be responsible for maintaining it. But many years were to elapse before this laudable object was attained. In 1881, the Town Council became responsible for the treatment of epidemics of infectious fever and acquired part of the buildings of the Royal Infirmary for that purpose, after the hospital had been transferred to its present position in Lauriston Place.

In the early part of the nineteenth century circumstances arose which made it desirable to change the term of service of the physicians-in-ordinary, to increase their number and to rearrange the distribution of the medical beds. It will be recalled that in 1751, with a view to terminating the defective system of attendance by rotation, two physicians were elected by the managers without placing any limit upon the period of their appointment, an arrangement which still remained in force more than seventy years later. When in 1823 James Hamilton, senior, appointed physician in 1775, and to whose services in Queensberry House reference has been made, resigned his post, the first important alteration was effected. The principle of a time limit was introduced and the term of service restricted to seven years: this was later extended to ten years, with re-election renewable at the pleasure of the

Board.[1] This arrangement remained as the basis of service till comparatively recent times when physicians (and surgeons) were appointed for five years with eligibility for re-election at the discretion of the managers for a second and a third term of similar duration, the whole period of office not to exceed fifteen years.[2] With the increase in the population of the city and a consequent unavoidable multiplication in the number of patients attending the Infirmary, it became imperative to reinforce the medical staff by adding to its number. Accordingly a third physician-in-ordinary was appointed in 1827 and a fourth in the following year.[3]

As narrated in Chapter IX (p. 139), permission was granted in 1829 to the ordinary physicians to give clinical lectures and, after the surgical patients had been transferred to the High School building in November 1832, a redistribution of the beds was made in the medical hospital and clinical teaching by the extra-academical members of the staff was rearranged. The medical cases were subdivided into three groups of equal proportions, the two senior or "permanent" physicians, as they are described in the minutes, being placed in charge of one-third of the patients, while the remaining third was in the care of the two junior physicians, each attending the hospital alternately for a period of twelve months. The delivery of clinical lectures by the senior of the two permanent physicians was optional, but was obligatory upon his colleague.

In 1854 the physicians-in-ordinary, like the professors of medicine in the eighteenth century, united to give a combined course of instruction, an arrangement mainly due to the influence of William—later, Sir William—Tennant Gairdner, after his appointment as physician to the Infirmary in 1853. Impressed with the wisdom of obtaining the services of every capable teacher, as a matter of principle, he persuaded the managers to allow his two junior colleagues, Alexander Keiller and James Warburton Begbie, to share in a combined clinical course, the students to attend with a joint-admission card.

[1] Minutes, Royal Infirmary, 16th February 1824 and 20th January 1840.
[2] Minute, Royal Infirmary, 18th January 1897.
[3] Minutes, Royal Infirmary, 12th November 1827 and 14th July 1828.

As Keiller was specialising in gynæcology he taught the diseases of women, while Gairdner and Warburton Begbie lectured on the medical cases. Years later, when addressing the members of the Royal Medical Society in 1893, on " Edinburgh in the 'Fifties," Gairdner said: " In the history of the Edinburgh School and Royal Infirmary I trust it will be recorded, that when, being already a lecturer in the practice of physic and a hospital physician, the privilege of clinical teaching fell to my lot, I was anxious then, as at all times since then, to share it with others, so that all the members of the staff should, as far possible, be partakers in the good work." [1]

Sir William Gairdner, in the same address, described a remarkable acoustic peculiarity which was constantly noticed on the stair, situated in the angle between one of the wings and the body of the old Infirmary and which led from the waiting-room on the first floor upwards to the three floors above, on each of which was situated one of his wards. The peculiarity was a loud booming sound or echo, much more pronounced in the lowest flight than in either of the other two, though to the eye all were precisely alike. The phenomenon elicited by an emphatic stamp of the foot upon one of the stone steps was identical in its musical pitch with the " amphoric echo " heard on auscultating the chest over a large cavity in the lung, and was therefore invaluable as an illustration of physical diagnosis. This particular part of the Infirmary received the nick-name of " Gairdner's Corner." " This was long before the day when Helmholtz's resonators were brought into play as illustrations of physiological acoustics, and perhaps, therefore, the familiarity with the phenomenon of ' Gairdner's Corner ' had a certain educating value to successive classes of students."

Among the physicians-in-ordinary during this period were men whose special qualifications for the post left no room for doubt and whose long and valuable services added considerably to the reputation of the hospital. James Hamilton, senior—thus designated to distinguish him from his namesake, the

[1] *Life of Sir William Gairdner, K.C.B., M.D.*, by George Alexander Gibson, M.D., p. 449. Glasgow: James Maclehose & Son. 1912.

professor of midwifery—and Thomas Spens were for many years the senior physicians. Hamilton, a link between the eighteenth and nineteenth centuries, appointed physician in 1775, resigned in December 1823 at the age of seventy-four, after forty-eight years of continuous service. To mark their appreciation of his work the managers invited him to sit for his portrait to Mr John Watson—later Sir John Watson-Gordon.[1] The picture still hangs on the walls of the Board Room of the Infirmary. With an implicit faith in the therapeutic value of blood-letting and purging, his pill of aloes and colocynth, which remains to the present day associated with his name, was a favourite prescription. On a page of one of Hamilton's old case books, preserved in the Royal Infirmary, appears the following terse record of one of his patients: "February 1778; male; aloes pill with relief of the pain of belly and headache"! A handsome and picturesque figure in the quaint costume of the period he retained a preference for the three-cornered hat which earned him the soubriquet of "cocky" Hamilton. He died in 1835. Thomas Spens, his colleague, was physician-in-ordinary for forty years, from 1802 to 1842. "Tall, slender, modest, almost shy, extremely kindly and a thorough gentleman in manner and disposition, he was a sound and successful practitioner, free from prejudice and hobbies, and always open to correction by experience." When he became the senior physician on Hamilton's retirement, the managers in recognition of his services and to compensate him for the pecuniary loss he had sustained by the withdrawal of a Government allowance, granted him a salary of £100 per annum, a sum regularly paid to him till his retirement.[2] When president of the College of Physicians in 1803-04 he took his seat on the Board of Management in terms of the Charter, although one of the active staff of the Infirmary.

On the retirement of Hamilton, after so many years in office, it was perhaps natural that some restriction in the period

[1] Minute, Royal Infirmary, 16th February 1824. James Hamilton was also painted by Sir Henry Raeburn.

[2] Minute, Royal Infirmary, 16th February 1824.

of service should be introduced, and the next physician, appointed under the new regulation, was James Buchan, selected from amongst other candidates with greater claims to recognition. A graduate of Edinburgh of 1792, he had been in charge of the French Plague Hospital in Egypt during Napoleon's campaign: "a little, fair-complexioned, near-sighted, soft-speaking, quiet, slow, hesitating man, several years on the wrong side of fifty," he resigned his appointment in 1827. Another former physician to the Forces, a successful candidate when the staff of physicians was increased to four, was Thomas Shortt, a graduate of 1815. He had been on duty at St Helena at the time of the death of Napoleon and was officially present at the *post-mortem* examination. Described as the beau-ideal of the successful, fashionable physician, "he arrived at the hospital in carriage and pair, or in a smart cabriolet with a high-stepping horse and a 'tiger' hanging on behind, or even on occasions riding on horseback with the tiger at a respectful distance in the rear."

A man of very different calibre was Robert Christison—later Sir Robert Christison, Baronet—a university professor for fifty-five years, in the chair of forensic medicine from 1822-32 and professor of materia medica from 1832-1877: he gave his services to the Infirmary during thirty years of that long period, first as a physician-in-ordinary and afterwards as a clinical professor and manager. Although occupying the chair of forensic medicine when appointed to the staff of the hospital in 1827, his professorial position did not entitle him to act as one of the clinical professors, the subject not being then obligatory upon medical students.[1] Of erect and commanding presence, endowed with an athletic frame which permitted his enjoyment of mountaineering among the Bens and Glens of his native land, he retained to the end of a long life the physical energy to satisfy this ruling passion. A man of strong force of character, with some of the qualities of a great soldier, he exercised a powerful influence upon his

[1] With his appointment to the chair of materia medica, in 1832, Christison resigned his post as physician-in-ordinary, but continued to serve the hospital as one of the professors of medicine.

colleagues on the Senatus Academicus and on the Board of the Royal Infirmary. Persevering in research and accurate in observation, Christison as a physician and toxicologist gained a European reputation, and as a medical jurist he was engaged on behalf of the Crown in all the important criminal trials for poisoning. " When he was lecturing on curare, the arrow poison of the South American Indians, he used to come to the University a quarter of an hour before the class met to practise with the blowpipe, so that during the lecture he might demonstrate how the natives made use of it. A target having been placed on one side of the classroom he stepped down on the other side, inserted the arrow, took aim and in a moment it was quivering in the bull's eye, and he returned to his desk amidst the rapturous applause of his class." He died in January 1882 at the age of eighty-four, and at his public funeral the solemn procession proceeded along the crowded streets from his home in Moray Place to his interment in the New Calton Burying-Ground.

Amongst Sir Robert's colleagues on the staff of the Infirmary was William Pulteney Alison, a grandson of John Gregory the physician, and the elder brother of Sir Archibald Alison the historian. As professor in the University for thirty-five years—1820-55—and the holder of three chairs in succession, forensic medicine, the institutes of medicine, and the practice of physic, he may be appropriately named a chair collector. As clinical physician in the wards of the Infirmary and in dispensary practice, he deservedly earned the appellation of " Beloved Physician." In his work amongst the poor of the city during the fever epidemics he became impressed with the fact that there was a direct connection between destitution and epidemic diseases ; and, as a result of his efforts, he was finally successful in securing amendment in the Poor Law of Scotland. Of Alison, Christison has written that " he dispensed his bottles on much the same principle as he gave away his sixpences to the crowd of beggars round his door in Heriot Row, as he left his home in the morning. Suffering humanity was ever too much for Alison : it was impossible for him to refrain from an immediate and often unwise demonstration of practical sympathy."

Instruction in clinical medicine was constantly hampered by the excessive number of students ; this state of affairs in the hospital gave rise to repeated criticism, it was unsatisfactory for the patients, inconvenient to the physicians in attendance and not conducive to the best type of teaching. The matriculation roll in the faculty of medicine during the decade 1823-24 to 1832-34 reached the high figure of 8564, the largest number in one year of the period reaching 935, the lowest 807, with an annual average of 856 ; and the annual income of the Infirmary derived from the sale of hospital tickets, while varying somewhat from year to year, reached in 1832-33 the substantial sum of £2613. At the end of the decade, in 1833, the qualifying period of medical study was prolonged from three years to four, and practical anatomy, with attendance at lectures on clinical surgery, midwifery and forensic medicine, was made compulsory. It is significant that a period ensued during which there was a notable decline in the number of medical students.

To avoid the evil of overcrowding an arrangement was made by which four of the professors of medicine should participate annually in the duties of clinical physicians and four wards were appropriated for their use, two of the professors attending at the same time and teaching for a period of three months.[1] But twenty years later, in 1848, the managers, being still doubtful of the efficiency of the system of clinical teaching, raised the question of the desirability of establishing a professorship of clinical medicine on the lines already adopted in clinical surgery.[2] As the professors of medicine were under no compulsion to lecture in the Infirmary, some of them indeed declining to do so, the existing arrangement on a purely voluntary basis did not promote efficiency. The teaching of clinical surgery, on the other hand, by an individual professor had proved a successful experiment and

[1] Minute, Royal Infirmary, 13th November 1826.

[2] Minutes, Royal Infirmary, 20th November 1848 and 9th April 1849.

there was every reason to believe that, with a suitable endowment, a corresponding chair in medicine would attract a number of well-qualified candidates. It was not the intention of the managers, in the event of the establishment of this chair, that those professors, who might consider it essential for the efficient teaching of their respective branches of medical science, should be deprived of the opportunity of giving clinical instruction in the hospital. But the proposal failed to obtain the concurrence of the medical faculty, and neither in 1849 nor again in 1851 when the matter was reopened was any positive step taken; and it was not till 1913 that a chair of clinical medicine was instituted.

Counter proposals, however, were made by the clinical professors for increasing the resources of the hospital and providing facilities for the special study of particular forms of disease. Thus it was thought desirable that wards should be set apart for diseases of the skin, for the diseases of women and infants and for such mental cases as were admitted into the Infirmary and, further, that beds for patients suffering from diseases of the eye should be instituted. Specialism in medicine was beginning to obtain a foothold in the hospital. The special wards suggested were to be assigned alternately to the care of the professors of medicine and the extra-academical teachers of clinical medicine.[1] More use was also to be made of the medical out-patient department. General agreement was reached upon certain of these proposals: beds for the treatment of diseases of the eye were to be reserved in the New Surgical Hospital shortly to be opened and, on 11th March 1850, an extra-physician for the diseases of women and infants was appointed, James Young Simpson being then elected to the staff of the Royal Infirmary. This appointment entitled him, if called upon, to give lectures upon the patients under his charge. It was further minuted that "no patient shall be placed in that ward until she has been made aware by the Treasurer-Superintendent or Matron that she will be under the charge of the said physician and may be more peculiarly the subject of attention to the

[1] Minute, Royal Infirmary, November 1849.

Lecturer and the students than she might be in a general ward."

Sir James Young Simpson's appointment to the Infirmary was not made in virtue of his office as professor of midwifery but as a personal tribute to his outstanding position in the medical profession. Elected in 1840 to the chair in the University, at the age of twenty-eight, this remarkable man on joining the staff of the hospital had already attained a world-wide reputation which attracted to Edinburgh not only patients but men of science from all parts of the globe. One of his colleagues in the Senatus, calling to see him while engaged in his practice at 52 Queen Street, thus describes the busy scene: "The two reception rooms were as usual full of patients, more were seated in the lobby, female faces stared from all the windows in vacant expectancy, and a lady was ringing the door-bell. But the doctor brushed through the crowd to join me and left them all kicking their heels at their leisure for the next two hours." His love of study, his thirst for knowledge and indomitable perseverance combined with an extraordinary power of concentration and an accurate and retentive memory, enabled him to accomplish what few other men were capable of doing. He could never be idle, and in archæological and historical research he found a source of recreation which occupied his hours of leisure. As one of the combative giants in that period of the history of the Edinburgh School, he found time also to take part in many a bitter controversy. He died on 6th May 1870, within a month of his sixtieth birthday and, notwithstanding the national desire that he should be interred in Westminster Abbey, he was buried in the Warriston Cemetery, Edinburgh, beside five of his children who had predeceased him, his funeral being one of the most memorable ever witnessed in Scotland.

James Matthews Duncan, an Aberdonian both by birth and education and intimately associated with Simpson in his experiments on chloroform anæsthesia, was appointed to the Infirmary in 1861, as a second extra-physician for diseases of women, thus becoming a colleague of Simpson. "The massive head, the rugged and impressive features with the firm mouth and square chin indicated great resolution of character and capacity for continuous work." He did much to place obstetrics on a sure scientific basis of ascertained facts. He regarded teaching, in which he was eminently successful, as a " daily intellectual gymnastic," to quote his own words, " as it taught him both his own ignorance and his knowledge and was an invaluable incitement to study." Regarded by many as the natural successor of Simpson in the chair of midwifery he failed in his object and, in 1877, in response to an invitation from St Bartholomew's Hospital, he proceeded to London to become the foremost exponent of the specialty in the metropolis.

A few years prior to the events just recorded—in 1839—the office of pathologist to the Royal Infirmary was created. The Board were then endeavouring to place the internal management of the hospital on a more satisfactory basis and the various steps taken to establish better supervision in the house will be told in a subsequent chapter on administration. But one of the early methods adopted was the appointment of a graduate in medicine in the dual office of Superintendent and Pathologist with residence in the hospital, although the duties, which the double position entailed, did not debar him from undertaking other work outside the Infirmary. The explanation of this somewhat unusual combination of offices is probably to be found in the fact that the Board had at their disposal a young man of great ability in John Reid, who had been giving very efficient service in the position of Special Clerk, thus gaining considerable practical knowledge of all the departments in the house.

In the past, the Board of Management had kept a close control over the regulations in force relative to the examination of the bodies of patients dying in the hospital. As early as 1742, an instruction was issued that " no body was to be opened unless the managers were first informed that some singularity in the symptoms of the disease during life had made it necessary and useful to do so " ; and permission to examine the body had to be given by five members of the Board.[1] An unusual incident was brought to their notice in 1759, when one of the surgeons, during his period of attendance at the hospital, examined a body in the operating theatre instead of in the mortuary, bringing with him several persons who had no hospital tickets. Having acted in contravention of the rules the surgeon was dismissed from further service in the Infirmary. In the statutes printed in 1778 it was definitely laid down that no physician or surgeon was permitted to perform a *post-mortem* examination without a licence signed by at least three of the managers.

The dual post of Superintendent and Pathologist was continued for five years, when further administrative changes were made dissociating the two offices.[2] The Infirmary has always been fortunate in the men selected as pathologists who, without exception, have attained eminence in the profession, the position serving either as a valuable stepping-stone to future promotion in the Infirmary or to advancement elsewhere. John Reid, a graduate of 1830, who was the first to hold the double appointment, was like James Young Simpson a native of Bathgate. He had been demonstrator of anatomy with Robert Knox and, in his early days in Edinburgh, as the intimate friend of John Goodsir, the anatomist, of Edward Forbes, the naturalist, and John Hughes Bennett, clinician and physiologist, he became along with them one of " The Brotherhood of the Friends of Truth," a small coterie that met nightly in the attic storey of 21 Lothian Street, the lodging of the Goodsir brothers. Reid brought to his duties at the Infirmary a love of science and a great desire to learn the truth. As the result of his experience during the fever epidemics he was able to describe the pathological changes found in typhoid fever, thus assisting in differentiating that disease from typhus. While acting as pathologist he lectured on physiology in the extra-academical school and, when a vacancy occurred in 1841 in the Chandos Chair at St Andrews, he was appointed professor of anatomy and medicine. His experimental observations on the functions

[1] Minute, 19th January 1742.

[2] Chapter XII, p. 204.

of the eighth cranial nerves, observations which will repay study today, extended his reputation amongst physiologists. Reid died in 1849 at the early age of forty. His successor at the Infirmary was Thomas Beavill Peacock, a graduate of 1842, elected to the staff of St Thomas's Hospital, London, in 1849, and afterwards becoming full physician to that Institution.

With the separation of the double office in 1843, John Hughes Bennett became pathologist to the Infirmary, retaining the appointment till his election to the chair of institutes of medicine in the University in 1848, when he became clinical physician in the hospital. A firm believer in the value of coordinating the teaching of physiology and clinical medicine, he was the last of the occupants of that chair to act as a "professor of medicine" in the Infirmary. "Vivid and telling as a clinical lecturer he was at his best at the bedside." His successor as pathologist was (Sir) William Tennant Gairdner, "a tall, slender youth, whose grave and thoughtful aspect was heightened by the use of spectacles." In his work as pathologist he laid the foundation of his great attainments as a physician. Promoted to the latter office in 1853 he lectured on medicine in the extra-academical school till 1862, when he was called to the chair of practice of physic at Glasgow. Daniel Rutherford Haldane, following in the footsteps of Gairdner as pathologist, gave thirty-four years of service to the Royal Infirmary; nine as pathologist, fifteen as physician-in-ordinary and ten as a manager. The sixth in the succession (Sir) Thomas Grainger Stewart, appointed pathologist in 1862, was for twenty-four years professor of medicine in the University. His students will recall the tall and dignified figure and the gift of language which enabled him to paint the descriptive word-pictures of disease, leaving an indelible impression on their minds.

The duration of the period of residence of patients undergoing treatment in hospital is a subject which must always cause some concern to those interested in its management: it bears a very close relation to the number of those on the waiting list desiring admission, as the more rapid the "turn over" in the wards, the more quickly the beds are vacated and new cases admitted. Little or no attention appears to have been directed to this question in the Infirmary till the year 1850 when, for the first time, reference was made to it in the annual report of the managers. It was stated that the average time spent in hospital by each patient was 36 days, there being no differentiation, however, between the medical cases, the surgical and those suffering from infectious fever. Obviously the period of residence must vary in these different groups. In the year 1853-54, a more detailed return was given, the two main departments of medicine and surgery being differentiated and special returns recorded of the patients in the fever and Lock wards. As a rule the average duration of residence in the fever wards was shorter than elsewhere in the hospital, while in the Lock wards the period greatly exceeded that in the rest of the surgical department.

One illustration may be given in the figures published in the report for the year 1854-55 :—

	Average Residence in Days.
Fever wards	30·2
Ordinary medical wards	35·3
Medical hospital generally	34·9
Ordinary surgical wards	42·0
Lock hospital	66·0
Surgical hospital generally	43·3

For many years the period of residence in the ordinary surgical wards exceeded that in the ordinary medical wards. It was not till 1880 that the position was reversed when, for the first time, the average stay in the surgical hospital was less than in the medical department. In 1854-55, convalescence after injuries and operations was still considerably retarded by complications such as long-continued suppuration and gangrene, complications which debilitated the patients and necessitated the frequent dressing of wounds. It was still the period "Before the Dawn," and the genius of Lister—house surgeon with James Syme in that year—had not yet revolutionised the practice of surgery. A comparison of the figures in the table above quoted with those given in 1934-35 will reveal at a glance how different the position has become :—

	Average Residence in Days.
Medical wards . . .	24·47
Surgical wards . . .	12·87

It was found on inquiry that the period of residence in the Royal Infirmary exceeded that in certain other institutions, such as the Glasgow Royal Infirmary, the General Hospital, Birmingham, and the Greenock Infirmary. This was attributed by the medical staff in Edinburgh mainly to four causes : (1) That the rules governing admission to the hospital were more liberally interpreted ; (2) that amongst the class of patients admitted the proportion of those with chronic organic disease was high ; (3) that there was an absence of any facility to enable the staff to keep the patients under observation outside the hospital ; and (4) that the number of patients attracted to the Royal Infirmary of Edinburgh from a distance necessitated detention for a longer period than would otherwise be required if their homes were within easy access. A weekly report of all those under treatment for more than forty days was insisted upon and every means adopted to make residence as short as possible, compatible with restoration to health.

One possible avenue of relief presented itself through the assistance furnished by certain benevolent persons who, combining as a committee, made arrangements to establish a few convalescent houses in the city : by using these as intermediate stations between the hospital and the home, an opportunity was provided to enable the patients to reach a more complete stage of recovery before their final discharge. In this lay the germ of the future Convalescent House of the Royal Infirmary. These houses first became available about 1857 and, although a decrease took place in the length of the period of residence in the Infirmary without any temporary fluctuations, it was somewhat difficult to assess the actual part they played in bringing about the reduction.

CONVALESCENT HOUSE AT CORSTORPHINE

In July 1864, a welcome offer was made by an anonymous benefactor to build and present to the Infirmary a Convalescent House, on the understanding that the managers undertook to maintain it. A suitable site comprising five acres of ground was obtained at Corstorphine, then a small village lying about two miles to the west of Edinburgh. Sheltered from the north by Corstorphine Hill, with an open southern frontage and with the Pentland Hills forming a distant background, the situation was ideal for the purpose in view. The plans of the house were prepared by Kinnear and Peddie, the architects, and the building was erected at the cost of £12,000, including the provision of the feu-duty; accommodation was found for nearly fifty patients. The House was formally opened in July 1867, when the name of the donor, William Seton Brown, was disclosed. A housekeeper, at a salary of £40, a gardener and a gatekeeper were engaged, and the minister of Corstorphine accepted the duties of chaplain. The care of the patients was placed in the hands of Thomas Annandale, junior assistant surgeon to the Infirmary.

In 1893, through a bequest of £13,000 from Mr James Nasmyth, the eminent engineer, two wings were added to the original building, thus giving the additional accommodation of forty beds. The Convalescent House, to which patients more or less able to look after themselves are sent for a statutory period of three weeks, undoubtedly relieves the pressure on the beds in the Infirmary. During the year 1934-35, as many as 1533 were in residence, the daily average number of beds occupied being 69·18, a number somewhat smaller than in previous years. The cost of upkeep was £3912, a sum which included the conveyance of patients from and to the Infirmary.

The main problem which besets the managers of the Infirmary today is more or less identical with that which faced their predecessors nearly a hundred years ago; and the remedies suggested and gravely considered for its solution are of a very similar nature. In both generations the same fundamental cause has existed, the eternal difficulty in making both ends meet—in balancing the annual expenditure with the revenue. Through many years the chief burthen of complaint reiterated in the annual reports, becoming almost monotonous in the regularity with which it was stated, is the tale of the deficit of receipts over expenditure. Occasionally, but at long intervals, a ray of sunshine has illuminated the shadows and dispersed the gloom, when the accounts balanced, or when the receipts placed a few pounds on the credit side.

For a number of years the annual contributions had been quite inadequate to meet the current expenditure, especially during the epidemics of fever and, without a steady increase from that source, it might become necessary to reduce the number of patients admitted to the hospital, a step which the managers were very unwilling to adopt, as it would react adversely on the interests of the hospital and medical school. During the period 1st October 1840 to 30th September 1848 the annual *average* deficit of ordinary revenue over expenditure was more than £1700. With the exception of three years during that time an annual deficit existed even after applying the legacies and donations which properly belonged to Capital. Moreover, in 1842, it had been deemed necessary again to encroach upon accumulated Capital by selling Stock in order to liquidate debt which was due to the Royal Bank of Scotland. The following figures are quoted as an example of the financial position during one year of the period under review: annual receipts from all sources other than legacies and donations, £9323; expenditure, £10,980; deficit, £1657; when the legacies and donations which amounted to £1562 were applied to meet the deficiency, a sum of £95 still remained as a debit balance.

In the report of the Committee of the Court of Contributors, 1850-51, a very instructive analysis threw some light not only on the sum derived from annual subscriptions but also, in the case of Edinburgh at any rate, on the number of persons subscribing. Subscriptions were then raised under two heads, those made through district collectors and those by means of Church-door collections: they were recorded from three areas, Edinburgh, Leith and Newhaven, and the Counties of

Scotland. The Church-door collections obviously could not be analysed as regards the number of individuals subscribing, but they realised the sum of £1512, of which Edinburgh contributed £1374, Leith and Newhaven £60, and the Country Parishes £78. In Edinburgh the subscriptions received by the collectors amounted to £1641 and were obtained from 4064 citizens. As the population of the city, revealed by a recent census, numbered 160,000 persons, only one-fortieth of the total contributed through that channel to the funds of the Infirmary. When the sum given by each of these individuals was submitted to analysis it was found that more than two-thirds of the subscribers gave less than one pound each. From Leith and Newhaven the collectors received £277, and from the Country Parishes £632: hence the sum received from the three areas amounted to £2550, which, added to the Church-door collections, gave a total sum of £4062. As the number of patients treated in the Infirmary during the same year was 4637—from the city, 3367, from Leith and Newhaven, 340, and from the country districts, 930 [1]—the conclusion previously reached that the hospital was not receiving from the public the financial support that its claims undoubtedly deserved, seemed to be justified. If it were to remain "an open door" to those really qualified for the charity, increased liberality was certainly required.

In May 1856, six medical and nine surgical wards—in all, 144 beds—were closed as a precautionary measure, the state of the annual contributions making no other course possible.[2] It was fortunate that owing to a more healthy condition of the community less demand was being made upon the accommodation in the hospital, and in no instance was a case of acute illness denied admission nor any requiring active remedial treatment. The public had been repeatedly warned that this drastic step might become necessary if financial assistance was not forthcoming and, without sufficient support, the responsibility no longer rested with the managers. On

[1] The number 930 included 30 patients from England and Ireland.

[2] In the following autumn forty beds were restored to facilitate clinical teaching.

the principle that the coat should be cut according to the cloth there seemed to be no other course than to close some of the wards, until the finances permitted of their reopening.

The situation thus created raised the further question as to the desirability of utilising the vacant beds by admitting a class of patients who could afford to pay a small board for their maintenance. It seemed reasonable to argue, and with some truth, that the normal resources of the hospital were being wasted by declining to receive paying patients when accommodation remained unused through lack of funds. But doubt being expressed as to how far it was practicable to combine under one roof a charitable institution and one in which payment was exacted, the managers decided against their introduction. Yet in the eighteenth century the two systems had worked smoothly side by side for many years when payment had been received for the maintenance of soldiers and sailors, domestic servants, the insane and the lying-in woman ; and even in 1856, the Parochial Boards were annually contributing a considerable sum for the care of pauper patients, and the managers were then considering the propriety of exacting a still higher remuneration from these Boards both in the towns and country districts.

An application for Government Grants and the adoption of a measure of compulsory local assessment also came under consideration. Although it was felt that the Infirmary conferred more good upon the community generally than any other institution of a similar kind, and therefore had strong claims to national support, considerable doubt was expressed as to whether any such appeal to Government would prove successful, or indeed ought to be made. The Infirmary was essentially a charitable Institution, hitherto supported by the voluntary contributions of the public, a means of support which it was hoped the hospital would continue to receive so as to maintain its full efficiency. Local taxation, if instituted, would probably terminate the voluntary and charitable contributions of the public and forfeit their interest in its support. It would eventually increase the cost of maintenance of the hospital by depriving it of the gratuitous services of its medical and surgical staff, for which payment would require to be made, and it would lose the assistance of a body of efficient managers voluntarily conducting its affairs. Moreover, the admission of patients would be restricted to those living in the city and suburbs and lead to the exclusion of those residing outside these boundaries, thus destroying the national character of the Royal Infirmary.

Such were the views then held and the decisions reached by the managers on the important question of hospital policy : times and circumstances have changed, but the problem of the maintenance and of the efficiency of the Infirmary is none the less real today.

CHAPTER XI

EXTENSION OF THE ROYAL INFIRMARY IN THE NINETEENTH CENTURY, 1800-1853

NEW WING ATTACHED TO THE ORIGINAL HOSPITAL—THE OLD HIGH SCHOOL OF EDINBURGH AS THE SURGICAL HOSPITAL, 1829—SURGEONS' SQUARE AND THE EXTRA-ACADEMICAL SCHOOL—PROFESSOR JAMES SYME AND THE CHAIR OF CLINICAL SURGERY, 1833—THE SURGICAL STAFF OF THE INFIRMARY—THE NEW SURGICAL HOSPITAL, 1853—CHLOROFORM ANÆSTHESIA, 1847.

FROM time to time, as opportunity arose, house property in the immediate vicinity of the hospital had been acquired with a view to providing the means of future extension. But it was not till the last decade of the eighteenth century that the first addition was made to the Infirmary, not however by utilising any of the houses previously purchased, but by attaching a wing to William Adam's original building. Two questions had then come under the consideration of the Board, a proposal to transfer the maternity cases from the hospital to a separate house, and the provision of more beds for sick and injured sailors. The first of these problems solved itself, when in 1793 the Edinburgh Lying-in Hospital was opened as a special institution by Alexander Hamilton, the professor of midwifery.[1] The solution of the second problem, more beds for sailors, was arrived at when the managers added a new wing, containing three wards, to the west gable of the Infirmary.[2] The exact position of this wing is shown in Ainslie's Map of Edinburgh, published in 1804, but no detailed information concerning its internal arrangements is given in the minutes of the managers. But patients suffering from infectious fever were transferred from the fever ward to the upper floor of the wing, as the surgeons complained that during the summer months the air was frequently rendered

[1] Chapter VII, p. 100.

[2] Minutes, Royal Infirmary, 31st January 1791 and 4th June 1792.

so impure in the vicinity of the fever ward that the recovery of patients after operations was often retarded and that sometimes, indeed, it led to fatal results! The ward thus vacated was used for operation cases. It is somewhat difficult to find an adequate explanation of the action of the Board in erecting a new wing when a number of the beds in the hospital were unoccupied, and even the allowance provided by Government for the treatment of sailors scarcely seemed to justify this further outlay on construction.

Although the finances of the Infirmary had been subjected to considerable strain in connection with the early epidemics of fever, the prospective disposal of the High School, at the head of the High School Wynd and in close proximity to the hospital, compelled the managers in 1827 to face some financial sacrifice in order to protect the amenity of the Infirmary. The growth of the New Town had accentuated the need of establishing a school for boys in a more convenient situation than that provided at High School Yards. Many of the residents in the New Town considered that a second school had become necessary and, accordingly, the Edinburgh Academy was incorporated by Royal Charter in 1823 and, under the management of a board of directors, had been opened on the north side of the city. The Town Council, however, being of the opinion that the community would be best served by placing their school in a more central position, eventually decided to rebuild the High School upon the southern aspect of the Calton Hill, a site certainly more salubrious and more picturesque than that which it had so long occupied. The foundation stone of the new school was laid in 1825 and, in 1829, the pupils were transferred to Thomas Hamilton's classic edifice on the Calton Hill.[1]

Prior to this event the managers of the Infirmary, realising that the old building would probably be sold, and fearing the possibility that no limitation would be placed upon the height of new houses erected on the site, petitioned the Lord Provost and Magistrates to place some restriction upon their elevation.[2]

[1] *The History of the High School of Edinburgh*, by William Steven, D.D. Edinburgh, 1848.

[2] Minute, Royal Infirmary, 22nd January 1827.

They drew attention to the need of a constant circulation of fresh air around the hospital and referred to the fact that some alarm had already been expressed in consequence of the height of the buildings previously erected between the Infirmary and University on the west side, and in Drummond Street on the south side of their property. If this were to be repeated on the east side, ventilation would be still further interfered with. When the school was eventually advertised for sale a committee of the Board of Management of the hospital were appointed to attend the proceedings; but the upset price being fixed at £9000 no offer was made.[1] A second upset price of £7750 again brought no response. Finally, in May 1829, the managers offered a sum of £7500 with the proviso that the Town Council would agree to pay the whole of the auction duty along with that on the feu charter. Although failing to obtain a rebate of more than half of the auction duty they purchased the property for the sum of £7609, nearly all of which, contrary to the provisions of the Charter, was provided by the sale of investments and from a cash deposit in the Bank of Scotland. In the following year a site adjoining the High School was also bought for £1300 [2] so that the total sum withdrawn from the Capital Stock in connection with these transactions amounted to £8909, thus making a considerable drain upon the future annual revenue of the hospital derived from investments.

Having acquired the High School the managers decided to convert it into a surgical hospital, complaints having been made of the inconvenient overcrowding of the surgical wards in the original building. Plans were prepared and submitted for the consideration of the surgeons, and estimates for reconstruction of the building amounting to £3138 were accepted. In addition, an operating theatre capable of accommodating four hundred students was attached to the east wall of the building, so that the total expenditure upon the surgical hospital amounted to a sum slightly exceeding £12,000. In adapting the building for its new purpose many of the partitions

[1] Minutes, 5th May 1828, 20th April, 11th May and 27th July 1829.
[2] Minute, Royal Infirmary, 4th January 1830.

were removed, and a long corridor was constructed on each floor; but the walls separating the corridors from the adjacent wards were not carried to the roof throughout their entire length, thus permitting of a better circulation of air between the wards, the corridors and staircase. Baths on improved principles were introduced and rooms were added for the use of nurses and resident house surgeons. The external walls were left untouched and, indeed, remain today as they were originally erected in 1777, solid and but little weathered with the passing of time.

In response to an appeal from Dr Carson, the Rector of the High School, a stone, on which were carved the Arms of the City and the dates of the reign of James VI, was removed from the east gable of the janitor's lodge for transference to the new High School. The stone had occupied a prominent place in the wall of the School built in 1578, and was therefore an interesting relic of bygone times and worthy of preservation in the new school on the Calton Hill.

While the surgical patients were still being entertained in the original Infirmary building, operations were not infrequently performed on Sunday morning during the hours of service at Lady Yester's Church on the opposite side of Infirmary Street.[1] The minister of the Kirk, a popular preacher and interested in the welfare of the students, attracted the more serious-minded who occupied the gallery in considerable numbers. When the clang of the Infirmary bell, signalling the commencement of an operation, resounded throughout the church, he deemed it wiser, as the result of experience, to stop his discourse and resume his seat in the pulpit till the unceremonious clatter of feet accompanying the rapid emptying of the gallery had ceased. The lure of the operating theatre prevailed over the eloquence of the preacher!

The Surgical Hospital was opened in November 1832 providing accommodation for seventy-two patients but, in the years following, the number of beds was increased to eighty and then to one hundred and three. All the surgical cases

[1] *Edinburgh Medical Journal*, vol. xxix, "Harveian Oration," 14th April 1884, by Alexander Keiller, M.D.

were transferred to it with the exception of those patients suffering from erysipelas, so that separate medical and surgical houses were thus instituted.[1] Nearly forty years later, an inmate of the surgical house, a patient of Joseph Lister, has thus recorded his impressions of the hospital :—

And lo, the Hospital, gray, quiet, old,
Where life and death like friendly chafferers meet

. . . . . .

A tragic meanness seems so to environ
These corridors and stairs of stone and iron,
Cold, naked, clean—half workhouse and half jail.[2]

Following closely upon the purchase of the High School, with its conversion into a surgical hospital, the managers, in June 1833, came into possession of old Surgeons' Hall, built in 1697, and recently vacated by the surgeons on occupying their new premises in Nicolson Street. The managers of the Infirmary, apparently still obsessed by the fear that high buildings would be erected on the site of the Hall, then in a somewhat ruinous condition, if it were disposed of in the open market, made an offer for it and the adjoining ground. The property consisted of the Hall and the ground on its north frontage ; the house built as a lecture room by John Bell, the surgeon ; and the feu-duties of a number of houses in Surgeons' Square, of the annual value of £45. The College of Surgeons agreed to sell the several properties for a sum of £2100, taking £600 as the price of the Hall, £500 for John Bell's house and £1000 for the feu-duties at twenty years purchase.[3]

Slowly but surely the Infirmary was acquiring the whole of the area once occupied by the monastery and the other conventual buildings owned by the Black Friars in Pre-reformation days. Surgeons' Square was both the birthplace and the nursery of the extra-mural or extra-academical school of medicine. Although the Square has long lost its identity and its name is no longer written on the map of the city, the

[1] Minute, 17th January 1833.
[2] *A Book of Verses*, by William Ernest Henley. David Nutt. London, 1888.
[3] Minute, Royal Infirmary, 24th June 1833.

area must always remain of historic interest to the medical profession of Edinburgh, as the early home of its school of anatomy and surgery. Occupying the ground on the east side of the Infirmary and the High School and between them and the Pleasance, the houses in the Square during many years served various useful purposes.[1] In Surgeons' Hall, Alexander Monro, *primus*, in 1720 as previously narrated, commenced his distinguished career as an anatomist and, in the Square in the later part of the eighteenth century, John Bell associated with his younger brother Charles, before the latter migrated to London, taught anatomy in its application to surgery. There too John Barclay and Robert Knox, during the professorship of the third Monro in the University, lectured on anatomy to many hundreds of students, and the teaching of surgery was in the hands of such able exponents as John Thomson, John William Turner and John Lizars, successively professors of surgery in the Royal College of Surgeons.[2] There Robert Liston and James Syme demonstrated anatomy with John Barclay and, as young men, together conducted a class of anatomy and surgery. Amongst others, at a later date, were Allen Thomson, John Struthers—afterwards Sir John—and William Sharpey teaching anatomy; and in the session of 1838-39 James Young Simpson delivered his first course of lectures on midwifery.[3]

After the purchase of Surgeons' Hall the managers granted a lease of the building to Robert Knox who, as the successor of Barclay, had at first occupied his rooms on the west side of the Square. As a teacher of anatomy, "*primus et incomparabilis*," Knox in 1833[4] was still attracting many students to his lecture theatre, but for him "the tide was on the ebb, and the growing animosities of his contemporaries rendered the ebb more and

[1] The area is designated as Surgeons' Square in Kincaid's Map of Edinburgh published in 1784; and in the city directory of the same year the Square is given as the address of a Mrs Porter who kept boarders: it is sometimes designated Surgeon Square.

[2] *The Edinburgh School of Surgery before Lister*, by Alexander Miles. A. & C. Black, Ltd. London, 1918.

[3] *The Edinburgh Medical Journal*, March 1882. "Some of the Older Schools of Anatomy," by Charles W. Cathcart, F.R.C.S.

[4] Minute, Royal Infirmary, 3rd August 1833.

more apparent." In 1826, anatomical dissection had been made a compulsory part of the medical curriculum bringing with it increasing difficulty in securing the necessary material for the instruction of so many students. In Edinburgh the violation of graves, an old-standing means of supply, had been recently superseded by actual murder, as the crimes of the notorious Burke and Hare had disclosed to an astonished and indignant community. "Fifteen times the 'deil's luck' befriended them: the sixteenth turn of the wheel proved fatal to the murderers." [1] For twelve months they had carried on their nefarious traffic in the city till the murder of the old woman Docherty, whose body was recognised in Knox's dissecting room, revealed the tragedy. In 1829, William Burke was executed for the West Port murders and William Hare, having turned King's Evidence, fled the city. Knox never regained the confidence of the public and, a few years after his occupancy of Surgeons' Hall, he found it necessary to turn his back upon the scenes of his former triumphs. He died in London in 1862 in comparative destitution, "one of his last occupations being that of lecturer, demonstrator or showman to a travelling party of Ojibbeway Indians." [2]

In the course of the next few years the remaining houses in the Square were purchased. These included the house immediately to the west of the old Hall formerly used by John Thomson when teaching surgery. The accommodation in it had also proved useful during the recent epidemics of fever. Finally, the Hall of the Royal Medical Society adjoining John Barclay's anatomical theatre, the foundation stone of which had been laid by William Cullen in 1775, was purchased in 1851, thus preparing the way for further extension of the Royal Infirmary.

Today only two buildings remain to mark the site of the old Square; the greatly altered Surgeons' Hall, of three storeys instead of the original two, now the Headquarters of the University Officers' Training Corps and, in the north-east

[1] *The Sack-'em-Up Men*, by James Moores Ball, M.D. Oliver & Boyd. Edinburgh, 1928.

[2] *The Life of Sir Robert Christison, Bart.*, vol. i, p. 311. William Blackwood & Sons. Edinburgh and London, 1895.

corner a tall and renovated house which, in its time, had served various purposes, but is now part of the establishment of the University Settlement at High School Yards.

The opening of the Surgical Hospital in the autumn of 1832 and the transference of the surgical patients from the old building necessitated a rearrangement of the beds and a new distribution amongst the members of the staff. It may be recalled at this point that, in 1800, the old system of attendance by rotation had been abrogated and six surgeons were elected by the managers; three groups of two, each in succession, took charge of the wards for a period of two years, the individual surgeons, however, being eligible for reappointment four years after the expiry of their previous period of service. But in 1818, although maintaining the same number of surgeons, a subdivision of the staff was made into three classes, the Consulting, the Acting, and the Assistant Surgeons, two being placed in each group. At the end of every biennial period thereafter, a change was made in each group: the senior consulting surgeon retired, the senior acting surgeon became a consulting surgeon, and the senior assistant surgeon was promoted, but this latter step "was not to be regarded as a matter of course, far less of right."[1] A new junior assistant surgeon was then elected. In the event of any vacancy occurring from death or resignation during the biennial period, it was filled by election. This was still the method of staffing when the Surgical Hospital was opened.

While the managers were considering the allocation of the beds, James Russell announced his resignation of the chair of clinical surgery[2] and James Syme was appointed his successor. In a letter to the Infirmary dated 23rd March 1833, intimating his election, Syme stated that an offer of his services to the hospital might facilitate the arrangements which would be necessary, in case it was the desire of the managers that the course of lectures delivered by the occupant of the chair should continue to be connected with the Royal Infirmary. As

[1] Minute, Royal Infirmary, 14th December 1818.

[2] Chapter IX, p. 145.

" mature and anxious deliberation " by the Board was necessary in reaching a final decision upon the plans to be adopted in the Surgical Hospital, the reply of the managers was not communicated to the Senatus Academicus till 8th May, when it was presented in the following terms :—

The Managers of the Royal Infirmary beg leave to assure the Senatus that they feel the same desire to maintain an intimate connection between the Hospital and the University as their predecessors have constantly done. In regard to the present application they have to inform the Senatus, that they consider that it is not only *ultra vires*, but would be improper were it not so, to form any permanent arrangement for the Professor of Clinical Surgery, or put any part of the establishment committed to their superintendence beyond their control.

They beg leave, however, to acquaint the Senatus that they have appointed Mr Syme, the Professor of Clinical Surgery, Junior Assistant Surgeon, by which he will, if nothing unforeseen occur, be connected with the Hospital for a long series of years ; and in consequence of his filling the Chair of Clinical Surgery in the University they propose to put immediately under his charge three of the smaller wards capable of containing thirty beds, with the privilege of giving clinical lectures upon such patients as may come under his care.

It must be left for the Managers of the day to determine what arrangement ought to be made for the Professor of Clinical Surgery when he shall cease to be an Assistant Surgeon, by which time they shall have had the experience of some years to guide them. The Managers think it necessary to add that they at all times reserve to themselves the power of making such changes in their arrangements as any emergency may require.

Syme expressed his satisfaction with what had been done and, as junior assistant surgeon in the Infirmary, he commenced his distinguished career in the chair of clinical surgery. As an old High School boy he was to become a " Master " in the building in which he had formerly sat as a pupil. Although only thirty-three years of age when appointed to the chair, he had already established his fame as a surgeon. Foiled, in 1829, in his attempt to obtain an assistant surgeoncy in the Infirmary, Syme founded his surgical hospital in Minto House, once the town residence of the Elliots of Minto. A three-storeyed building surrounded by garden, it stood on the east side of Argyle Square, overlooking the Cowgate and within a stone's throw of the University.[1] There he gathered around him an ever increasing number of patients and students, enhancing his reputation as an operating surgeon and as a teacher.

When he joined the surgical staff of the Royal Infirmary in 1833, his colleagues were Sir George Ballingall and John Campbell, the consulting surgeons; Robert Liston and John Lizars, the acting surgeons, along with John William Turner, the professor of systematic surgery, as the senior assistant surgeon. Turner, promoted acting surgeon, died in November 1835 and the vacancy on the assistant staff was filled by the appointment of William Fergusson. In the hands of these accomplished men, all of whom had served their apprenticeship in the dissecting room, following the tradition of the Edinburgh School at that period, surgery then stood on a very high plane in Edinburgh. It was still the pre-anæsthetic period when a combination of coolness, dexterity and rapidity of action was essential for the performance of a successful surgical operation. It was still the pre-Listerian age. The range of surgery was thus restricted, and major operations consisted largely in amputation of limbs, in the removal of stone from the bladder and in the ligation of arteries in the treatment of aneurysm, an operation which is now relatively infrequent. It was the period too when infections frequently supervened on surgical interference, a complication which often terminated in the death of the patients from hæmorrhage, septicæmia or pyæmia.[2]

Sir George Ballingall, a man of military bearing and a capable surgeon, knighted on the occasion of the accession of William IV, had served as a surgeon in the army in France and in the Far East. Elected to the staff of the Infirmary

[1] Old Minto House was demolished when a city improvement scheme carried Chambers Street through Argyle Square. The present Minto House is a comparatively modern building now occupied by departments of the University.

[2] *Joseph, Baron Lister, Centenary, 1827-1927.* "Before the Dawn," by Alexander Miles, M.D., LL.D. Oliver & Boyd, Edinburgh, 1927.

in 1822, he was appointed regius professor of military surgery in the University, retaining the chair and his position as consulting surgeon in the Infirmary till his death in 1855.[1] John Campbell was consulting surgeon till 1838 when he joined the Board of Management of the hospital. A good and reliable surgeon, he was never classed like some of his colleagues as brilliant. Robert Liston and John Lizars were men of a different stamp. Liston, whose bust has a place in the Board Room of the Infirmary today, was a son of the manse: he has been described as "a tall man, powerful in form, dressed in a dark bottle-green coat with velvet collar, double-breasted shawl vest, grey trousers and Wellington boots," and one of the boldest and most dexterous operators of his day. While still a student and acting as one of the surgeons' clerks he had criticised the surgical practice of the hospital and, being found guilty of interfering improperly with the arrangements of the department, he was prohibited from entering the wards and the operating theatre. Some years later he tendered his apology to the managers and was reinstated. When appointed assistant surgeon in 1828 his reputation was already established but, being defeated by Syme in the contest for the chair of clinical surgery in 1833, he resigned his position as acting surgeon in the following year and accepted the chair of clinical surgery at University College, London, and the surgeoncy at the North London Hospital, later named University College Hospital. John Lizars who held the professorship of surgery in the College of Surgeons of Edinburgh was "bold and fearless, almost reckless, as an operator." He was the first in Scotland to tie the innominate artery in the treatment of an aneurysm and the first in Britain to perform ovariotomy. John William Turner was "a timid, shy man who seemed fitted by nature for anything rather than the duties and responsibilities of an operating surgeon." In William Fergusson the hospital secured for five years the services of a remarkably dexterous and skilful surgeon. A man of handsome and commanding presence, he became, after Liston's death in 1847, the leading operating surgeon in London, as in

[1] The chair of military surgery was abolished in 1856.

1840 Fergusson had left Edinburgh, having accepted the chair of surgery at King's College, London, and the surgeoncy at King's College Hospital. Created a Baronet in 1866 he was made Serjeant-Surgeon to Queen Victoria. A word-picture of him in the operating theatre of King's College Hospital has been left to posterity : it describes him as a tall dignified figure, carefully dressed in black frock coat, wearing a black bow tie and with his feet encased in " Bluchers "—half-boots, no laces or buttons, square-toed and highly polished. With a white apron tied over his coat and, with his voluminous wrist-bands turned well upwards, he was then ready to commence operations.[1]

With the departure of Liston and Fergusson from Edinburgh London gained the services of two of the most distinguished surgeons of the period. But James Syme remained in his native city, " in all supreme, complete in every part."[2]

For a brief span one further contemporary figure, Sir Charles Bell, took his place on the stage of the Royal Infirmary, pre-eminent amongst his colleagues, not as a brilliant operating surgeon, but as an anatomist, physiologist, pathologist, surgeon and artist, to whom the term genius may be assuredly applied. Reference has already been made to his migration as a young man from Edinburgh to London, in 1804.[3] There, as a pioneer, " he formulated a working conception of the nervous system at a time when all was in a state of chaos, a conception which stands today and has served as a basis of all subsequent inquiry and progress."[4] On the death of J. W. Turner in 1835, Charles Bell was invited to fill the vacant chair of systematic surgery at Edinburgh, and his appointment was received with general acclamation. His departure from his beloved Middlesex

[1] *British Masters of Medicine*, edited by Sir D'Arcy Power, K.B.E. London : " The Medical Press and Circular," 1936, p. 104. Article by Mr Cecil P. G. Wakeley, F.R.C.S.

[2] *Horæ Subsecivæ*, by John Brown, M.D., LL.D. A. & C. Black, London, 1897. Quotation from Joseph Lister's estimate of his master.

[3] Chapter VIII, p. 129.

[4] *Edinburgh Medical Journal*, 1935, vol. xlii, p. 252. Professor Edwin Bramwell, " Harveian Oration," 15th June 1934.

Hospital, at the very commencement of its life as a medical school, and his resignation of the surgical chair in the University of London were regarded by his colleagues in the nature of a calamity ; but the step was not lightly undertaken.

Bell was then sixty-two years of age, too old to make a fresh start in life : but, " London," he wrote to his brother, " is a place to live in, not to die in," and the opportunity thus offered to return to his native city must have made a very strong appeal. On his return to Edinburgh in 1836, Charles Bell was elected one of the consulting surgeons to the Royal Infirmary and, along with his colleagues Sir George Ballingall and John Campbell, he served the hospital in that capacity till his death in 1842. He died at Worcester while on a visit to friends and was buried in Hallow Churchyard.

When Syme in due course became one of the acting surgeons to the Infirmary the managers proceeded to redistribute the surgical beds, then 103 in number : 43 were given to Syme, 40 to the senior and 20 to the junior acting surgeon.[1] As there were then 280 beds in the medical hospital the full complement of beds in the Infirmary was 383, but all were not in daily occupation. In 1841, as the surgeons were unanimous in their opinion that the wards were overcrowded, the number of surgical beds was reduced by thirty, thus reverting to the accommodation for which the surgical hospital had been designed. An improved system of ventilation was at the same time introduced, this and the reduction of beds being very necessary alterations when septicæmia and pyæmia were so prevalent in the surgical wards of the hospital. It is unfortunate that in the annual report of patients under treatment in the Royal Infirmary no differentiation of medical and surgical cases was made till the year 1849-50 ; but in that year, of the 3633 patients under treatment, 1764 were ordinary medical cases, 1349 were surgical, and 520 were fever cases. Although there was no general epidemic in the city, the number of patients suffering from infectious fevers still remained abnormally high.

[1] With the promotion of the professor of clinical surgery to the position of acting surgeon there were thus three acting surgeons.

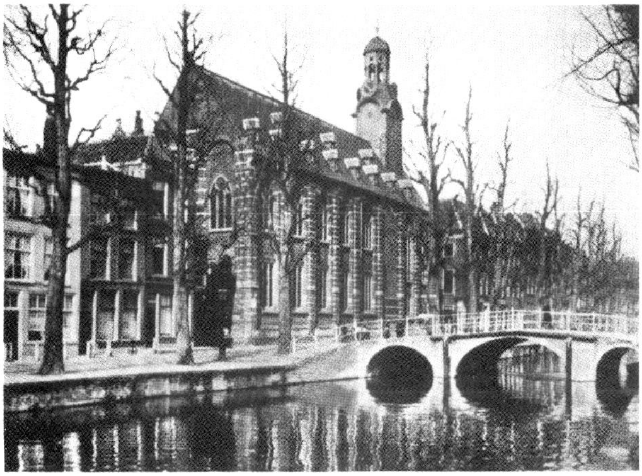

The University of Leiden on the left bank of the Rapenburg Canal: the University dates from 1575

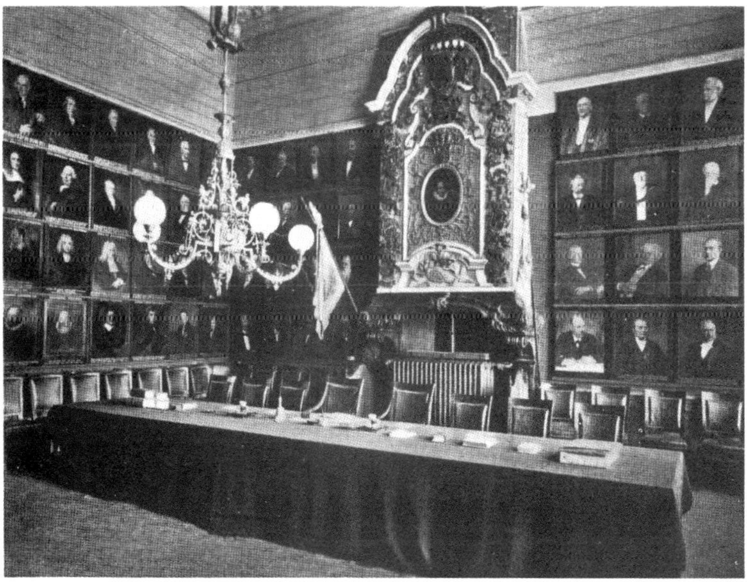

The Senate Room in the University of Leiden: formerly the lecture room of Professor Hermann Boerhaave

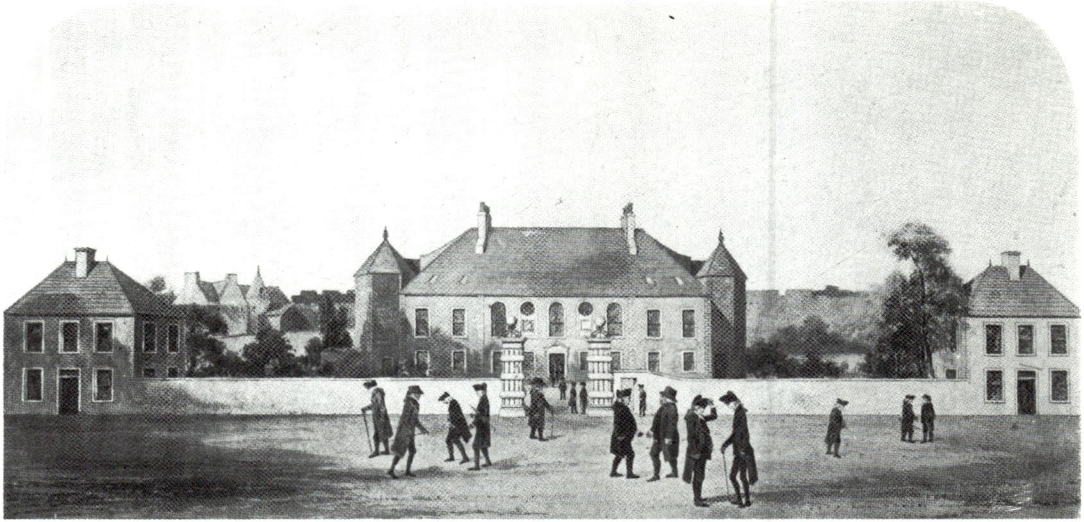

The Surgeons' Hall of 1697: the building, facing north, formed the south side of Surgeons' Square.
In the background is part of the Flodden Wall constructed in 1513

(*From a Sketch in the Royal College of Surgeons of Edinburgh*)

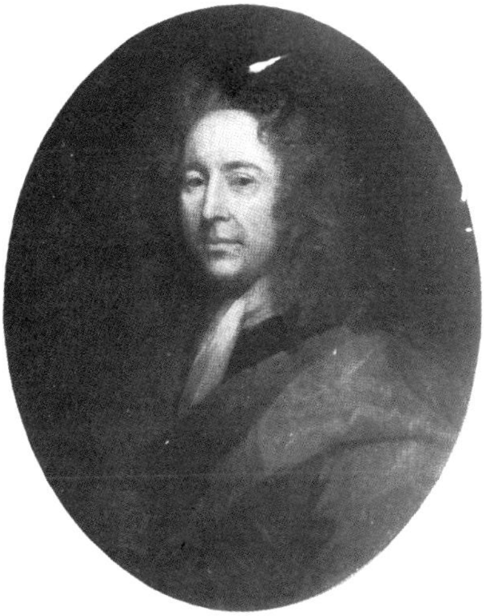

1.—JOHN MONRO

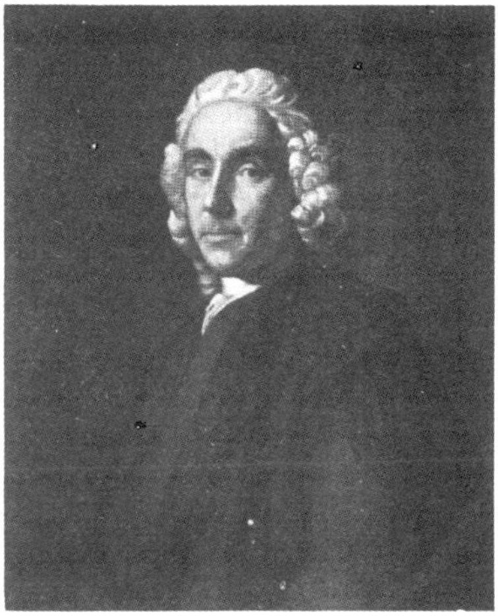

2.—ALEXANDER MONRO
(*Primus*)

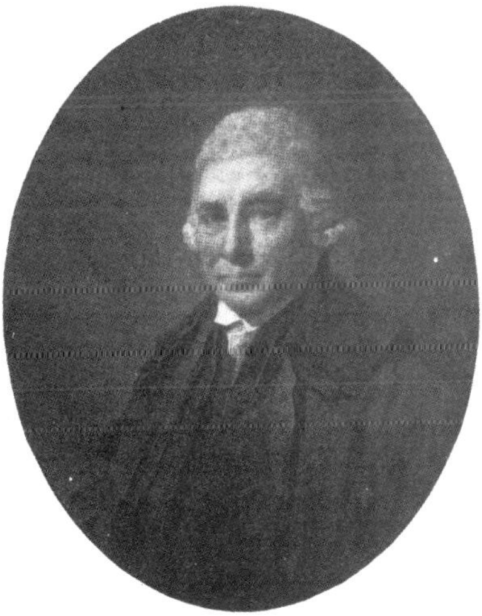

3.—ALEXANDER MONRO
(*Secundus*)

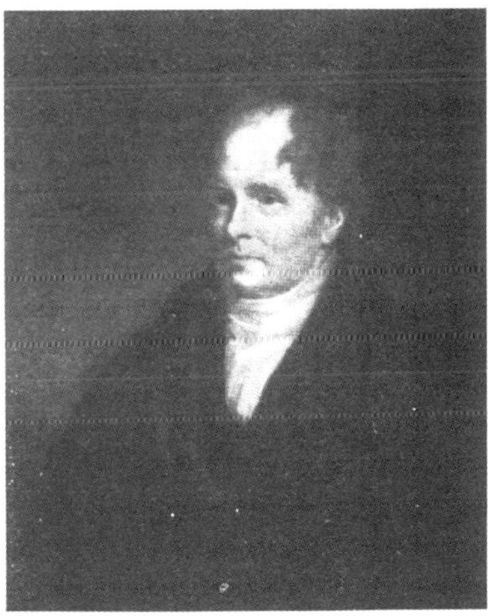

4.—ALEXANDER MONRO
(*Tertius*)

Four Generations of the Family of Monro

(*Nos.* 1, 2 *and* 4 *from portraits in the Royal College of Surgeons of Edinburgh. No.* 3 *from engraving by James Heath from portrait by Sir Henry Raeburn*)

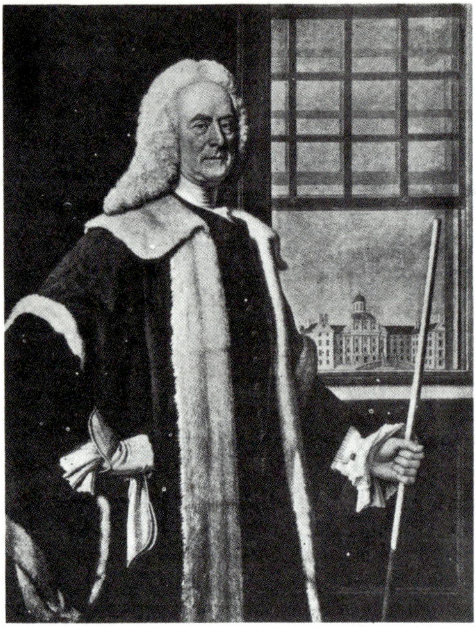

GEORGE DRUMMOND
Six times Lord Provost of Edinburgh

(From the portrait by J. Alexander in the Board Room of the Royal Infirmary)

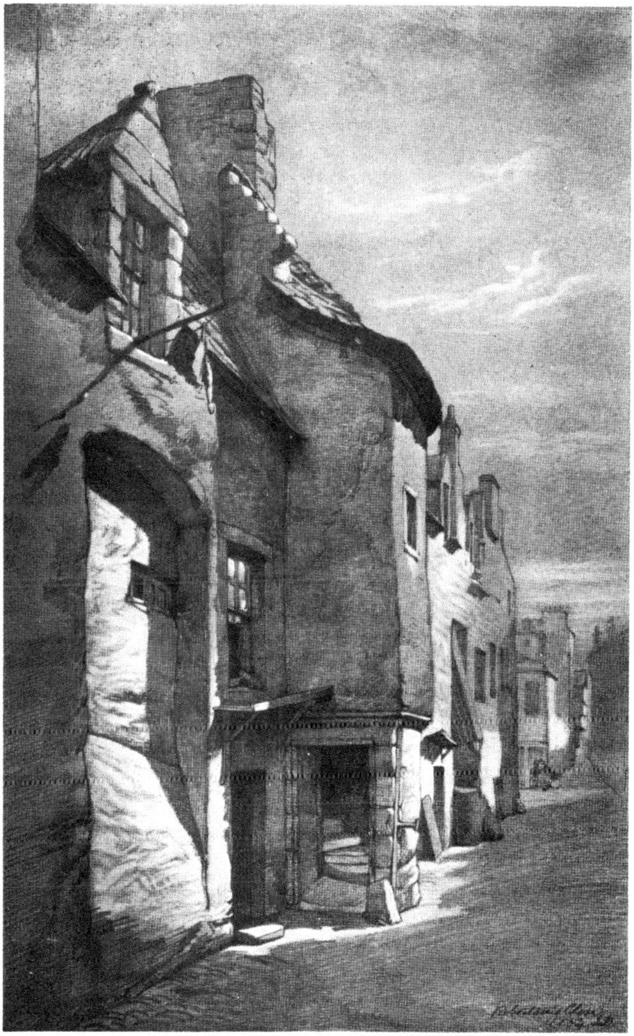

View of Robertson's Close from the Cowgate, showing the old houses on the east side

(*From a drawing by Mr James Drummond in 1854*)

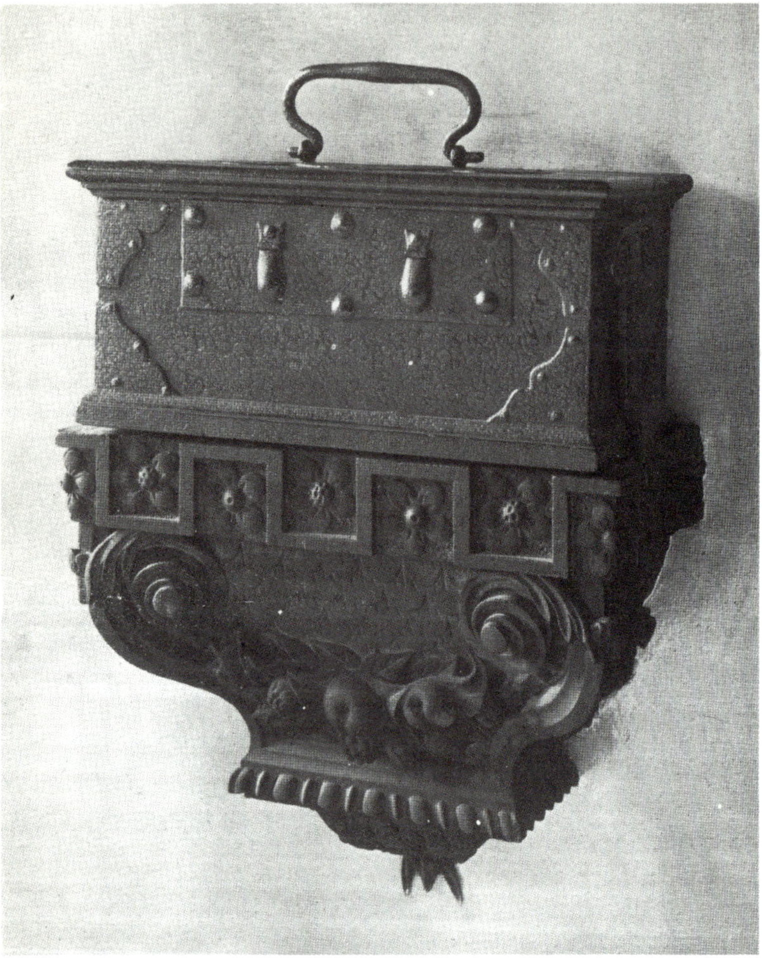

The Charity Box, a relic of the original Hospital in Robertson's Close, now in the entrance hall of the Royal Infirmary

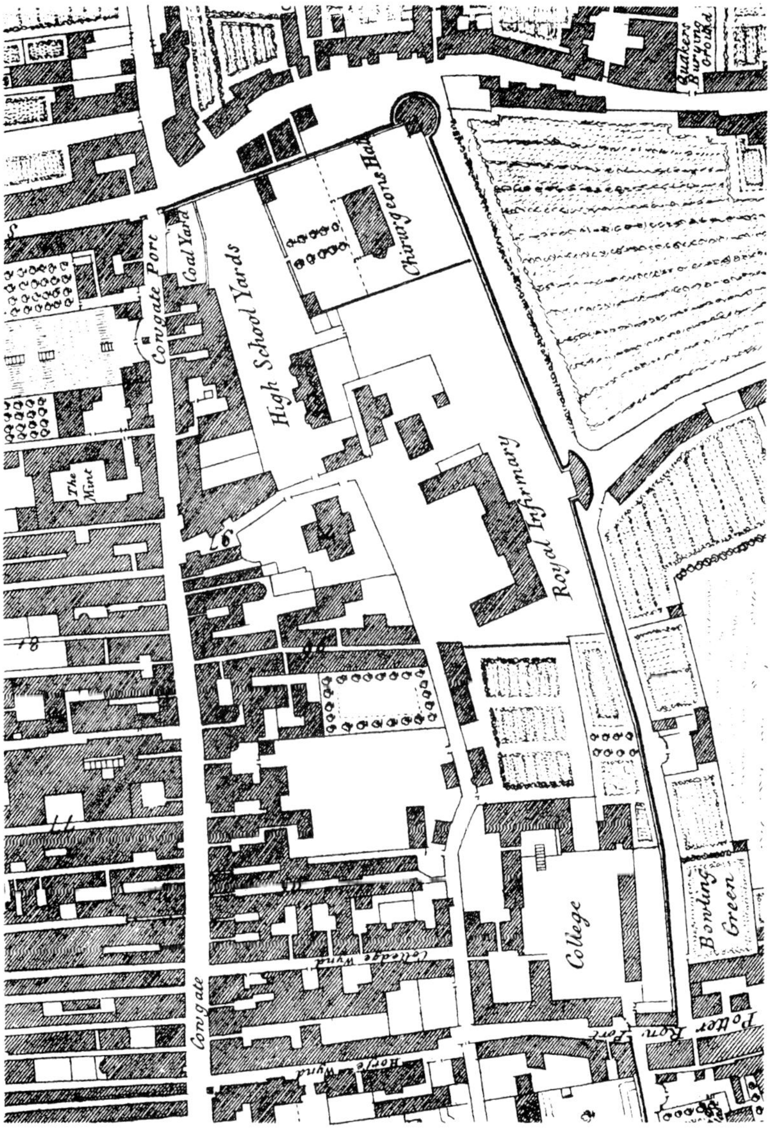

Section of William Edgar's Plan of Edinburgh, 1742

Royal Infirmary opened December 1741; the High School of 1578; Surgeons' Hall of 1697.
96. Robertson's Close. 97. High School Wynd. K. Lady Yester's Church of 1647.

The open space between the College and the Royal Infirmary is the College garden

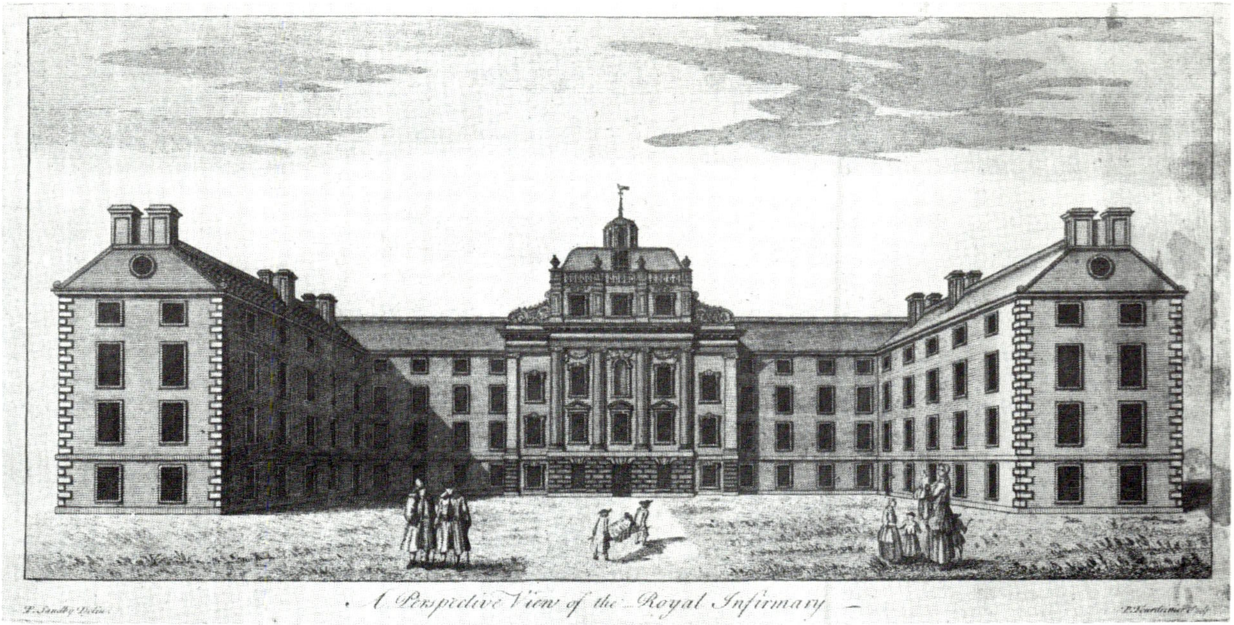

Engraving by Paul Sandby of the Royal Infirmary founded in 1738.

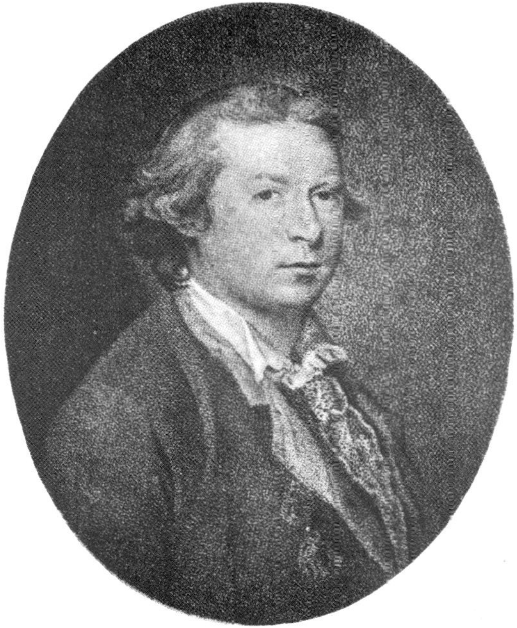

JOHN GREGORY
Professor of Practice of Physic, 1766-1773
(*From a portrait by F. Cotes*)

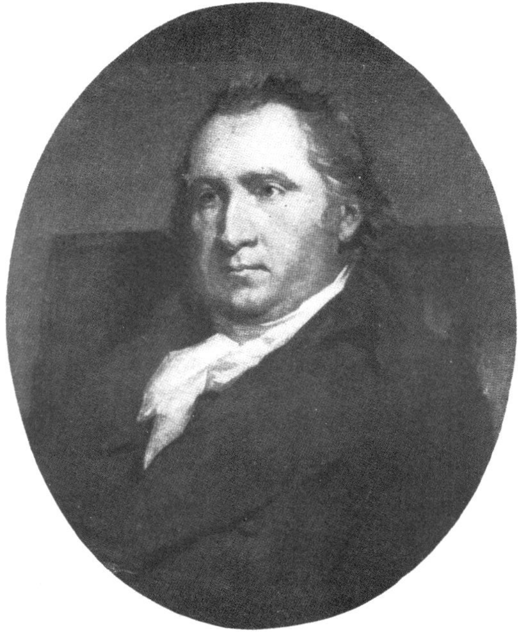

JAMES GREGORY
Professor of Institutes of Medicine, 1776-1789
Professor of Practice of Physic, 1790-1821
(*From a portrait by Sir Henry Raeburn*)

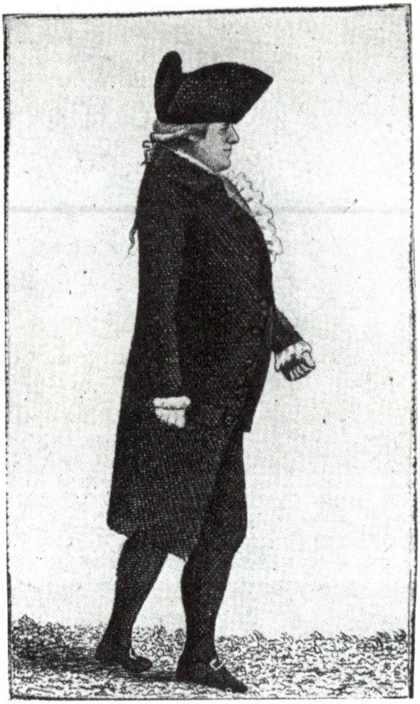

JAMES HAMILTON, Senior
Physician to the Royal Infirmary, 1775-1823
(*Reproduced from John Kay's " Original Portraits "*)

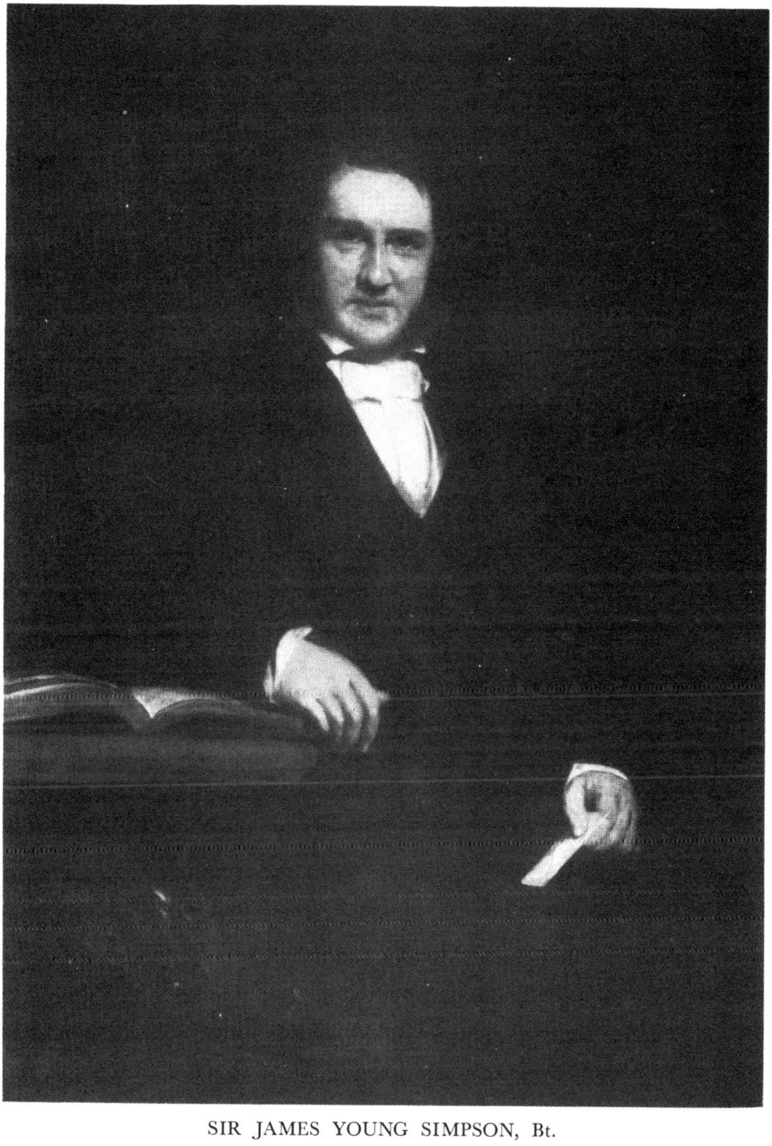

SIR JAMES YOUNG SIMPSON, Bt.
Professor of Midwifery, 1840-1870

(Reproduced by kind permission of Professor R. W. Johnstone, from a portrait ascribed to Sir John Watson Gordon, P.R.S.A., R.A.)

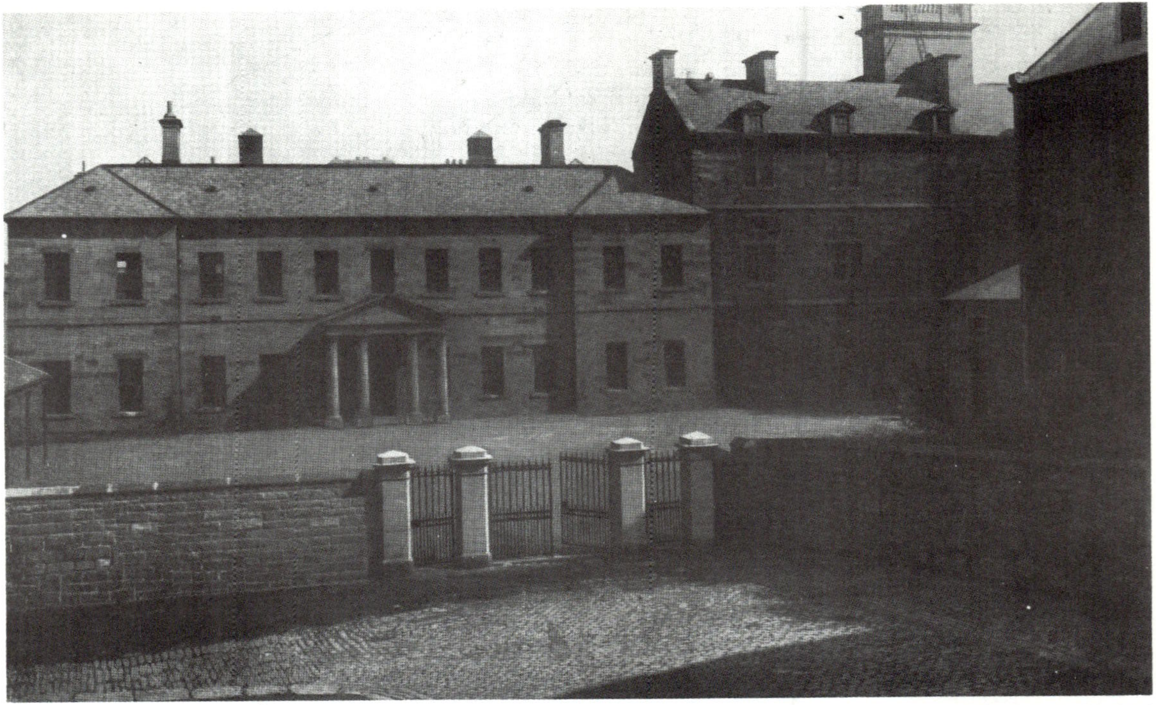

Photo by] [*Mr F. C. Inglis, Edinburgh*

The Old Surgical Hospital opened in 1832 : it was previously the High School erected in 1777 to replace the School of 1578 which occupied an adjacent site. The building is now used as the Department of Geography of the University

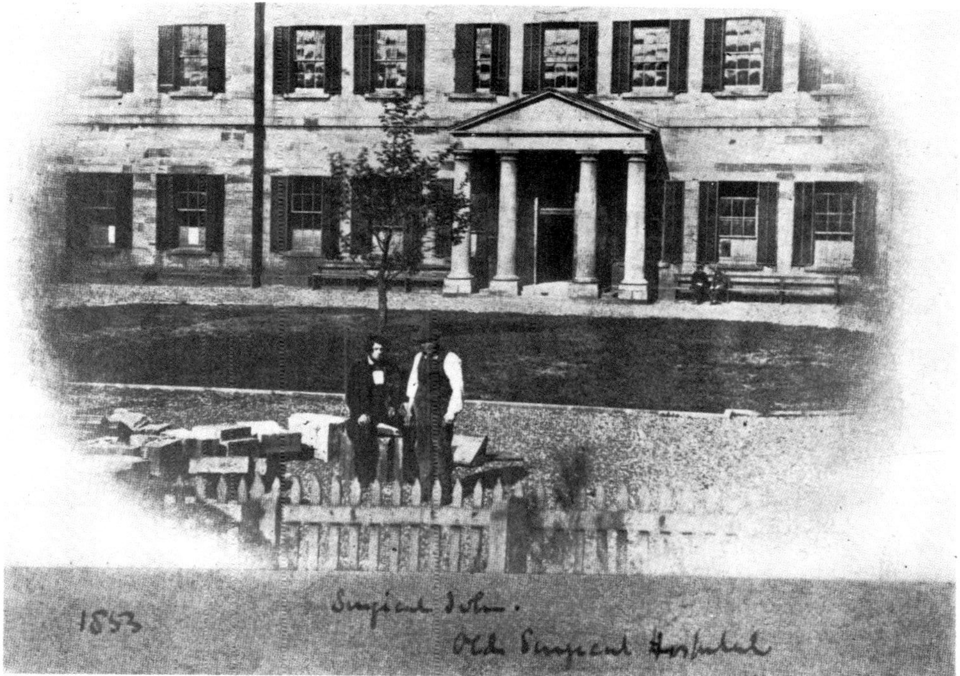

The façade of the Old Surgical Hospital during the period when James Syme was in charge of the wards : in the foreground is the figure of John, the surgical porter

(From an old photograph dated 1853, lent to the author by Mr Andrew Whyte, the Steward, Royal Infirmary)

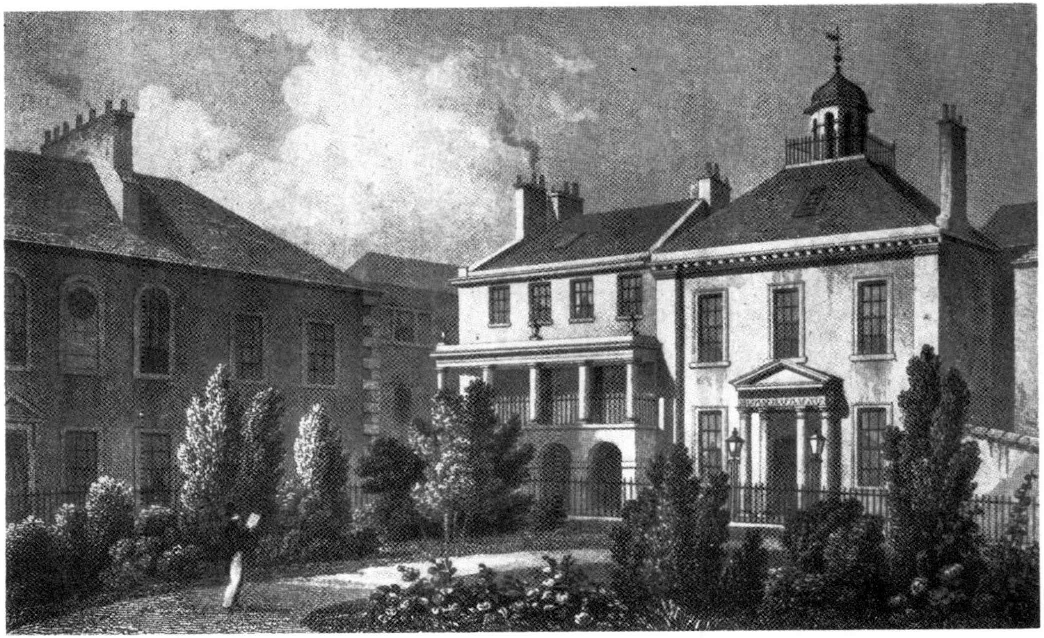

South-west corner of Surgeons' Square: on the left is Surgeons' Hall, on the right the Hall of the Royal Medical Society, and in the centre the building with the pillars contained the Lecture Room of the anatomists, Barclay and Knox: in the building between it and Surgeons' Hall is the Lecture Room of John Thomson

(From a Drawing by Shepherd, published in 1829)

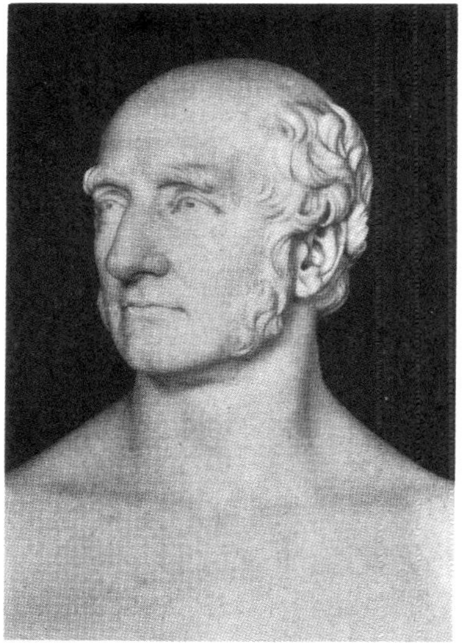

ROBERT LISTON

Surgeon to the Royal Infirmary and Professor of Clinical Surgery, University College, London

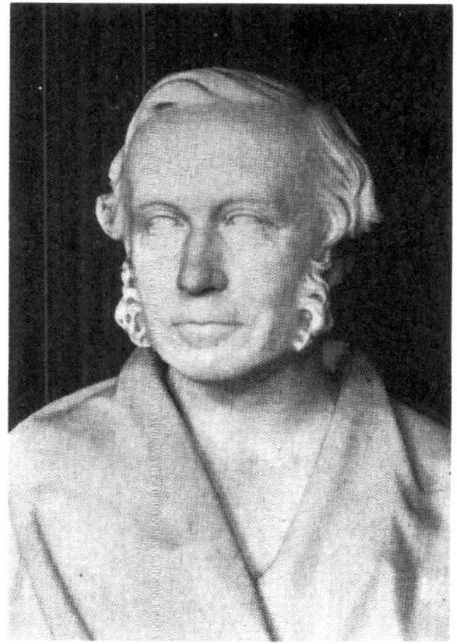

JAMES SYME

Surgeon to the Royal Infirmary and Regius Professor of Clinical Surgery, Edinburgh

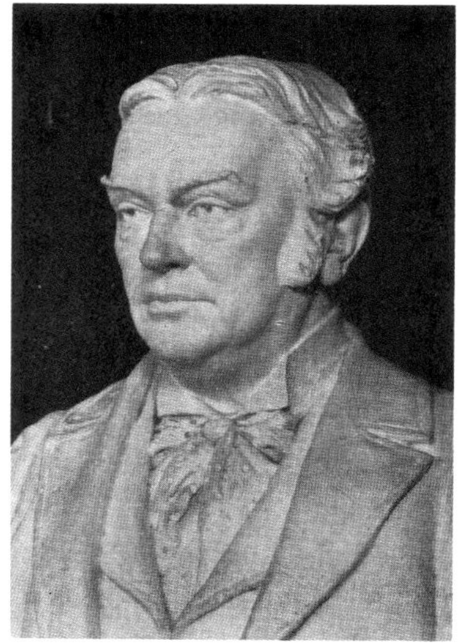

THOMAS ANNANDALE

Surgeon to the Royal Infirmary and Regius Professor of Clinical Surgery, Edinburgh

(Photographs of the Busts in the Board Room of the Royal Infirmary, by kind permission of the Managers)

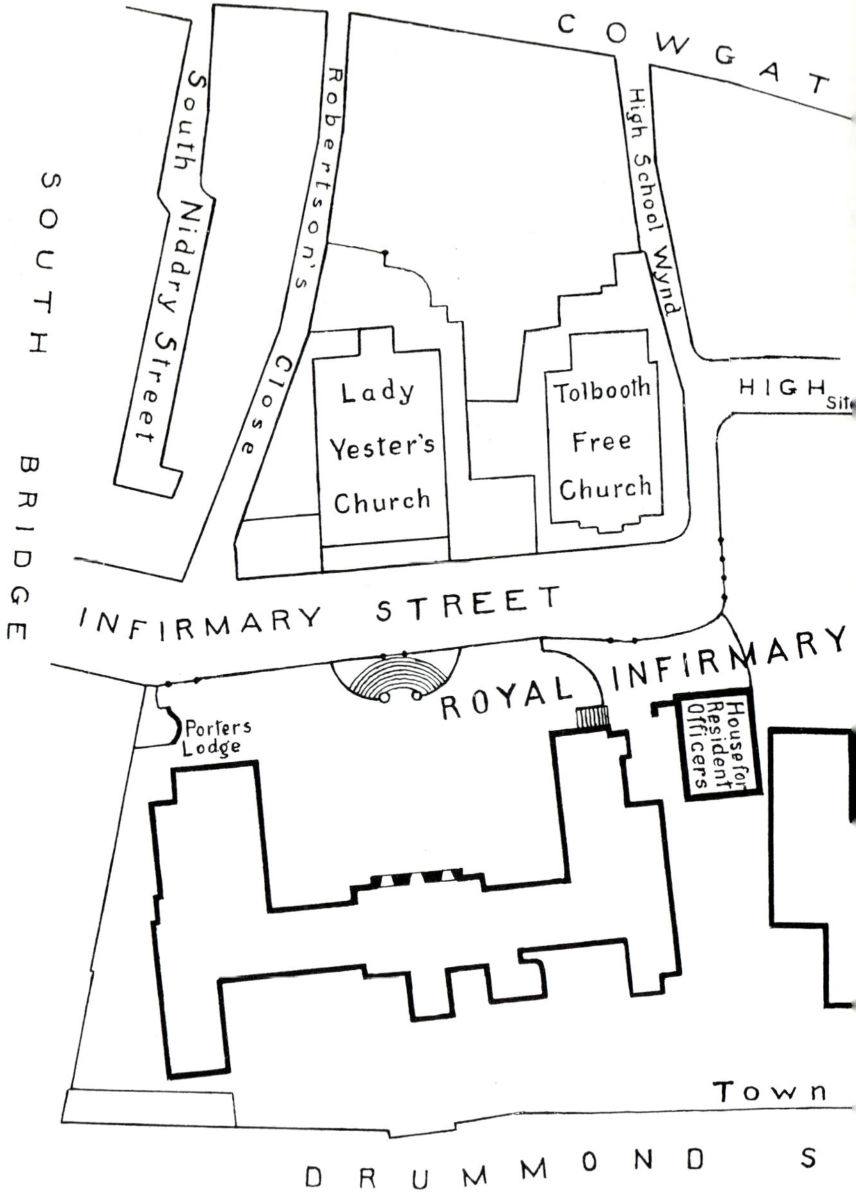

PLAN OF INFIRMARY AREA OF THE CITY IN 1853 AFT

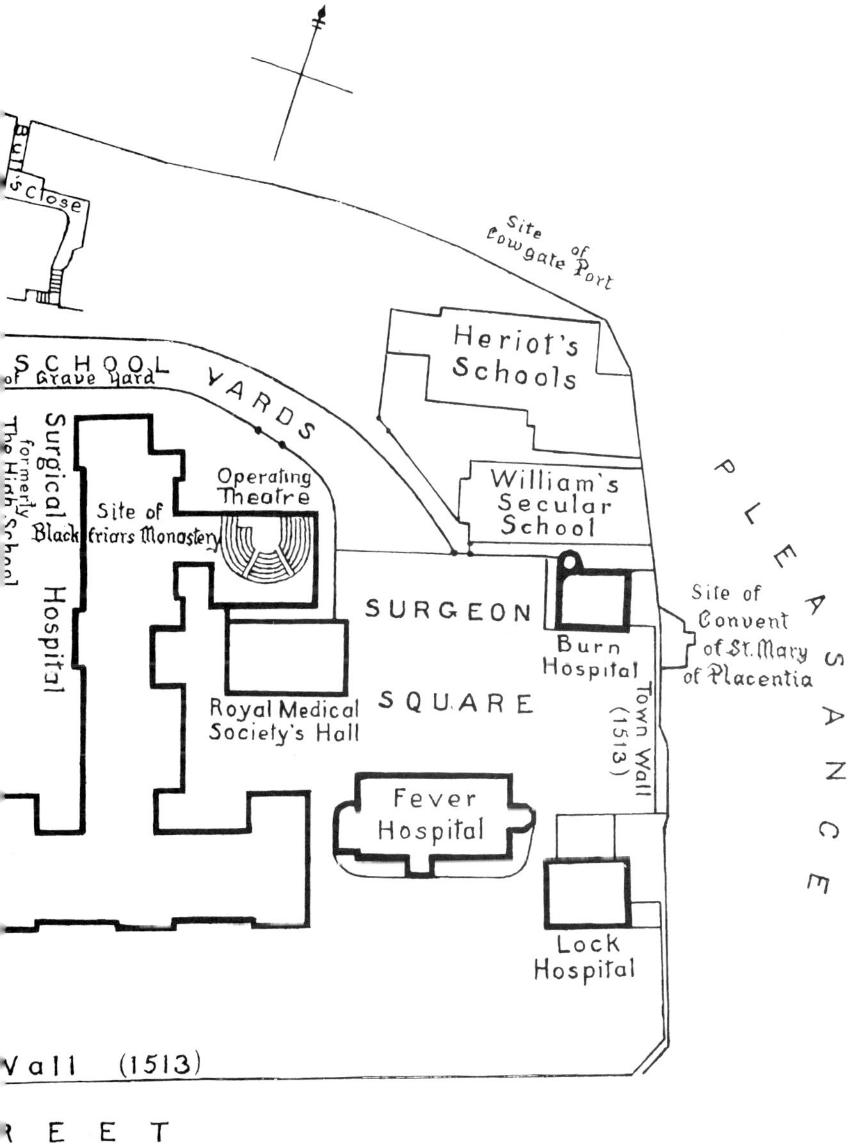

THE ERECTION OF THE NEW SURGICAL HOSPITAL

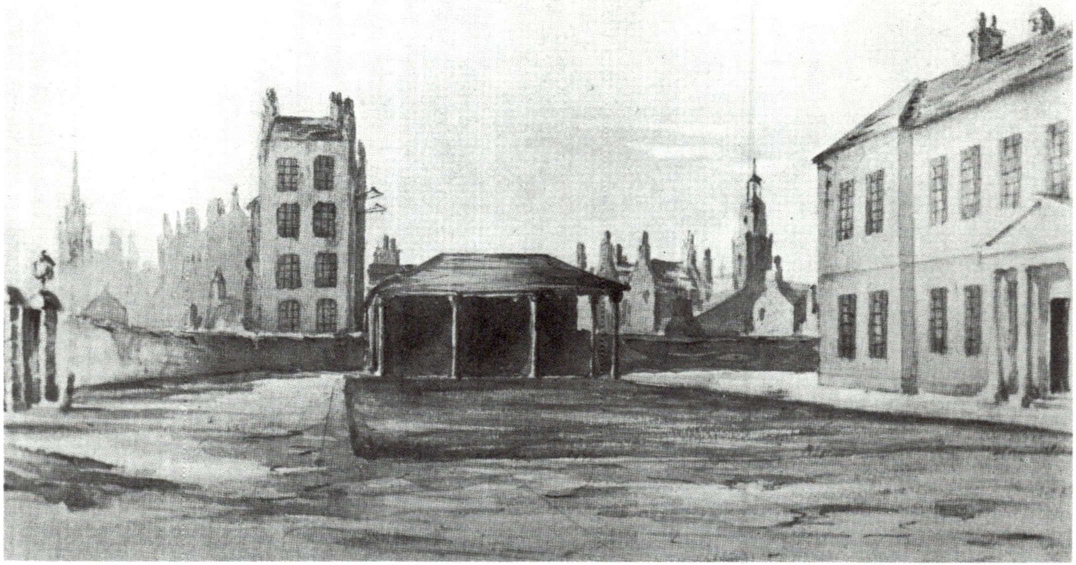

The forecourt of the Old Surgical Hospital, formerly the High School, with the carriage shelter in the centre of the picture : on the left is the spire of the Tron Church, on the right that of St Patrick's Roman Catholic Church. The tall house stands at the corner of High School Wynd and High School Yards

(*Reproduced from a water-colour sketch lent to the author by Professor Sir John Fraser,* K.C.V.O.)

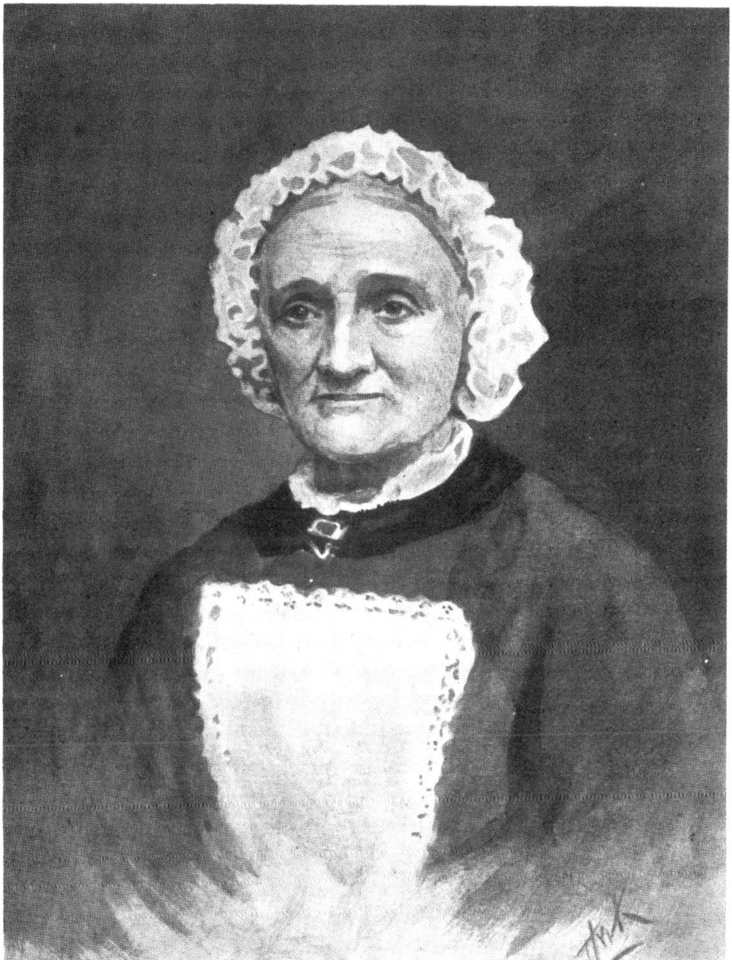

JANET PORTER

Died 10th February 1890, aged 80 years. For 47 years she gave her services as Nurse in the Royal Infirmary of Edinburgh

(From a portrait subscribed for by members of the Nursing Staff associated with her during her years of work)

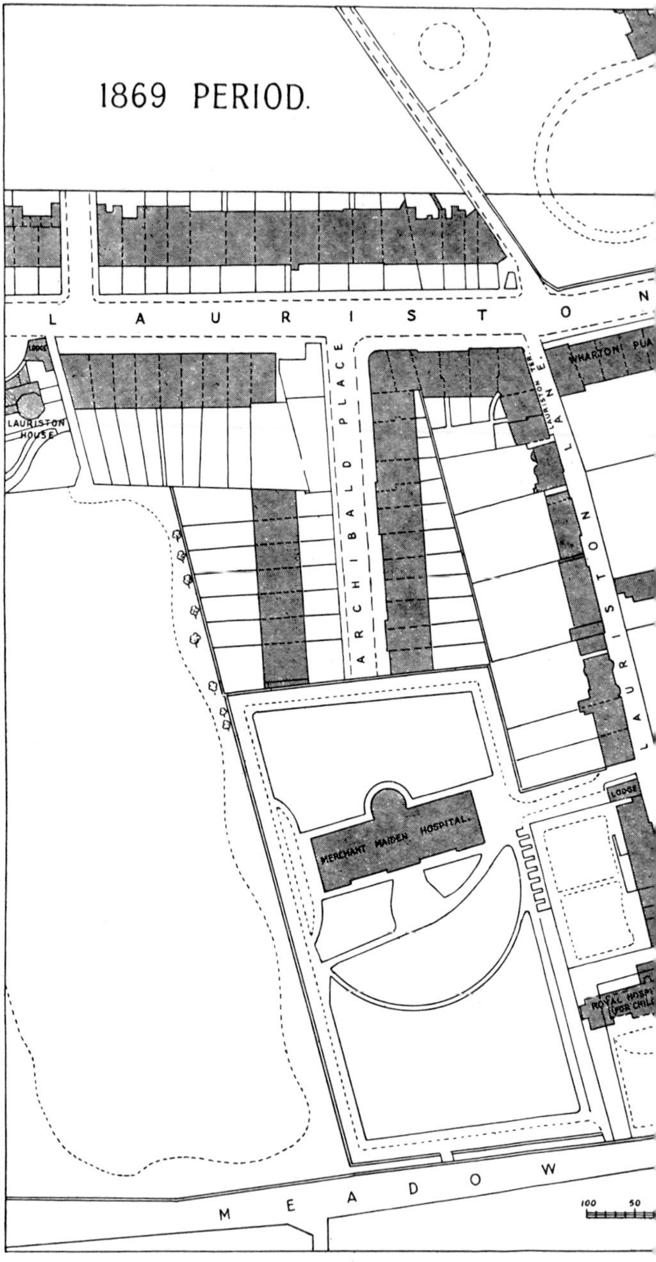

PLAN OF SITE IN LAURISTON PLACE SELECTED IN 1

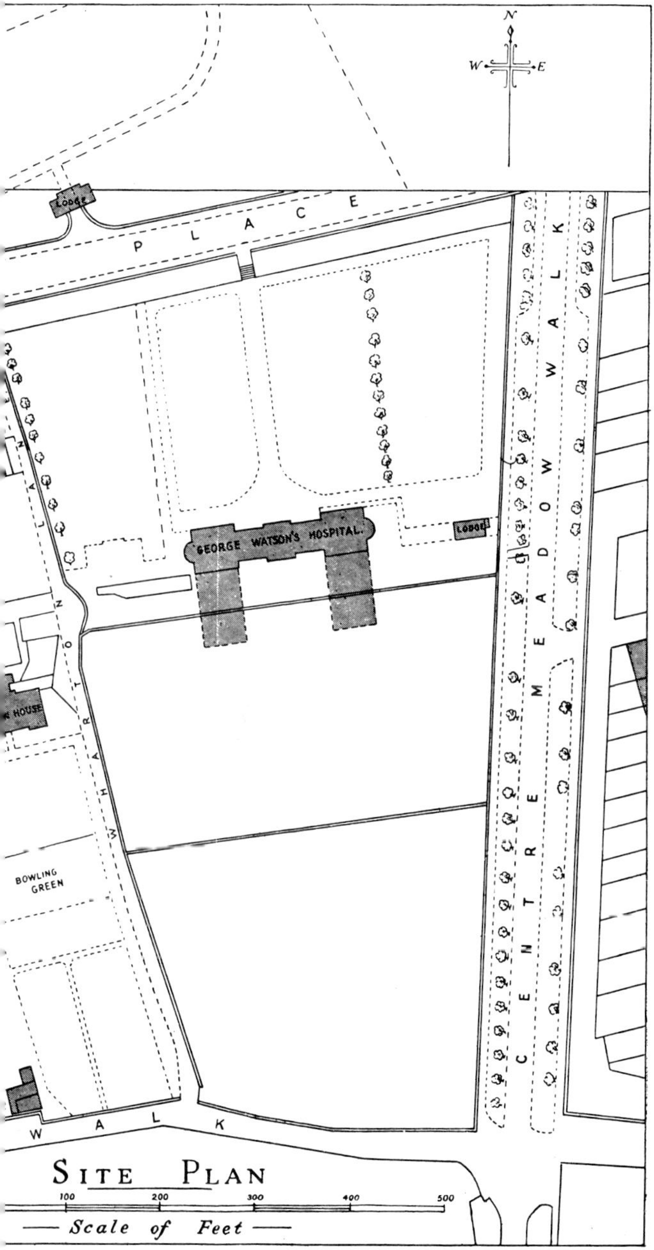

R THE ERECTION OF THE NEW ROYAL INFIRMARY

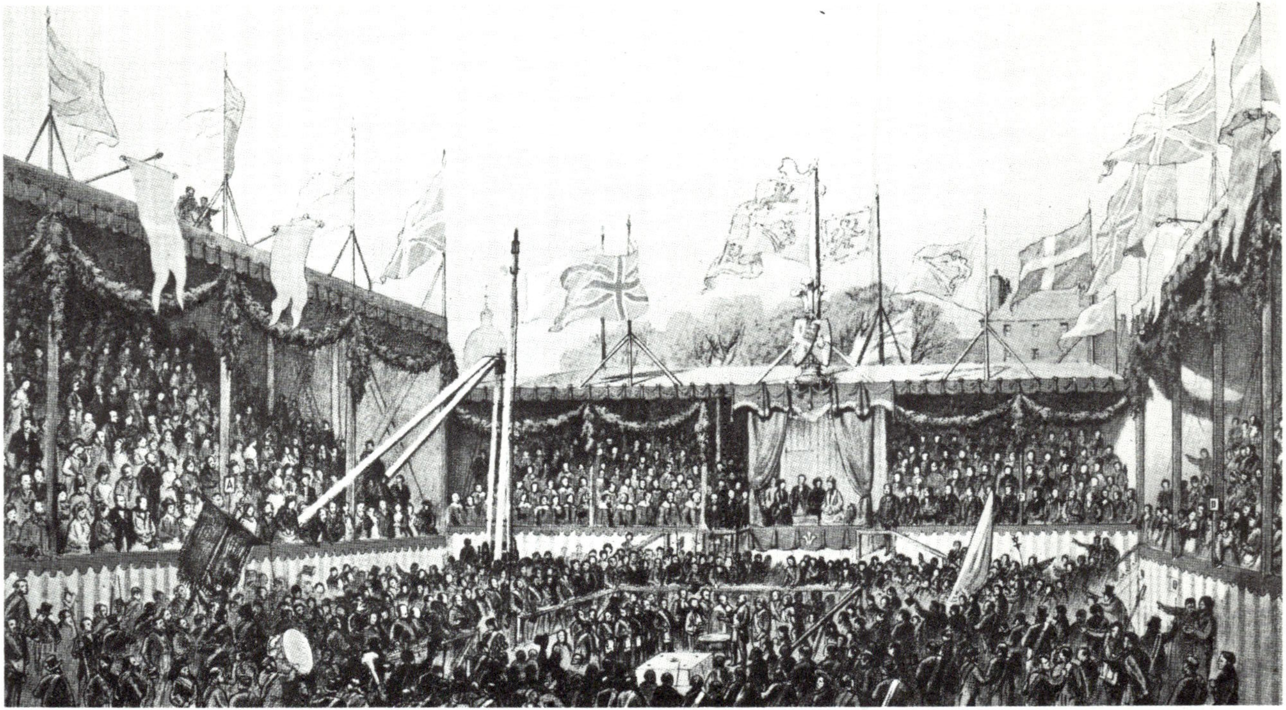

H.R.H. ALBERT EDWARD, PRINCE OF WALES

Laying the Foundation Stone of the New Royal Infirmary, 13th October 1870

(From an old coloured lithograph)

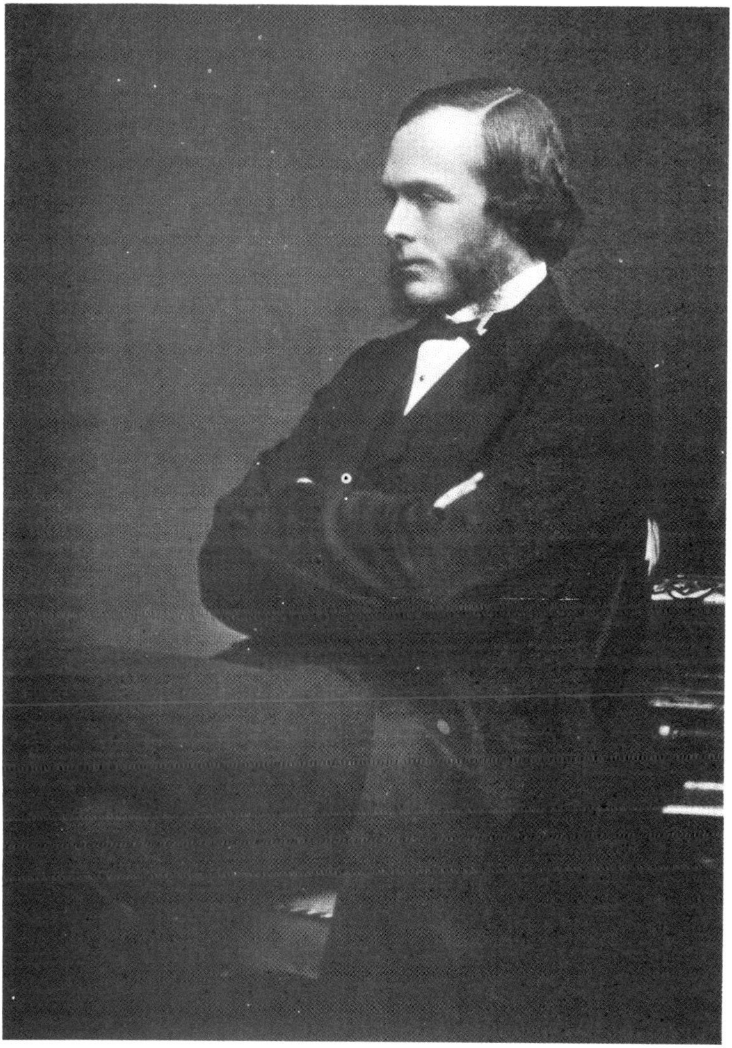

JOSEPH LISTER

Photograph taken during his first period of residence in Edinburgh, 1853-1860

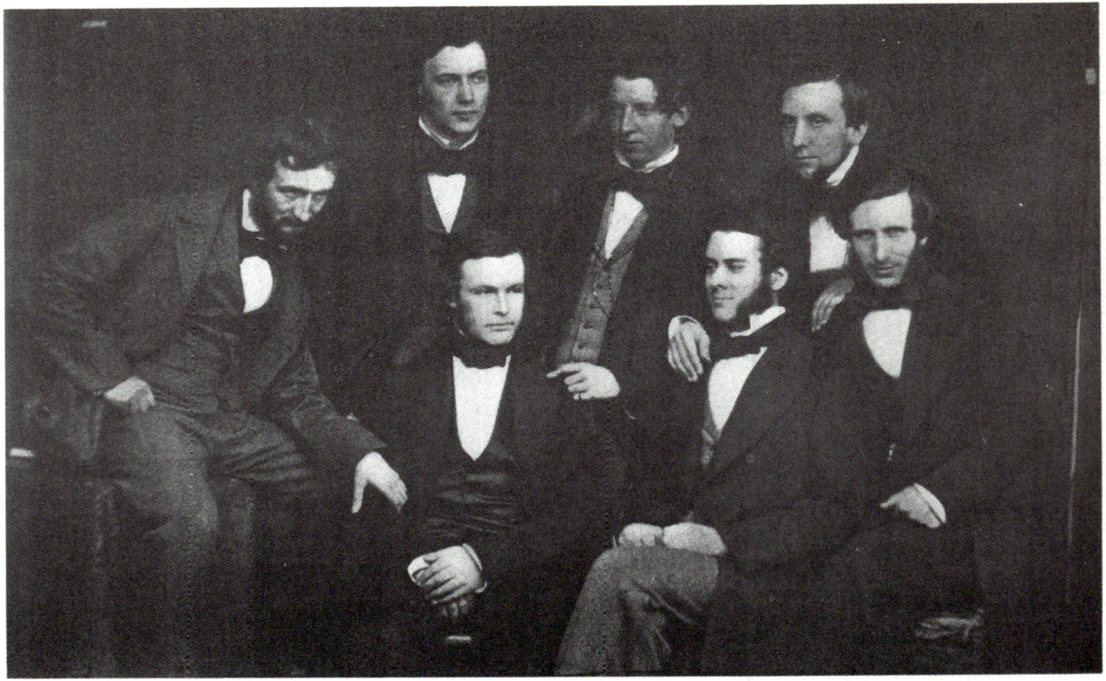

Back Row—John Kirk. George Hogarth Pringle. Patrick Heron Watson
Front Row—John Beddoe. Joseph Lister. David Christison. Alexander Struthers

JOSEPH LISTER AND HIS FELLOW-RESIDENTS, OLD ROYAL INFIRMARY, SUMMER, 1854

(*From a photograph in " The Residency," Royal Infirmary*)

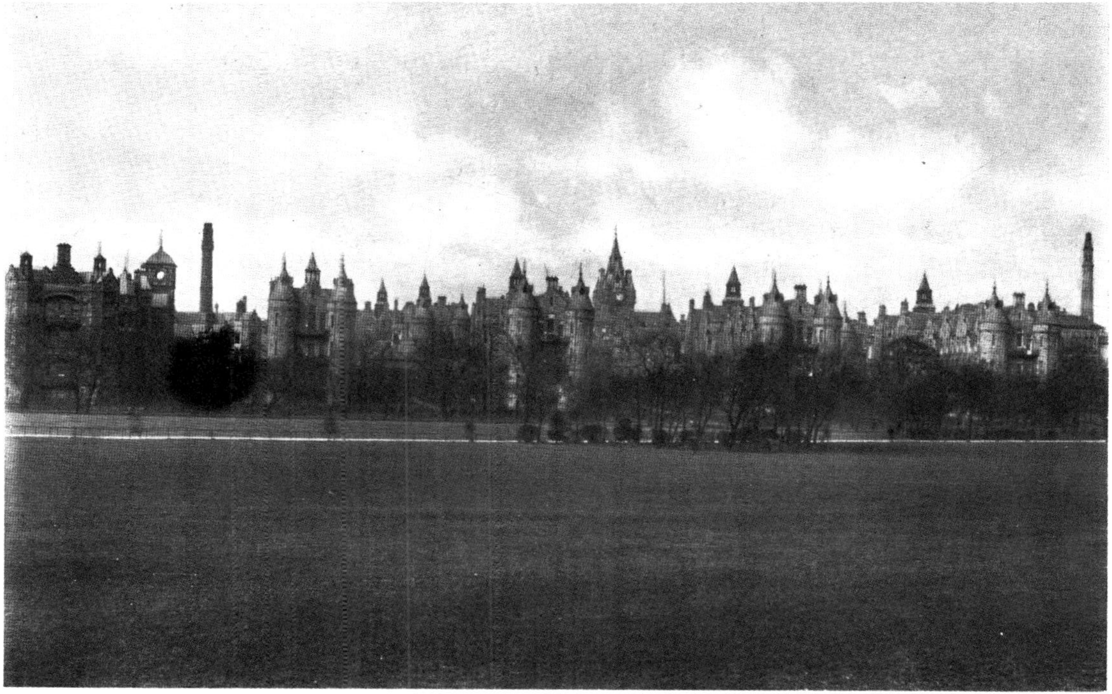

Photo by] [*William Dickson, Edinburgh*

The Medical Pavilions of the New Royal Infirmary viewed from the Meadows, that on the left being the Diamond Jubilee Pavilion. On the extreme right is the tall chimney of the University New Buildings (Medical School)

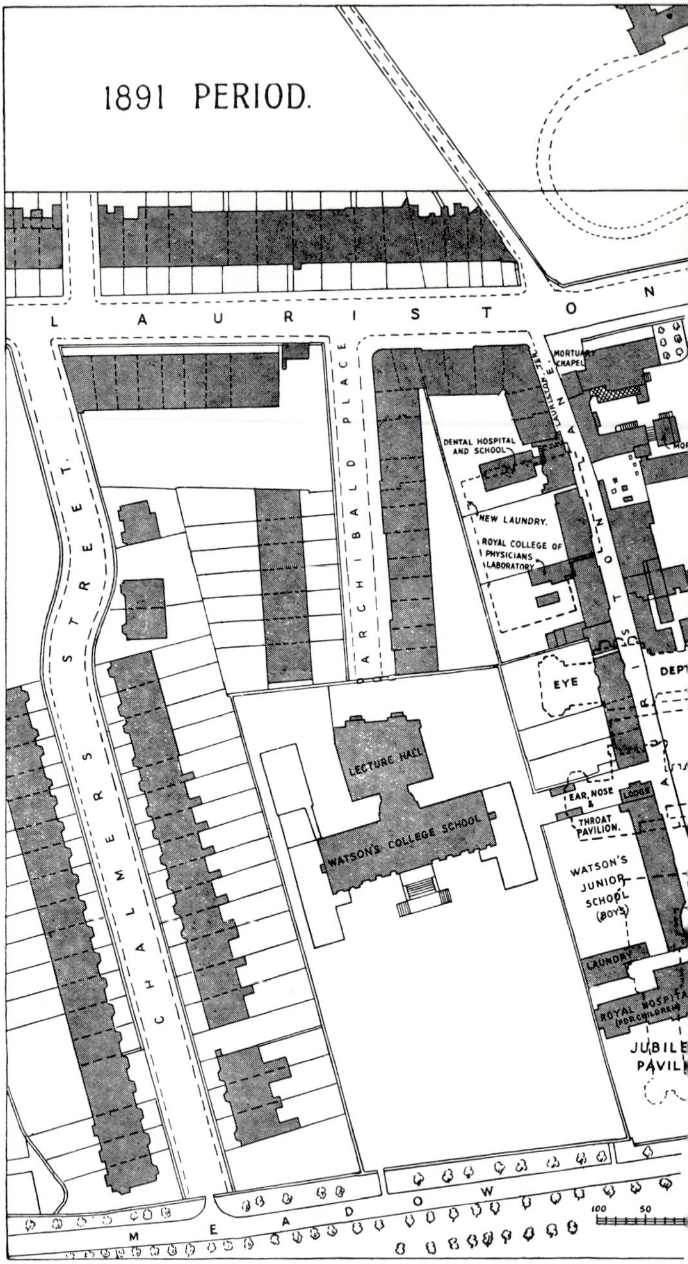

PLAN OF EXTENSIONS OF THE ROYAL

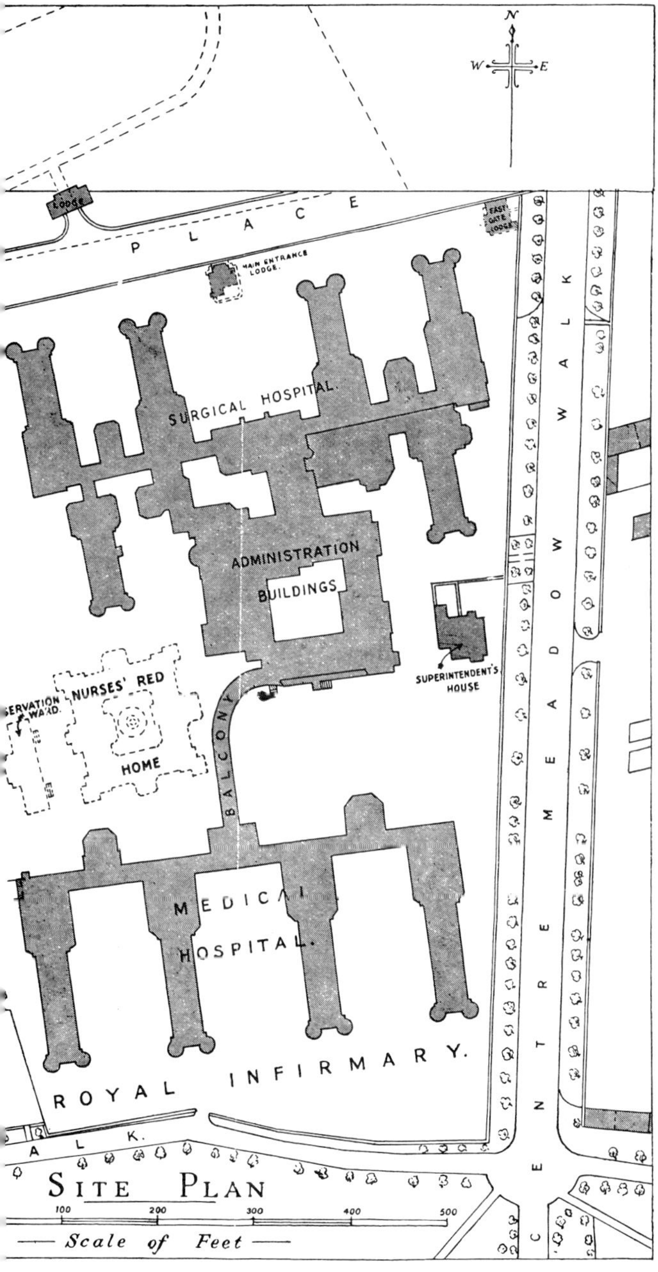

NFIRMARY DURING THE PERIOD 1891-1904

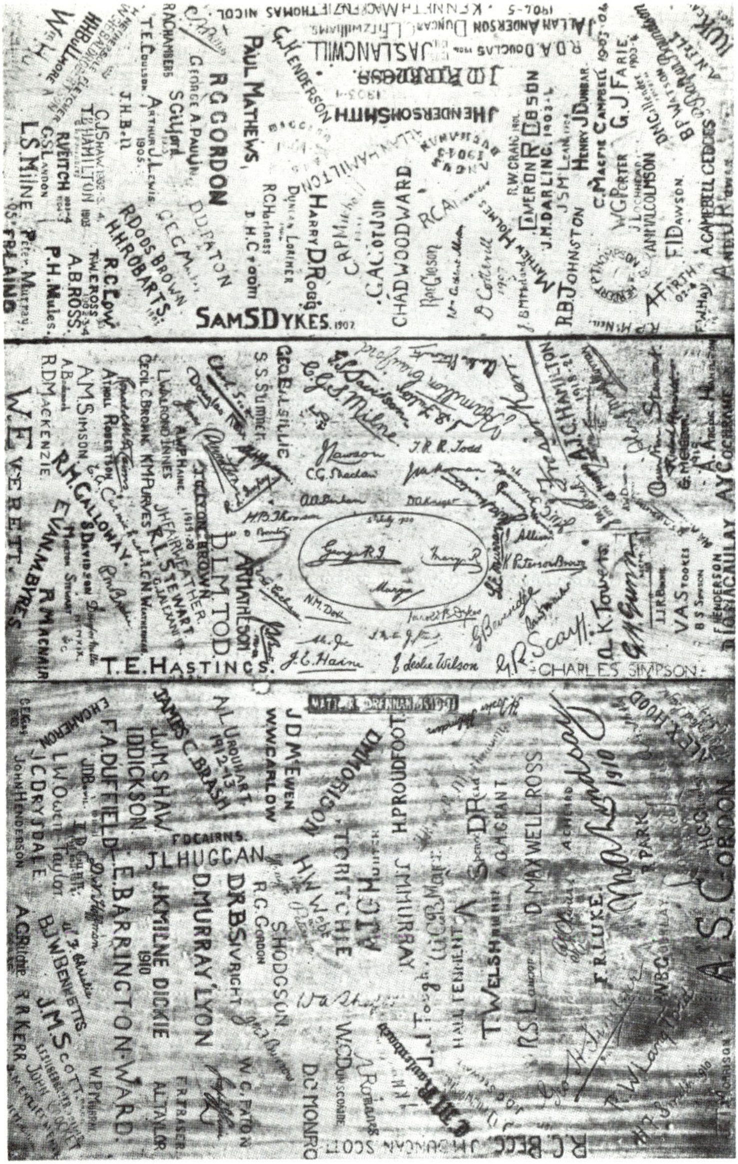

Photograph of part of the Dining-Room Table in the Residency of the Royal Infirmary on which are carved the names of past and present house physicians and house surgeons. On the centre leaf are the signatures of Their Majesties King George V. and Queen Mary and of H.R.H. Princess Mary, commemorating their visit to the hospital on 5th July 1920.

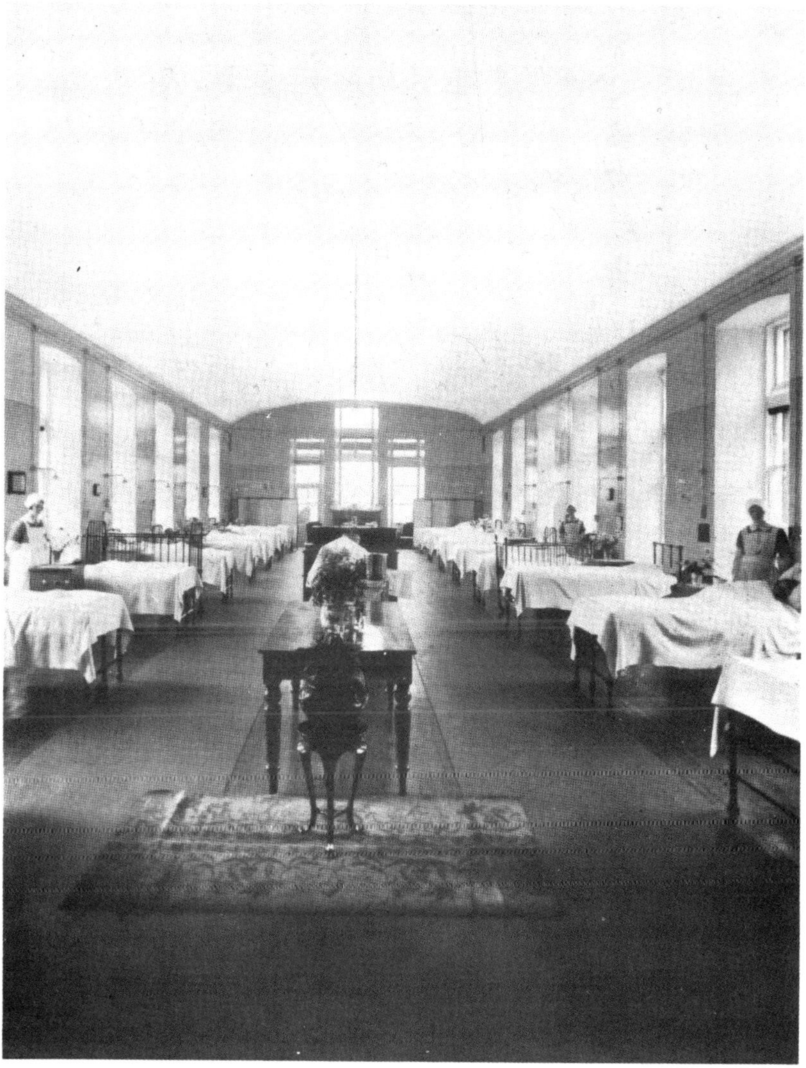

WARD IN THE MEDICAL HOUSE, ROYAL INFIRMARY

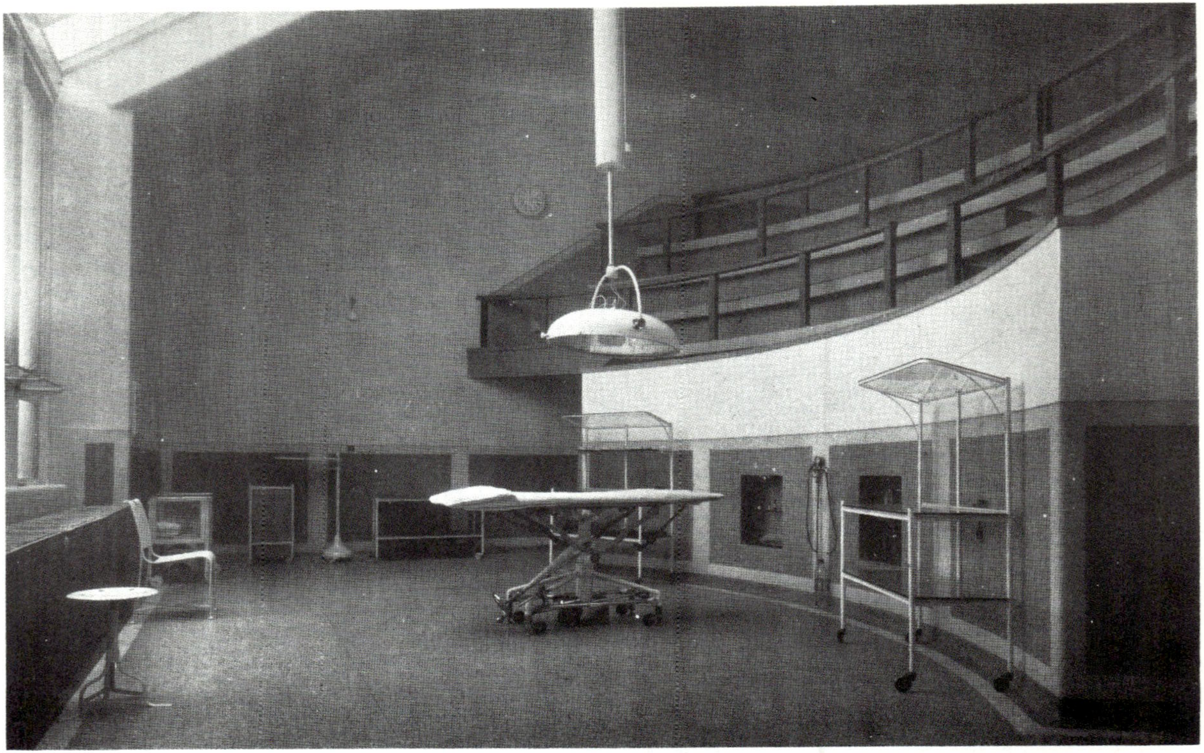

A MODERN OPERATING THEATRE IN THE ROYAL INFIRMARY

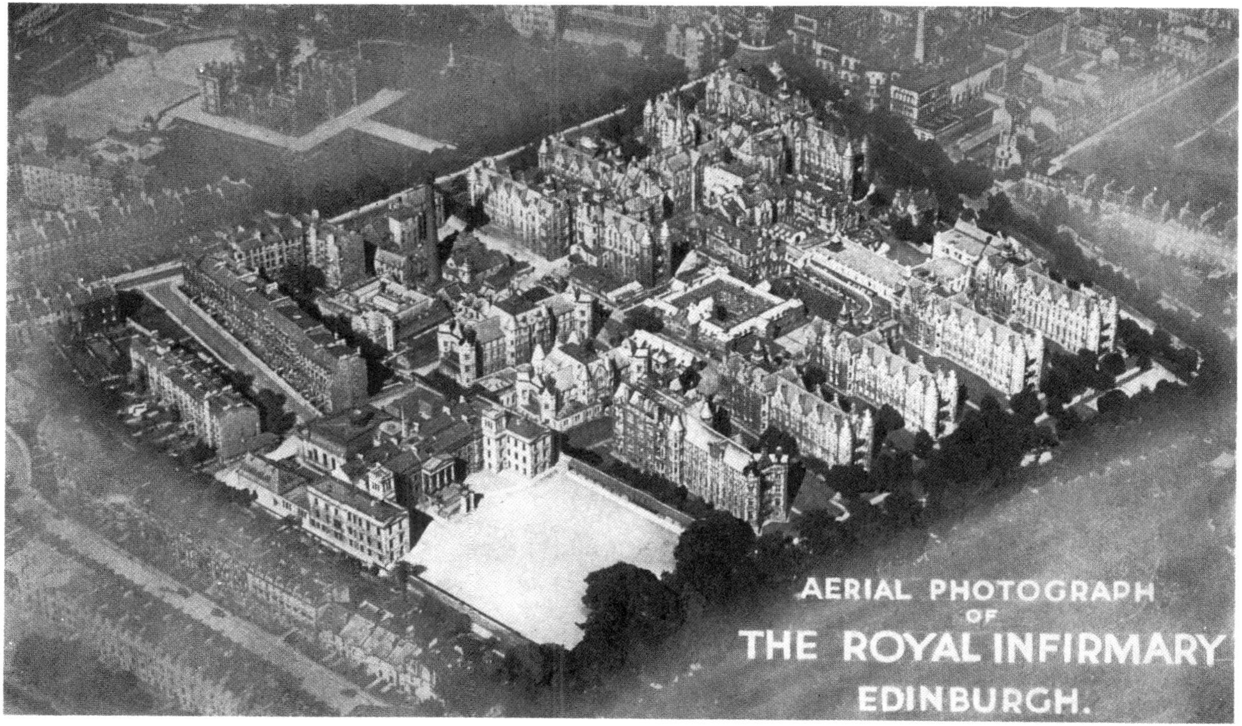

Aerial Photograph of the Royal Infirmary showing in the south-west corner George Watson's College for Boys and the playground, the site purchased for the erection of the Simpson Memorial Maternity Pavilion and the Florence Nightingale Home for Nurses

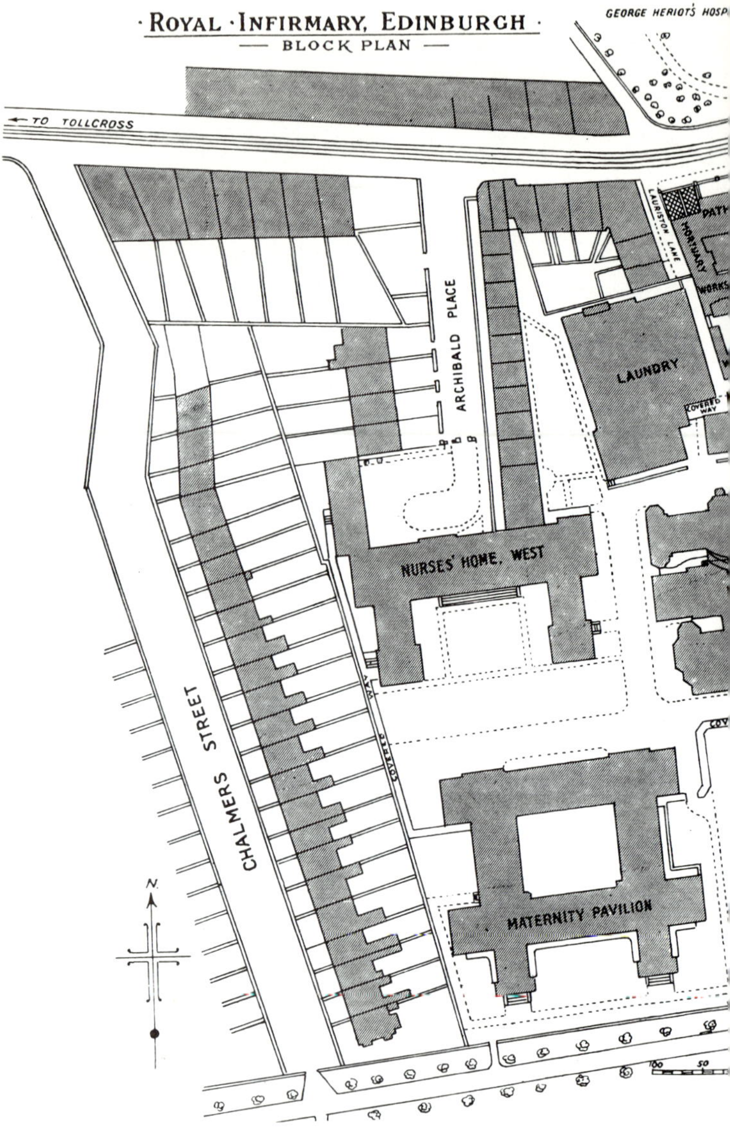

A.—Surgical Out-patient Department, and Wards 7 and 13.
A 1.—Surgical Out-patient Theatre.
B.—Wards 2, 8, 14 (Surgical), Dietetic Department.
C.—Ward (Casualty), Diagnostic Theatre, and Operating Theatre for Wards 13 and 14.
D.—Operating Theatre for Wards 7 and 8.
E.—Wards 3 (Delirium), 9 and 15 (Surgical).
F.—Administrative Offices, Wards 19 and 20.
G.—Wards 4, 10, and 16 (Surgical).
H.—Operating Theatre for Wards 9 and 10.
J.—Operating Theatres for Wards 11, 12, 17, and 18.
K.—Wards 1, 5, 11, 17. Operating Theatre, Wards 5 an
L.—Wards 6, 12, and 18 (Surgical).
M.—Chapel and Administrative Departments.

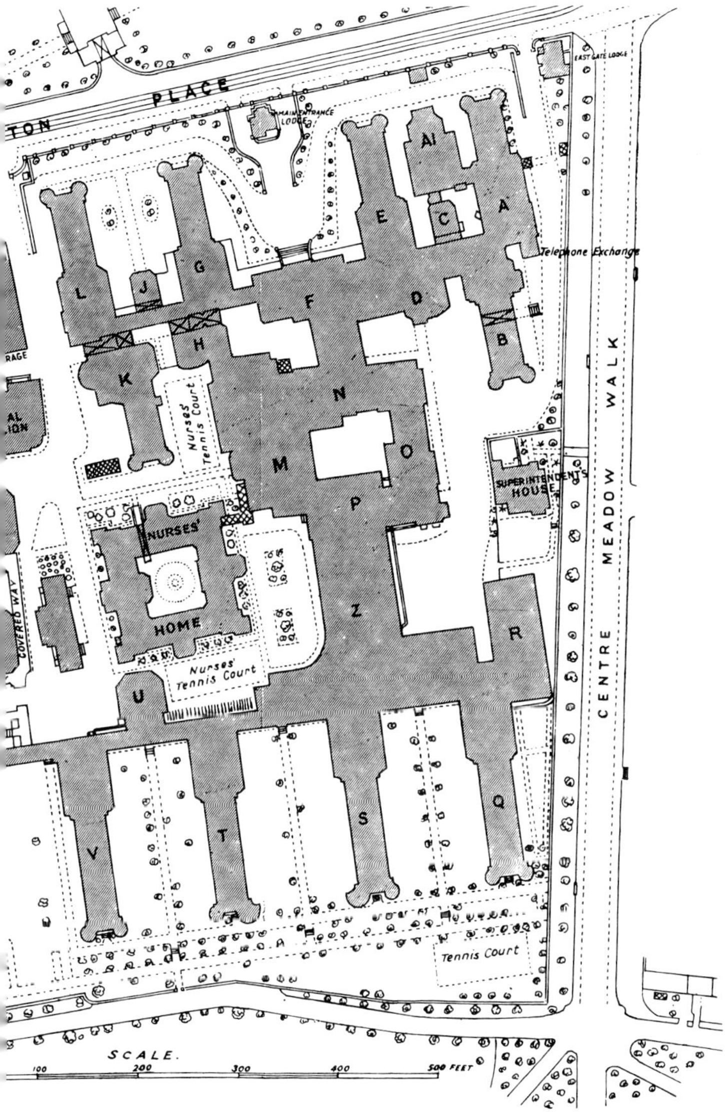

N.—Large Theatre and Administrative Departments.
O.—Medical Out-patient Department and Residency.
P.—Dispensary.
Q.—Wards 22, 23, and 24 (Medical).
R.—Clinical Medicine Laboratory, Ward 21 (Dietetic), etc.
S.—Wards 25, 26, 27 (Medical).
T.—Wards 28, 29, 30 (Medical).
U.—West Medical Lecture Theatre.
V.—Wards 31, 32, and 33 (Medical).
W.—Wards 34, 35, and 36 (Gynæcological).
X.—Ear and Throat Pavilion.
Y.—Ophthalmic Pavilion.
Z.—Radiological Department.

It soon became necessary to consider the erection of a second surgical hospital, the construction of a new kitchen, laundry and washing-house to serve the needs of the whole establishment, an extensive drainage system and much needed repairs upon the medical hospital, then more than a century old. For these and other reasons the financial situation continued to cause anxiety, as the future maintenance of a greatly enlarged Infirmary could not be viewed with equanimity. In December 1848, Syme had drawn attention to the deficiency in the surgical accommodation, so that patients requiring relief had to be rejected while convalescents were often prematurely discharged. The beds in the Surgical Hospital, therefore, had been supplemented by utilising the fever hospital—the old Surgeons' Hall—by erecting a shed in Surgeons' Square and by transferring the cases of burns from the existing surgical wards to a house on the east side of the Square, which became designated the Burn Hospital.[1] The Lock patients also were housed in the building which formerly contained John Bell's lecture room.

Plans for the New Surgical Hospital and the other extensions were prepared by Mr David Bryce, architect, and a building fund was opened: larger legacies and donations followed the announcement of the projected new hospital. The site selected was situated on vacant ground to the east of the Medical Hospital between it and Surgeons' Hall. The building was of three floors with attics: its south frontage faced Drummond Street and, on its northern aspect an extension was constructed so as to communicate with the first Surgical Hospital, the waiting rooms being placed in the portion connecting the two buildings. Accommodation was thus provided for 128 surgical beds along with additional 19 beds for patients suffering from diseases of the eye.

The hospital was opened on 30th April 1853. This permitted of a rearrangement of the whole surgical department with the assembling of the patients in two buildings structurally

[1] Burn Hospital was No. 9 Surgeons' Square and was formerly called the Cottage; it was the janitor's house in the time of the High School, and as stated on p. 187, the building is now part of the establishment of the University Settlement at High School Yards.

adapted for their care and treatment, while the various outbuildings above described were dispensed with. As ten of the beds in the old Surgical Hospital were reserved for special emergencies or as "relief" beds, when a ward or wards required to be cleaned, there remained 62 beds in daily use in the old High School building. In the New Surgical Hospital, provision having been made for 128 surgical patients, there was a total of 190 available beds in the two hospitals. The professor of clinical surgery, ranking as an acting surgeon, was given 72 beds—62 in the old Surgical Hospital and 10 in the new building: the remaining 118 in the New Surgical Hospital were allotted to the senior and junior acting surgeons-in-ordinary in the proportion of 72 to the former and 46 to the latter. The patients suffering from affections of the eye were at first placed under the care of the surgeons admitting them but, in 1855, William Walker was appointed the first ophthalmic surgeon to the Royal Infirmary. Walker became surgeon-oculist to Queen Victoria and was president of the Royal College of Surgeons of Edinburgh in 1871. He commenced a course of lectures on diseases of the eye in 1858. Thus was established the second of the special departments in the Infirmary.[1]

James Dunsmure, senior, and Richard James Mackenzie were the two acting surgeons-in-ordinary when the hospital was opened, James Spence and James Donaldson Gillespie being the assistant surgeons. Mackenzie was a surgeon of great promise but his career was unfortunately cut short by his premature death at the early age of thirty-five. Having volunteered for service in the Crimea he died of cholera in September 1854, shortly after the battle of the Alma. His place as acting surgeon was filled by the promotion of James Spence: "a tallish, slightly stooping figure with a slow semi-swinging walk, his rather pronounced features, with their thoughtfully anxious, half-sad expression, earning for him the soubriquet of 'dismal Jimmy.'" "I shall never forget," writes one of his contemporaries, "when walking on one occasion with William Walker, the ophthalmic surgeon, we

[1] Diseases peculiar to women in 1850.

met Spence with his most dismal expression, all clothed in black and crape, 'Seeing some of your work home, Jamie,' said Walker, and a grim smile illuminated his features as he shook his stick at us and passed on." As a demonstrator of anatomy with Alexander Monro, *tertius*, for seven years, and afterwards as a lecturer on anatomy at Surgeons' Square, Spence laid the foundation of a perfect knowledge of anatomy which pre-eminently distinguished his work as an operator in later years.

The projected arrangement of beds in the New Surgical Hospital was slightly modified before the house was actually ready for occupation, in consequence of a petition in 1849 from the medical faculty of the University requesting that James Miller, the professor of systematic surgery, should have beds permanently committed to his care, an application which met with considerable opposition in more than one quarter and which was refused on more than one occasion.[1] James Miller, a son of the manse and a native of Angus, had studied Arts at St Andrews and afterwards, as a medical student at Edinburgh, had been a pupil of Liston and his private assistant. Appointed assistant surgeon to the Infirmary in 1840, he was promoted acting surgeon in 1842 and, in the same year, succeeded Sir Charles Bell as professor of surgery. Handsome in appearance, a fluent and eloquent speaker, he was a popular and attractive lecturer and as a hospital surgeon a bold and dexterous operator. Having completed his period of five years as surgeon and having thrice been given an extension of one year, the managers then resolved that in justice to the other surgeons on the staff no further extension could be allowed: they accordingly elected him consulting surgeon. In the autumn of 1852, James Miller renewed his application for beds on the ground that it was necessary for the efficient discharge of his duties as a teacher that he should have patients in the hospital, whereby he might quote to his pupils examples of surgical diseases. He made no claim to act as a clinical teacher in the hospital or to interfere with the

[1] Minutes, Royal Infirmary, 31st December 1849, 14th October 1850 and 20th September 1852.

duties of his colleague, the professor of clinical surgery. After considerable discussion the Board of Management finally resolved by a majority to grant the request, allotting to the professor of surgery three wards or eighteen beds in the New Surgical Hospital, twelve being deducted from the charge of his professorial colleague and six from the senior acting surgeon-in-ordinary.

This action of the Board of Management was adversely criticised by some of the Fellows of the Royal College of Surgeons and, at a subsequent meeting of the College, it was decided by a majority of those voting to memorialise the managers of the Infirmary.[1] In their memorial attention was drawn to the fact that the three wards allotted to James Miller would no longer be available for clinical teaching and that the permanent establishment in the hospital of the two professors of surgery would tend to injure the interests of the extra-academical school. But the managers, conscious that there was nothing in the old agreement of 1738 between the Infirmary and the Incorporation of Surgeons to prevent their making any reasonable change which they deemed advisable, considered that it was within their power to appoint the professor of systematic surgery to the charge of a small number of beds. No further action was taken and the professors of systematic surgery continue to enjoy the privilege of the charge of wards during the whole tenure of their professorship. Many years later, in 1905, the University Court on the recommendation of the faculty of medicine and the Senatus appointed the professor of systematic surgery as a lecturer in clinical surgery, thus enabling him to give a separate course of clinical lectures in the Infirmary qualifying for graduation. The managers gave their approval to this step.[2] In 1854 the period of office of the acting surgeons-in-ordinary was extended from five to eight years, and subsequently in 1860 to ten years.

A few years prior to the opening of the New Surgical Hospital two events occurred almost simultaneously, neither of which can be omitted from the history of the Infirmary.

[1] Minute, Royal Infirmary, 11th July 1853. [2] *Ibid.*, 4th September 1905.

After Liston's death in London in 1847, Syme was offered the vacant chair of clinical surgery at University College. It was a great honour and the position presented many attractions, but it was not without a struggle that Syme with his unrivalled position as a surgeon in Scotland finally accepted the offer. He left Edinburgh on 13th February 1848, only to return, however, five months later. Although warmly welcomed by his colleagues and students in London he found that, in addition to his duties in the chair of clinical surgery, those of the chair of systematic surgery were also to be imposed upon him. Consequently he tendered his resignation, returned to Edinburgh on 3rd July and was reappointed to the chair of clinical surgery. In a letter, dated 6th July, to the Managers of the Infirmary he wrote, " If reinstated in the Royal Infirmary it will be my earnest and increasing endeavour to prove deserving of your confidence." As the arrangements made in the hospital after his retirement had been merely of a temporary character his request was immediately granted and he was reappointed surgeon to the Infirmary.

The other event exercised a much wider influence on the future course of the practice of surgery involving, as it did, the introduction of the use of chloroform as a general anæsthetic. In the first half of the nineteenth century surgeons were giving considerable thought to the problem of relieving or preventing pain during operations. The effect produced on the mind of the youthful onlooker at some of these grim scenes may be gauged by quoting the impression left on Charles Darwin while a student of medicine at Edinburgh in 1828. In his autobiography he relates how he " attended on two occasions the operating theatre in the hospital at Edinburgh and saw two very bad operations, one on a child, but I rushed away before they were completed. Nor did I ever attend again for hardly any inducement could have been strong enough to make me do so ; this being long before the blessed days of chloroform. The two cases fairly haunted me for many a long year." In 1798 Sir Humphry Davy experimented upon himself with nitrous oxide, " the laughing gas," and believed that it might be used to deaden pain in surgical operations. In 1828, Henry Hickman a young practitioner in Ludlow successfully anæsthetised animals with the same gas, but his work being disregarded no further advance was made, until in America in 1844 Horace Wells employed nitrous oxide in dental surgery. In 1842, Crawford W. Long and Charles T. Jackson independently recognised the anæsthetic property of the vapour of sulphuric ether and, in 1846, William T. Morton of Boston extracted teeth painlessly under its influence. Early in the century chloroform as a chemical compound had been discovered by several observers and in 1847 Flourens, the French physiologist, demonstrated in his experiments on animals that it could induce general anæsthesia by inhalation. In the same year, James Young Simpson, in his endeavour to find a drug free from some of the inconveniences and objections pertaining to ether, which he had been using following Morton's success, experimented on himself in his house, 52 Queen Street, with the vapour of chloroform along with his assistants, James Matthews Duncan and George Keith.

Satisfied that in chloroform he had obtained a drug which would serve his purpose in maternity practice, Simpson administered chloroform on a pocket-handkerchief to the first patient anæsthetised with the vapour in the Royal Infirmary, with James Miller as the operator. Amongst those in the crowded theatre on that memorable occasion was Professor Dumas of Paris, one of the French chemists who had established the chemical composition of the drug. The patient, a boy about five years of age, after a few inspirations ceased to cry or struggle and passed into a sound sleep. The shaft of one of the bones of the forearm—the necrosed radius—was removed through a long incision without the slightest evidence that pain had been inflicted. The child was then removed to the ward, sleeping quietly and, half an hour afterwards, he awoke " with a clear merry eye and placid expression of countenance wholly unlike what is found to obtain after ordinary etherisation." The boy, who could speak only the Gaelic, on being questioned by a Gaelic interpreter found amongst the students, stated that he had felt no pain nor was he conscious of any on awaking.[1] Robert Liston, who had performed the first painless operation in England under ether anæsthesia, thus wrote to James Miller in November 1847, "The chloroform is a vast advance upon ether. I have tried it with perfect success. . . ."

[1] *Memoir of Sir James Y. Simpson, Bart.*, by J. Duns, D.D. Edinburgh: Edmonston & Douglas, 1873.

CHAPTER XII

CHANGES IN THE SYSTEM OF ADMINISTRATION

COMMITTEE OF ENQUIRY INTO ALLEGED MISMANAGEMENT, 1818—ESTABLISHMENT OF STANDING COMMITTEES OF THE BOARD, 1823—DEVELOPMENT OF THE ADMINISTRATIVE SYSTEM, 1837-1871—APPOINTMENT OF THE SUPERINTENDENT, 1871—THE OLD AND THE NEW SYSTEMS OF NURSING—EDINBURGH ROYAL INFIRMARY ACT, 1870—CHANGES IN THE CONSTITUTION OF THE COURT OF CONTRIBUTORS AND BOARD OF MANAGEMENT.

THROUGHOUT the greater part of the period covered by the events narrated in the two previous chapters, embracing more than the first half of the nineteenth century, questions relative to the internal management of the Infirmary and to its general administration came from time to time under consideration. There were several reasons why these matters had assumed greater prominence. The recurring epidemics of fever commencing in 1817, with the provision of temporary arrangements necessary to cope with the large increase in the number of patients, had dislocated the normal life of the hospital, and the continued acquisition of more property, with the expansion of the work of the Infirmary in more than one direction, had undoubtedly added to the labours and the responsibilities of its permanent officials. Since its opening, nearly a century earlier, no additional assistance had been given either to the Treasurer or to the Clerk to the Corporation, neither of whom gave whole-time service to the Institution. It was also becoming increasingly evident that someone having authority should reside in the house so as to exercise a general superintendence and be responsible to the managers for its good order.

The desirability of appointing a resident official was brought somewhat prominently to the notice of the managers in consequence of a series of complaints as to alleged abuses and irregularities—for example, the lack of cleanliness of the beds and bedding, the poor quality of some of the food supplied to the patients, defective ventilation in the wards and the need of nurses with a higher standard of qualification. A committee of the Board elicited the fact that there was a substratum of truth in some of these allegations, especially in regard to the bedding, and orders were at once given for the erection of a washing and drying house to which all linen and blankets should be frequently sent. Other defects were also rectified and the question of the appointment of a House Governor was considered, the committee of enquiry being of the opinion that a medical man, preferably one who had had experience in a military or naval hospital, should be chosen for such a post.[1] Unfortunately, in one sense, considerable publicity had been given in the Press to these complaints [2] and, at the annual meeting of the Court of Contributors held in January 1818, one of the members of the Court stated at great length the alleged abuses existing in the management of the Infirmary and moved the appointment of a committee of enquiry. Although the managers considered that the motion exceeded the powers vested in the Court, they willingly accepted the proposal: a strong committee was formed and an exhaustive enquiry was instituted. At the adjourned meeting of the Court in March it was reported that, as the result of careful scrutiny, no abuse in the management had been discovered and "that such instances of inattention as had accidentally crept in had been discovered by the managers themselves before the committee of the Court had been appointed or the enquiry thought of: that the managers be thanked for their uniform and zealous attention to the interests of the charity and that the fullest confidence be placed in their desire to rectify any occasional defects that might from time to time arise." A motion on these lines was proposed and seconded but, as some objection was raised, a vote was demanded and the roll called. The resolution was then carried by a majority of 143 votes, 175 voting in its favour and 32 against the motion.

[1] Minute, Royal Infirmary, 4th August 1817.
[2] *The Scotsman*, 20th September 1817.

Following upon these incidents, improvements were introduced designed not only to facilitate the discharge of the routine administration of the hospital but also to strengthen the supervision of its internal management. One of the earliest was the establishment of Standing Committees of the Board. Hitherto, when any particular line of enquiry was deemed necessary, a committee was temporarily constituted to make the desired investigation and in due course to report to the Board of Management. But the managers decided that it would be a distinct advantage if regular standing committees were elected to which any questions relative to particular aspects of the affairs of the hospital might be referred, each committee submitting the result of its enquiry to the General Meeting of Managers.[1] As the result of this decision the following five committees were elected, their special duties being sufficiently indicated by their titles :—The Medical Managers' Committee, the Finance, the Building, the House, and Law Committees. The Nursing Committee, which today is an important standing committee, was appointed at a later date when the Nursing Department was established. The Building Committee, which for obvious reasons at that period was one of the original standing committees, was in after years reconstituted from time to time as the occasion demanded.

In the light of the comparatively recent election of a permanent chairman of the Board of Management, it is not without interest to note that the expediency of making such an appointment had first engaged the attention of the managers as far back as 1843. The Lord Provost was *ex officio* chairman of the Board, but in his unavoidable absence it was customary to call to the chair the senior manager on the monthly list of those visiting the hospital. Although no action was taken the opinion was expressed that, if one member was made chairman for the year, he would be of considerable assistance to the Clerk to the Corporation in adjusting the minutes and in preparing the important business which came before the Board.

At the meeting of the Board of Management on 6th October 1930, the question of the appointment of an official who would

[1] Minute, Royal Infirmary, 3rd March 1823.

be in close touch with the work of all the committees and in a position to coordinate the many activities of the hospital was again raised. As there was nothing in the Royal Charter or in any subsequent Act of Parliament to prevent such an appointment being made Sir Thomas B. Whitson, then the Lord Provost, moved, "That the managers appoint one of their number to be Chairman of the Board of Managers at the first meeting of the Board following the Annual Meeting of the Court of Contributors each year ; such Chairman to be an *ex-officio* member of all Committees, but not to be eligible for re-election as Chairman for more than three years in succession." The resolution having been carried without dissent the Lord Provost then moved the election of Harriet, Lady Findlay, D.B.E., to the office of Chairman of the Board, and the motion, duly seconded, was unanimously adopted and Lady Findlay became the first permanent chairman. When, at the end of 1932 she left the Board, Sir Thomas Whitson was elected chairman, and the rule limiting the appointment to the period of three years being repealed in January 1936, he was again elected for a fourth and a fifth year.

Although as early as 1817 opinion was strongly in favour of introducing a resident-superintendent with a general control over the internal economy of the house, it is difficult to understand why this appointment was not made till twenty years later. The managers, "deeply sensible that the prosperity of the Institution depends upon the regularity of the internal management, cleanliness and comfort of the patients, are of the opinion that that can only be effected by the appointment of a respectable and intelligent medical man to reside in the house, to be in charge of the apothecary's department and to have a general superintendence of the house." [1] Nevertheless, no active step was taken till 1837 when the office of House Governor and Chief Apothecary was advertised : "he must reside in the hospital, be unmarried, and not under 40 years of age. A medical gentleman who has served in the Navy or Army would be preferred." The final decision fell upon John Brown, M.D., with previous service in the Navy, and his

[1] Minute, Royal Infirmary, 4th August 1817.

salary was fixed at £120 per annum. His duties included the maintenance of discipline over the resident clerks attached to the physicians and surgeons and over the domestic staff, but he had no concern with the professional treatment of the patients. Before the expiry of twelve months John Brown fell a victim to typhus fever; the dual office was then discontinued and replaced by a new combination, that of Superintendent and Pathologist.[1] With the resignation of the second holder of this conjoint office, after five years' trial, it was discontinued. A really satisfactory solution of the problem of superintendent had not yet been reached and, in 1843, a non-resident House Clerk or Steward was appointed temporarily and made responsible for the stores and their distribution throughout the Infirmary. The post was a forecast of the present day Steward and is of further interest from the fact that Mr Peter Bell was selected to fill it, in which office he commenced his long and faithful service to the Infirmary throughout a period of forty years.[2]

The simultaneous resignation of the Treasurer and of the Clerk to the Incorporation, tendered in a conjoint-letter to the managers in October 1843, prepared the way for a further rearrangement of posts, both these officials being desirous of giving the Board this opportunity. They had found that the increasing expansion of the business of the Infirmary interfered with their own professional engagements, making it impossible for them to give the necessary time and application to their several duties. The resignations were accepted and both men were elected members of the Board of Management, Maxwell Inglis, the ex-Treasurer, being chosen by the Board from amongst the Contributors and James Hope, Writer to the Signet, the former Clerk, from the Society of Writers to the Signet.

Mr James Hope, D.K.S., born on 28th May 1803, the third son of the Right Hon. Charles Hope of Granton, Lord President of the Court of Session, was connected with the Royal Infirmary in more than one capacity—as Clerk to the Corporation from 1836 to 1843, as a manager for a number

[1] Chapter x, p. 170. [2] Minute, Royal Infirmary, 23rd January 1843.

of years and, finally, as Law Agent from 1873 to his death in February 1882. He took the deepest interest in its affairs and his sound common sense and wide professional experience, combined with his unvarying courtesy and zeal in the cause of charity, made him a valuable coadjutor in the management of the hospital. The present firm of Hope, Todd and Kirk, Writers to the Signet, of which he was the founder, has been associated with the legal business of the Infirmary for one hundred years. Following upon the death of James Hope the office of Law Agent remained in the hands of the Firm, passing later to the care of James Hope's grandson, James Arthur Hope, W.S., who held it from 1915 till his death in March 1925, when the present holder of the office, Mr Arthur H. C. Hope, W.S., the great grandson of Charles Hope of Granton, succeeded to his father. James Hope had the unique experience of being elected Joint Deputy Keeper of the Signet in 1828, at the early age of twenty-five, and became sole Deputy Keeper in 1850. The Right Hon. Charles Hope was a manager of the Infirmary for nearly half a century, resigning in 1842, the year prior to the election of his son James as a manager.

The two new appointments made in January 1844 implied whole-time service as essential if the work was to be satisfactorily conducted. Mr James Farnie was elected Treasurer, under the new title Treasurer-Superintendent, with a salary of £220 and was required to live in the hospital ; and, in addition to the duties previously delegated to the office of Treasurer, he exercised a general control over all the inmates and was responsible for the supplies and economy of the house. Mr Peter Bell was promoted from Steward to the position of Clerk to the Corporation, commencing with a salary of £100. His duties were also whole-time but he did not require to live in the hospital. On the death of James Farnie in 1846, Mr Alexander McDougall who had been apothecary for seven years filled the vacancy.

The double office of Treasurer-Superintendent was maintained for twenty-eight years, when once again the old idea of placing a medical man in the position of Superintendent was revived by a committee of the Board appointed in the spring of 1871 to enquire into the expenditure of the Infirmary. The work of the dual office was proving too great a strain upon one man. Moreover, the Treasurer, if freed from the burden of superintending, would be able to devote his time more thoroughly to the finances of the hospital and stimulate the work of collecting in town and country, while the internal economy and discipline would be better maintained by the type of man who combined a wise blend of firmness and tact with the power of control. The whole-time appointment of Superintendent was advertised in the autumn of 1871. The salary offered was £420 with an additional £80 till the house of residence in the grounds of the new Infirmary, then under construction, should be ready. One hundred and forty-six applications were received : a short leet of seven names was selected, three of them being proposed and seconded at the meeting of the managers. The final vote resulted in the election of Deputy Surgeon-General Charles Hamilton Fasson, Indian Medical Service, then attached to the Herbert Hospital, Woolwich.[1] In February 1872 he commenced his duties. As the chief authority within the Infirmary and the Convalescent House all questions concerning their internal arrangements were, in the first instance, to be referred to him. He was the intermediary between the medical and surgical staff and the Board and its several committees ; and he was responsible to the Board and more immediately to the House Committee for the good order and government of the household. He was to exercise a general superintendence over the whole establishment and see that the duties of all who were resident in the hospital were properly discharged.

One of the most serious defects in the conduct of the hospital was the inefficiency of the nursing system, and the Superintendent on his appointment was asked to prepare and present a report stating his views as to how this might be remedied. In the period following the suppression of the monasteries the art of nursing became neglected and, in so far as it had been organised on monastic and conventual

[1] Minute, Royal Infirmary, 18th December 1871.

lines, disappeared. For many years afterwards there was no one, in Britain at any rate, to take the place of the Mother Superior and the Nuns who had largely constituted the profession in medieval times. Consequently skilled nursing was totally lacking when the voluntary hospitals were founded at the beginning of the eighteenth century. But its tradition had never entirely died out and the titles of Matron and Sister were preserved as survivals of monastic days, when the city fathers assumed the control of St Bartholomew's and St Thomas's Hospitals in the reign of Henry VIII. The status of the nurse, however, sank to a very low level during the eighteenth and first half of the nineteenth centuries and there were comparatively few individuals really fitted or qualified for the posts they filled.

For years little attempt had been made by the governors and medical staffs of hospitals to improve the conditions in which these women worked : often untrained and ignorant of their calling they were poorly housed, ill-fed, underpaid and over-worked, and many of them were regarded as attendants and servants rather than as nurses. Yet it is important to emphasise that the evil reputation which the vocation acquired at this time was largely due to the character of the women who were called in to give occasional help in time of emergency, "the watchers," as they were sometimes named. There were many sisters and nurses who, although lacking in expert knowledge and training, were nevertheless valuable and indispensable members of the nursing staff of the hospitals.

Few references to the nursing establishment are made in the early minutes of the Infirmary in Edinburgh. In December 1792 an agreement was reached to raise the "wages" of the nurses, the day nurse to receive £5 instead of £3, 10s. per annum, while the payment of the night nurses, who slept outside the hospital and paid a rent for their rooms, was to be increased from fourpence to sixpence per night ; and "no nurse on any pretext whatsoever to receive gratuity in money or otherwise from any patient on pain of dismissal." When in 1811 an enquiry was instituted, a plea was advanced by the medical staff in favour of procuring nurses of a superior character along with higher wages for those engaged in the fever wards, and on the attendance of those patients who had undergone serious surgical operations. The question of pensions for those who had grown old and infirm in the service of the hospital was also discussed but without any decision being reached.

An instructive, though somewhat depressing, description of the nursing conditions prevailing in the Royal Infirmary in 1859-60 has been left for posterity to reflect upon by one who was then house surgeon with James Syme.[1] The conditions and personnel, while no worse than in other hospitals, were wholly inefficient. A staff of nine women were placed in charge of Syme's seventy-two patients distributed in six wards and six little rooms, an arrangement which greatly aggravated the difficulties of nursing. Two were staff nurses, each being responsible for thirty-six beds : the remaining seven were night nurses, a considerable part of whose duties was the cleaning and scrubbing of the wards and corridors. The staff nurses were Mrs Lambert and Mrs Porter, " wonderful women, of great natural ability and strong Scottish sense and capacity, of immense experience and great kindliness." The seven night nurses were of a different class, old and useless drudges, half charwomen, rarely retaining their places for any length of time, ignorant and not always sober. Their hours of work were long, their hours of rest and sleep all too short. Coming on duty each night at 11 o'clock, they did not retire till 5 o'clock on the following afternoon because, after the completion of their night duties, they prepared the breakfast, cleaned the dishes and the wards and assisted in giving the patients dinner and tea. It was little wonder that during the night watches serious operation cases were exposed to grave risks from unobserved hæmorrhages and other complications. Nor was it an uncommon thing in these circumstances for groups of student-dressers to volunteer for four-hourly shifts during the night. The conditions certainly called for a radical change.

[1] " The Surgical Side of the Royal Infirmary, 1854-1892," by Joseph Bell, M.D. *Edinburgh Hospital Reports*, vol. i. Edinburgh, 1893.

Mrs Janet Porter remained in the service of the Infirmary for forty-seven years. After the death of Syme she was Lister's staff nurse during his professorship of clinical surgery—1869 to 1877—and, after the new Royal Infirmary was opened in 1879, she continued to work in the wards of Thomas Annandale in the position of a " retainer " rather than as an active nurse till her death in 1890, aged eighty years.[1] W. E. Henley, while a patient with Lister in the old Infirmary, has with masterly touch drawn a vivid picture of this shrewd old Scotswoman :—

The sweet old roses of her sunken face ;
The depth and malice of her sly gray eyes ;
The broad Scots tongue that flatters, scolds, defies ;
The thick Scots wit that fells you like a mace.
These thirty years she has been nursing here,
Some of them under Syme, her hero still.
Much is she worth, and even more is made of her,
Patients and students hold her very dear.
The doctors love her, tease her, use her skill.
They say " The Chief " himself is half afraid of her.

A bed in Ward 9 was named the Janet Porter Bed and her portrait, subscribed for by the nurses who had been associated with her and presented to the managers in 1890, was hung in the main corridor of the surgical hospital in the vicinity of the ward.

In the meantime a new force had sprung to life, destined not only to revolutionise nursing in all its branches but to improve the hygienic and sanitary state of the hospitals. In July 1856 Miss Florence Nightingale returned to England at the end of the war in the Crimea. Trained by the Deaconesses at Kaiserswerth in the Rhineland and as a " Sœur de Charité " in Paris, she had offered her services to the War Office and proceeded with her group of nurses, in November 1854, to Scutari on the Bosphorus, where the medical arrangements of the British Army had completely broken down. Struggling against overwhelming difficulties " she brought order out of chaos in the Scutari hospitals." [2] The same indomitable

[1] Mrs Porter died when the writer was house surgeon with Mr Annandale.
[2] *Eminent Victorians*, by Lytton Strachey. London, 1918.

spirit, the same perseverance and tenacity of purpose that had reformed these hospitals and which, on her return, compelled the authorities to re-organise the army medical department and to dispatch to India a sanitary commission to investigate the condition of the troops, were now to be applied to the creation of the modern system of nursing. When a grateful nation paid its tribute to her services to the soldiers in the war and presented her with a monetary gift of £50,000 she applied the fund to inaugurate, in 1860, the Nightingale Training School for Nurses at St Thomas's Hospital. A new era had dawned.

The establishment of the training centre in London initiated a general movement which stimulated to action the members of the boards of management of hospitals, and aroused the lively interest of the public in the supply of competent nurses to attend the sick and injured in their own homes. A committee of enquiry appointed by the managers of the Infirmary were unanimously in favour of higher salaries to attract a better class of women to the profession, of a probationary period of training, the creation of a special training fund and the appointment of a superintendent of nurses.[1] In Edinburgh, public interest in the subject found practical expression in the formation of a School or Association for the Training of Nurses with the appointment of a Mrs Taylor to act as instructress, and the Association petitioned the managers of the Infirmary to set aside three wards under her charge for the training of a group of probationer nurses on the lines carried out in the London hospitals.[2] With the concurrence of the medical staff the proposal was accepted, the managers providing the nurses with their rations and accommodation, the Association being responsible for their salaries. Evidence that the experiment was attended with some measure of success is shown in the request of the physicians that the Fever Ward should also be entrusted to Mrs Taylor for the instruction of a small group of apprentice-nurses.

It was customary to give ale at mealtime to the Nightingale Nurses as probationers, with the view of lessening the risk of

[1] Minute, Royal Infirmary, 25th March 1861. [2] *Ibid.*, 29th December 1862.

private recourse to stimulants : as a higher salary had not been offered by the Edinburgh Association as an inducement to attract women from England, it was felt that at any rate the diet in hospital should be equally generous. Accordingly the Association proposed to provide each nurse with two quart bottles of ale daily, if the managers were not prepared to do so. A conference took place in the Board Room at which a committee of ladies and other representatives of the Association discussed the question of the supply and quality of the beer.[1] Placed on the table were samples of the ale provided for the English nurses and two kinds of beer used in the hospital, one in daily use for the Infirmary nurses, the other, Prestonpans beer, drunk by the resident medical officers. The gentlemen present at the conference having tasted the several samples pronounced in favour of the Prestonpans as most suitable for the nurses ; the ladies concurred. It was accordingly determined " that in future every nurse should have an imperial pint of good table beer daily to be drawn off from the cask at the time of its being consumed, a slightly milder Prestonpans beer being ordered."

Notwithstanding the satisfactory solution of the somewhat knotty question as to the relative quality of the ale and beer, this scheme for the training of nurses proved to be short-lived, as it could hardly fail to be when placed under two controlling bodies in the same Institution.[2] While the managers were preparing to advise the discontinuance of the system, the Association asked permission to withdraw Mrs Taylor from the management of the three wards that had been placed at her disposal. Thus the matter terminated to the mutual satisfaction of both parties after a trial extending over a period of thirteen months.

The annual expenditure incurred by the Infirmary on the consumption of alcohol, both at that period and for many years subsequently, formed a very large item in the yearly accounts. Beer was regularly supplied to the members of " the family " and was included in the returns made under the heading of articles of maintenance : in 1862-63 the sum of £161 was spent

[1] Minute, Royal Infirmary, 16th March 1863. [2] *Ibid.*, 8th February 1864.

on beer under this head. On the other hand, £842 were expended on such items as port wine, sherry, spirits, porter and ale, prescribed for the patients and entered by the apothecary in the accounts of the dispensary ; the number of patients treated in the hospital during the same year, 1862-63, was 4681 ! A great change has taken place in the attitude of the medical profession towards the use of stimulants in the treatment of illness. In striking contrast to the above figures are those provided in the accounts of 1934-35, in which the expenditure on wines and spirits supplied by the dispensary was £165, the patients treated in hospital during the same year numbering 20,695.[1] Beer is no longer supplied to the members of " the family " as a routine article of diet.

The temporary arrangement made with the Association for the Training of Nurses having failed in its object, the managers proceeded in 1866 to appoint a Superintendent of Nurses. Miss Anne L. Sidey, lately matron of the Shelter in the Grassmarket, Edinburgh, was selected at a salary of £50 and was sent to London to study the methods adopted in the hospitals of the metropolis.[2] But owing to a breakdown in health Miss Sidey was compelled to tender her resignation, which was finally accepted in February 1871. At this stage the Superintendent, Deputy Surgeon-General Fasson, presented his report. He advocated the appointment of a Lady Superintendent of Nurses and a probationary system ; and, on the recommendation of the House Committee, Miss Elizabeth Anne Barclay was elected the first holder of the office at a salary of £100.[3] Trained at St Thomas's Hospital in the school established under the Nightingale Fund and with further experience gained in German war hospitals during the Franco-Prussian campaign of 1870-71, her education and social position eminently qualified her to fill the post. She brought with her from London a small band of trained nurses long known as " the Nightingales."

Miss Barclay at once proceeded to draw up a scheme embodying the new system of training. Briefly, the staff

1 Report for the year, 1934-35.

2 Minute, Royal Infirmary, 16th July 1866.

3 *Ibid.*, 7th October 1872.

was to consist of the Lady Superintendent, responsible to the Nursing Committee, now established as one of the Standing Committees; four Assistant Superintendents, two for day and two for night duty, qualified as such by their previous training as nurses; day and night nurses of equal status as Staff Nurses; Assistant Nurses, partly trained, to assist the Staff Nurses, and eligible for promotion when regarded as qualified; and Probationers, women between the ages of twenty and forty years, to be thoroughly trained for day, night or special duty in preparation for hospital posts or as skilled nurses in private families in time of illness. A class of Ward Assistants was introduced to carry out the rougher work of cleaning and scrubbing in the wards. The hours on duty were long, those of the day nurses from 7 A.M. to 8.30 P.M., and of the night nurses from 8.30 P.M. to 9 in the morning. Every day nurse had one hour off duty each day, and an additional two and a half hours were set aside for three meals, the time being doubtless frequently curtailed by the exigencies of the situation. Each nurse was entitled to one half-day off duty every fortnight and to two weeks' holiday in the year. The salaries of the staff nurses commenced at £18 increasing by increments of £1 annually to £23, with a yearly premium of £2 as a reward of zeal and efficiency. The salary of the assistant nurses was £14, with the same premium on similar conditions. The ward assistants received £12 and were required to find their own lodgings.

At one period, prior to the appointment of the Lady Superintendent of Nurses, members of the visiting staff, sometimes a physician, sometimes a surgeon, made application to the managers for a rise in the salary of their ward nurses and as a rule these requests were granted. The response usually took the form of an additional £1 to the previous salary. There was clearly no Salaries and Wages Committee in those days! But in a Minute of 29th March 1869 it is evident that the managers became more cautious and changed their policy as they resolved that in future, before responding to the recommendations of the staff, a report should be received from Miss Sidey, the Superintendent of Nurses.

The following entries are inscribed on the pages of a Night Superintendent's notebook compiled in 1873: "20th July, none of the night nurses on duty are found sleeping": on the other hand, on more than one occasion it is reported that a nurse is asleep in the small hours of the morning either upon a vacant bed or wrapped in a blanket upon two chairs. Lack of sufficient time off duty is the probable explanation of this soporific state. Again there is a note, "the resident physicians and surgeons were rather noisy from midnight till 3 A.M.!"

The lack of suitable accommodation, which had for some time proved an obstacle to the introduction of the nursing scheme, was overcome by converting one of the houses in the grounds of the Infirmary into a Nurses' Home. As the fitting up of the Home and the training of the probationer-nurses entailed considerable additional expense, the managers, at the suggestion of Miss Barclay, established a special "Nursing and Training Fund" to which they directed the attention of the public. Largely through her influence donations amounting to nearly £500 were received and a list of annual subscriptions was opened. Under Miss Barclay's able administration a marked improvement took place in this department of the hospital and, early in the new régime, the Royal Infirmary was in a position to supply well-trained nurses for other centres in the country, thus establishing a reputation which has been maintained throughout the years. Miss Barclay held office, however, for a comparatively short period of time, being obliged to resign in January 1874 for reasons of health. Miss Angélique Lucille Pringle, who had come to Edinburgh with Miss Barclay, was appointed her successor in the same year.

Florence Nightingale never lost her interest in the Royal Infirmary and she gave practical help to those engaged in selecting the nursing staff for the new Infirmary opened in Lauriston Place in 1879. Amongst the documents preserved in the hospital of historical interest to the department of nursing is a copy of a series of letters, and a few that are original, written by her to her intimate friend Miss Pringle.

One of them, dated 29th December 1873, contains a message to Nurse Janet Porter ; it reads, " please give Mrs Porter my kindest Christmas wishes and tell her I remember her perfectly and her care of me, sixteen years ago, when Mr Syme took me over the Infirmary. How long ago ! "[1] Florence Nightingale, who received the Order of Merit, died in 1910, at the advanced age of ninety years. A link between her and the Royal Infirmary is now perpetuated in " The Florence Nightingale Nurses' Home," the foundation stone of which was laid on 20th May 1936.

Many changes have taken place in the Nursing Department since the Superintendent and Miss Barclay introduced their schemes in 1872. The great increase in the number of patients has of necessity led to an augmentation of the staff, so that in 1935-36 the average daily attendance of nurses on duty was 446, while the highest number on any one day in the year reached 460. The ratio of nurses to patients has also undergone a change ; while formerly there was an average of one nurse to every five patients, the ratio has now become one to two and a half patients. One of the most important developments, however, has been the establishment of the Preliminary Training School for Nurses, introduced in 1924 with the object of providing a course of instruction for candidates seeking entry as probationer-nurses. The course necessary for qualification as a nurse is now four years, of which three months constitute the probationary period, seven weeks being spent in the Training School and six in the wards. At the end of this period those who are accepted for training sign an agreement to continue in the service of the hospital and complete the full term.

Prior to entering the Preliminary Training School each selected candidate, who must not be under 20 or over 31 years of age on entry, must pay a fee of £5, 5s., part of which is applied to the fees of the State Examination. On an average 15 probationers attend each course, and the number passing through the School during the year varies from 90 to 100, selected from 700 to 800 applicants. The instruction,

[1] Miss Nightingale visited the old Royal Infirmary in 1857.

which devolves mainly upon two Sister Tutors and an Assistant Sister Tutor, is both theoretical and practical in such subjects as anatomy, physiology, hygiene, practical nursing, first-aid and cooking, while on Sundays there is a brief attendance in the wards. The training concludes with a written and oral examination, when the successful candidates pass to the wards to complete their probationary period. The probationers then receive £20 for the first year: in the second year as Assistant Nurses they are in receipt of £25, in the third year £30 and in the fourth, £40.

When, in the later 'sixties of the nineteenth century, the decision was reached to erect a new Infirmary upon another area of ground than that which it had so long occupied, it became necessary to obtain the authority of Parliament "to remove the buildings to a more suitable position, and to acquire for that purpose the site of George Watson's Hospital and adjacent lands; and for other purposes." Amongst these "other purposes" there were included in the preparation of the new Bill certain sections which, by amending the Constitution of the Infirmary Corporation as previously set out in the Royal Charter of 1736, affected the future administration of the hospital. These special sections embodied in the Edinburgh Royal Infirmary Act, 1870, made provision to alter the former Constitution in two particulars; in the qualification necessary for membership of the General Court of Contributors, and in the number and the mode of election of the managers of the Infirmary.

In the terms of the Charter it was necessary for membership of the Corporation and of the General Court that the contribution should be "five pounds sterling each, or more, towards the said Infirmary," but, as amended under Section 16 of the Act, 1870, such qualification

> shall be the contribution by the person desiring to be a member thereof of an amount not less than five pounds in one sum, or the continuous annual contribution of an amount of not less than one pound after such annual contribution shall have been made during three consecutive years.

Further, the Charter had granted to members of the Court, or a majority of them assembled,

> full power and authority to make and constitute such by-laws, ordinances and regulations for the management and government of the affairs of the said Corporation, as to them shall seem meet, so that such by-laws, ordinances, and regulations be not contrary to the true intent and meaning thereof, nor repugnant to the laws of our realm.

But in Section 22 of the Infirmary Act it was laid down that

> the General Court of Contributors shall not have any executive powers in the management of the Infirmary, or of the affairs of the Corporation, which shall be managed exclusively by the managers appointed . . . provided always that the General Court of Contributors may from time to time make any suggestions or recommendations which to them may seem proper, and the managers shall consider, and, if they think proper, may adopt any such suggestions or recommendations:

while Section 23 enacted that

> the General Court of Contributors may from time to time alter any of the Statutes of the Corporation, or make new statutes in relation thereto, but so that such new or altered statutes shall not be inconsistent with the provisions of the said Royal Charter as amended by this Act.

The difficulty in drawing a distinction in every case between what constitutes the executive powers of the Board and the powers of the Court of Contributors to alter the statutes of the Infirmary Corporation as expressed in these two Sections of the Act, was illustrated some years later. An old By-law passed by the Court, subsequent to the date of the Charter, provided that the preses or chairman of the Board of Management should have only a casting vote at meetings of the Board. But the managers in 1886 proposed an alteration in the by-law so as to give the chairman both a deliberative and a casting vote, a change which, in the opinion of the Law Committee of the Board at that time, it was in the power of the managers to make. The Committee of the Court of Contributors in their report upon the management of the Infirmary during that year, while entirely approving of the proposed alteration, thought it advisable in order to protect the rights of the Court, should any discussion afterwards arise, to " add a saving clause in respect of the right claimed " by the Board. As the by-law now being altered by the managers had been passed by a General Court of Contributors subsequent to the Charter, it was clear that it could be altered only by that body, the Charter having authorised that the Court, " or a majority of them so assembled, shall have full power and authority to make and constitute such By-laws, Ordinances and Regulations for the Management and Government of the affairs of the said Corporation. . . ."

Some doubt, however, had apparently arisen as to the interpretation of the terms in the two Sections of the Infirmary Act, 1870, just quoted. If the by-law in question, or any other by-law is held to fall under the exercise of the " executive powers " of the Board in Section 22, then it would be in the power of the managers themselves to alter it. If, on the other hand, such powers are to be regarded as " Statutes of the Corporation " referred to in Section 23, then the by-law could be altered only by the General Court of Contributors. Thus the matter was left with the rights of both parties sufficiently protected by the foregoing statement.[1]

The essential changes in the Act of 1870, amending the previous procedure as regards the election of managers, were as follows : (1) The membership of the Board was increased from twenty to twenty-one : all were to be ordinary managers, and the quorum to be seven ; (2) with the exception of the Lord Provost of the city of Edinburgh, a manager *ex officio*—or in his absence the Dean of Guild—the managers were to be appointed annually and not, as formerly, elected by the managers themselves, but by the several bodies qualified under the Act to return representatives, each body making its own rules as to the manner of choosing its representative or representatives ;[2] (3) no manager was to be eligible for

[1] The Constitution and Rules of the Court of Contributors have been printed and can be obtained from the Secretary and Treasurer of the Royal Infirmary. Extracts of the Rules relative to membership of the Court, to the attendance of members at meetings of the Court and to their privilege of voting at meetings are contained in Appendix VIII.

[2] The selection of one Minister of the Gospel in Edinburgh was an exception, he being elected by the managers as had been done previously under the Charter.

re-election by the same body for a longer period than five years unless an interval of one year was allowed to elapse after his fifth election, when he again became eligible for annual re-election during another period of five years ; (4) if qualified, however, by his profession or business to represent another of the bodies, qualified under the Act to return a representative, he was at once eligible for election by that body. It was thus possible for an individual to have a seat on the Board for many years, either for periods of five years with intervals of one year, or without interruption.

The Act also introduced other changes, thus (5) the number of Fellows of the Royal College of Physicians of Edinburgh eligible to sit on the Board was reduced from five to two ; (6) the Professor of Anatomy in the University of Edinburgh was no longer entitled, as such, to a seat ; (7) four new bodies or "classes" in the city were given representation, the Senatus Academicus of the University, two ; the Company of Merchants of the City, one ; the Chamber of Commerce and Manufacturers of Edinburgh, one ; and the Society of Solicitors before the Supreme Courts of Scotland, one.[1]

In the event of any manager dying during his year of office, or for some other reason being unable to continue his membership, the vacancy thus created was to be filled by the body who had previously elected him, the new member to be in office during the remainder of the period for which the late manager had been appointed. All the qualified bodies, with the exception of the Court of Contributors, were required to elect their representatives in the month of December of each year, each representative assuming office from the first Monday of the following January. Of the six managers chosen by the Court of Contributors, two required to be members of the Infirmary Corporation and, at the same time, subscribers to the Convalescent Home belonging to the Corporation. These managers were elected at the meeting of the Court held on the first Monday of January in each

[1] The Town Council continued to have two representatives, the Lord Provost and one other ; the latter under the Charter had been the Deacon Convener of the Crafts of the City, but in the Act of 1870 any member of the Town Council might be chosen as the second representative.

year, or at some adjournment thereof, and they continued as managers from the time of their election until the next annual election by the Court.

The Edinburgh Royal Infirmary Act, 1870, still governs the qualification necessary for membership of the General Court of Contributors and the procedure of election of managers, but further legislation has introduced two important changes, one altering the date of the annual meeting of the Court in certain circumstances, the other providing for an increase in the number of members of the Board of Management. Many years were to elapse before either of these changes was made, yet it is appropriate to chronicle them at this point in the narrative, although it interrupts the chronological sequence of events.

As from time to time the first Monday of January coincided with New Year's Day, a public holiday, it was considered expedient to alter the date of the annual meeting of the Court. Power to do so was therefore sought under Section 94 of the Edinburgh Corporation Act, 1913, in which the necessary permission was obtained :

> when in any year the first Monday of January is a public holiday the annual meeting for the election of managers and the annual meeting of the General Court of Contributors of the said Corporation may be held on any day between the first and seventh days of January in each year, both days inclusive, and may be adjourned to such other day within or beyond that period as the meeting may determine.[1]

Fifty years after the Act, in 1920, the second change was carried into effect and the number of managers was increased from twenty-one to twenty-six by the addition of five members to represent certain of the large working-class organisations, the Edinburgh and District Trades Council responsible for organising the annual contributions from the employés in public works and other establishments in the city and neighbourhood, and the Coal-Mining and Shale-Workers Associations.[2] As

[1] Appendix IV.

[2] The Edinburgh and District Trades Council was, in 1932, named The Edinburgh and District Trades and Labour Council.

the former body, having sought representation on the Board, had been successful in securing two seats, the miners, although satisfied with the *status quo*, felt that, if representation was to be favourably considered, they also were eligible in virtue of their annual contributions to the hospital.

The Infirmary, situated more or less in the centre of a large and busy mining district embracing the three Lothians, part of the counties of Stirlingshire and Lanarkshire and, across the Firth of Forth, the counties of Clackmannan, Kinross and the western area of Fife, provided medical and surgical service to the miners and their dependents. Prior to 1906, their contributions had yielded about £1800 annually to the funds of the hospital; but, following the appointment of Mr Russell Paton as Organising Secretary for Subscriptions to the Infirmary, a campaign was opened with the object of increasing the contributions from the coal and shale-fields districts. As the result of his organising ability and untiring efforts these steadily increased and, ten years later, totalled the sum of £6000, the highest figure hitherto reached. By doubling the weekly subscriptions and by placing them on a permanent basis the sums collected in 1919, when the subject of representation had come under discussion, amounted to £8500. It was therefore a fitting and just recognition of the response of the miners that they also should have a seat on the Board of Management; consequently, the Miners' Association of Fife and Kinross, the Miners' Association of Mid and East Lothian and the combined Coal and Shale Miners Associations of West Lothian were each represented by one member.[1] The sanction of Parliament to increase the number of managers from twenty-one to twenty-six was obtained through the courtesy of the Town Council of Edinburgh who inserted the necessary clause in the Edinburgh Corporation Order Confirmation Act, 1919,[2] a courtesy again extended by the Town Council in 1930 when the managers were in that year further increased. In 1917 the county of Clackmannan was

[1] The two Coal and Shale Miners' Associations of West Lothian chose a representative alternately.

[2] Appendix v.

added to the Miners' Association of Fife and Kinross and the new title assumed was that of the Fife, Clackmannan and Kinross Miners' Union.

In 1920, the total contributions from the coal-fields and from the operatives in the shale and oil-works reached £11,250 and, in 1924 the peak year, a sum of £14,669 was collected from the same sources. At least 50,000 employés in these industries are subscribing annually to the funds of the Infirmary, and the number, including the wives and dependants who are treated in the hospital, average 2700 annually.

The membership of the Board was again augmented in 1930, when the workers' representation was increased by two representatives of the League of Subscribers which had been formally inaugurated in 1918. This attempt to provide a steady and constant stream of contributions from the working-class members of the community, to whom the benefits of the Infirmary were extended in time of sickness, was not an entirely new movement. It had first been suggested as far back as 1849 and, though its activities were on a somewhat limited scale, it had met with a moderate degree of success. The opinion was then expressed that, if the united efforts of employers and employés were systematically organised on a permanent basis, through such union a more secure source of annual revenue would be established than that provided by the donations of the wealthier part of the community. The League was formed in 1918 for the purpose of co-ordinating on a still larger scale, a more systematised scheme of obtaining financial assistance, on a purely voluntary basis, from the employés engaged in public works and business establishments, and from the staffs of schools, banks, insurance, Government and other offices in Greater Edinburgh and the provincial districts. The membership of the League is conditional upon the payment of a subscription of one penny per week for adults and one half-penny for apprentices and junior members, the members authorising his or her employer to deduct from the weekly wages their contribution to the League Fund for the Infirmary. The success of the scheme, therefore, is closely associated with the friendly cooperation of the employers who undertake the work of collection through the pay offices.

The membership of the League in 1929 had grown to 100,000 and, during the eleven years in which the scheme had been in operation, the aggregate sum of £201,996 had been collected and paid over to the funds of the Infirmary. The annual receipts during that period, while varying slightly from year to year, were approximately £20,000. Its established position and the excellent work which it had accomplished entitled that body to representation on the Board of Management, and two representatives joined the Board in January 1930. The necessary authorisation was obtained in an amending clause to the Edinburgh Royal Infirmary Act, 1870, which was placed in the Edinburgh Corporation Confirmation Act, 1930.[1]

In 1896, Miss Louisa Stevenson was elected the first lady manager as one of the six representatives of the Court of Contributors. Since that date the Board of Management has continued uninterruptedly to have one or more lady members, as many as four having had seats at one time. Miss Stevenson had a seat on the Board for nine years. She took a prominent part in all measures directed to promote the welfare of the community and the advancement of higher education amongst women, and from the University of Edinburgh she received the honorary degree of Doctor of Laws.

[1] Appendix VI.

CHAPTER XIII

"THE BATTLE OF THE SITES," 1864-1869

INFIRMARY STREET OR LAURISTON PLACE?—PROFESSOR JAMES SYME AND THE FINAL DECISION—DEATH OF JAMES SYME—THE FOUNDATION STONE OF THE NEW ROYAL INFIRMARY—THE DISPOSAL OF THE OLD INFIRMARY BUILDINGS.

FOR some years the state of the fabric of that part of the Infirmary, known as the Medical Hospital, had been a source of anxiety to those responsible for its preservation and upkeep, and they recognised that considerable repairs would soon be required if the building were to remain in a thoroughly efficient condition. In the long interval of a century and a quarter which had passed since its foundation-stone was laid, new ideas had been conceived regarding hospital construction, and more modern methods of ventilation were in use. Before a final decision was reached as to the expediency of remodelling or of rebuilding the whole structure it was deemed advisable to obtain the opinion of an expert. Accordingly, Mr David Bryce, the architect, was requested to prepare and present a report upon the condition of the medical hospital.

In October 1864, the financial position of the Infirmary and the accommodation it was able to provide for both medical and surgical patients might be described as satisfactory. The sum of £81,903 represented the value of the Capital Stock invested in good securities and in certain properties. The ordinary revenue for the year 1863-64 derived from all sources amounted to £13,190, and the total expenditure on the ordinary account was £15,408, thus giving an excess of expenditure over income of £2218, an excess, however, which was reduced to £1186 by providing from the capital account a sum of £1032 to meet a small outlay on building and repairs. The number of patients entertained in the Infirmary, although varying slightly from year to year, continued to show a progressive increase and in 1863-64 totalled 4594: of these, 4253 were admitted during the year and 341 remained in hospital from the previous year. The average number of occupied beds was 386, the highest in use at any one time being 438, and the lowest, 306. Of the 4285 patients treated and discharged during the year 1863-64, 1955 were ordinary medical cases, 1837 were surgical, and 493 were fever and smallpox cases. The managers in seeking an expert opinion were not influenced by any pressing need to increase the beds, but wished merely to learn the truth as to the actual condition of the fabric of the medical house.

The architect in his report presented on 19th December 1864 referred to several defects, the result of wear and tear, and especially to the weak condition of the timbers forming the floors of the wards, which would have rendered the latter unsafe for occupation had additional support not been from time to time supplied. The low position of the ceilings was also adversely commented upon as not in keeping with the modern ideas of ventilation; the baths placed in the basement were far removed from the wards and approached through cold draughty passages; and the rooms assigned for the administrative offices were too small and low in the ceiling. He objected also to the close proximity of the hospital to the high buildings in South Bridge and Drummond Street as interfering with the free circulation of air. In concluding his report he said: "I am of the opinion that as little money as possible should be spent on the present house as I am afraid that, if a large sum were expended in attempting to remedy so very defective an arrangement, it would prove unsatisfactory. In fact, my opinion is that nothing short of a new building will answer the purpose." It was obvious, therefore, that some drastic step was necessary.

The managers, the medical and surgical staff and the Committee of the Court of Contributors were in complete agreement with Mr Bryce's opinion. Therefore full power was given to him to examine the most approved modern hospitals and to prepare the plans and estimates for the construction of a new medical hospital in proximity to the two surgical hospitals, regarding the condition of which no serious complaint had then been made. A Building Fund was opened and a special appeal was issued to the public for contributions. In anticipation of the occurrence of a situation of this kind, the managers for some years past had annually added to capital account all legacies and donations exceeding £100, not ear-marked for special purposes ; and a considerable sum free from all restrictions had thus accumulated, part of which they proposed should now be set aside as a nucleus.[1] In addition to these they proposed to apply to a similar purpose a legacy of £6000 bequeathed, in 1865, by Miss Ann Cranstoun Fryer, late of Reading, permission to do so having been obtained from her executors.

Two plans were submitted by the architect, one representing the new medical hospital on the existing site, the other, with the new hospital in the same position, but with the proposal to acquire the ground and houses on the east side of South Bridge directly opposite the frontage of the University. This suggestion was made, not with the object of extending the hospital westwards as far as the street but, by the demolition of the houses, to secure a free circulation of air and at the same time to effect a city improvement, the more open space thus acquired between the hospital and the University giving a better view of the entrance and east façade of the Old College. The proposal was also made that the cost of this improvement should be met by assessing the citizens and, "that the small rate of one penny per pound on the valued rental of Edinburgh for ten or twelve years would accomplish the object."

At this stage of the deliberations—January 1866—the medical and surgical staff were unanimous in their condemnation of the unhealthy condition of the New Surgical Hospital opened in 1853. James Syme, while expressing satisfaction with the state of his own wards in the old High School building, affirmed that the other surgical hospital had been constructed on a faulty principle. This expression of opinion

[1] Minute, Royal Infirmary, 23rd October 1865.

by the staff fell like a bombshell on the managers and put an entirely new complexion on the situation. It was no longer merely a question of rebuilding the medical hospital : if two hospitals were required, would the existing site be the most suitable ? A Joint-Committee of the managers and of the Court of Contributors were appointed and early in the inquiry steps were taken to dispose, temporarily at any rate, of the complaints arising in connection with the New Surgical Hospital by carrying out extensive alterations upon it.

The question of the best site for the Royal Infirmary was then explored and many witnesses were examined. Two requirements appeared to be essential : first, that all the departments of the Infirmary should be centralised, so that if the medical hospital were removed from Infirmary Street the surgical hospitals should follow ; and, secondly, that the Infirmary should be in close proximity to the University and Surgeons' Hall so as to maintain the centralised character of the medical school. Two possible sites were considered by the Joint-Committee, that of the existing Infirmary and the site of George Watson's Hospital—later designated George Watson's College for Boys—situated on Heriot's Croft, an area lying between Lauriston Place and the Meadows, the latter an open expanse of ground, once the Burgh or South Loch.[1] The consensus of opinion of the medical and surgical staff favoured the existing site, as the improvements made in the New Surgical Hospital nine months previously were giving satisfaction ; the surgeons in charge desired its retention, though some of the witnesses examined expressed doubt as to whether the real effect of the alterations could be fully ascertained till a longer period had elapsed. James Syme had no improvements to suggest in the old Surgical Hospital which he regarded as probably the healthiest in Her Majesty's dominions. In the event of the present site being retained the committee recommended that the houses facing the University should be removed.

[1] In a Provisional Order of 1869 permission was granted to convert George Watson's Hospital from a boarding school into a day school with the title of George Watson's College for Boys.

Various objections were raised to the alternative site in Lauriston Place; in particular, its distance from the University, but especially its proximity to the Meadows which, because of imperfect drainage, might prove detrimental to the health of the inmates of the Infirmary, an objection, however, which was not considered insurmountable. On the other hand, the site had much to recommend it, but, in order to obtain a sufficiently large area for all the buildings required, it would be necessary to purchase in addition a strip of ground on the west side of George Watson's Hospital, on which stood the houses forming Wharton Place and the mansion and gardens of Wharton House. Taking all the circumstances into consideration the Joint-Committee concluded their report as follows: "Being now in possession of a site which is perfectly healthy, and into which more light and air may be let in the manner suggested—with buildings erected on it sufficient for the whole surgical department, of great pecuniary value, and probably as healthy and as suitable for all practical purposes as any other that might be erected—and the site, moreover, in the most favourable position with reference to the University and the Extra-Mural Medical School—the Joint-Committee are unanimously of opinion that, even on the supposition that the situation of George Watson's Hospital is on the whole preferable, there is no such superiority in it as would justify the pecuniary sacrifice implied in the removal of the Infirmary there, and therefore that the present site should be retained and the new Medical Hospital erected thereon."

In view of the decision of the Court of Contributors, in March 1867, to adopt the above report, a fresh appeal for funds to build on the existing site was issued. It was largely through the exertions of two men, Mr Thomas Jamieson Boyd, the convener of the committee, and later Lord Provost of the City, and of Councillor Colston, the City Treasurer who acted as secretary, that the large sum finally raised to erect the new Royal Infirmary was obtained. Within six months of the issue of the appeal the response had yielded £68,000, which, added to the sum of £40,000 apportioned by the managers from the Capital Stock, brought the total to £108,000. A Bill was introduced into Parliament to enable the Infirmary to acquire the ground and houses facing the University as part of the scheme. Although complete unanimity with the decision to erect the new hospital on the existing site was scarcely to be expected among all the members of the community interested in its future, satisfactory additions were made from time to time to the building fund.

On 19th October 1868, Syme wrote a letter to the Board of Management, the purpose of which entirely altered the whole situation. After recapitulating the course of events he went on to say that the sanguine expectations entertained from remedying the defects in the New Surgical Hospital, while certainly procuring considerable improvement, had not been realised, and pyæmia—the scourge of unhealthy hospitals—was still distressingly frequent. The inter-communication which had been made between that hospital and his wards in the old High School had greatly increased "the tendency to serious derangement" in them. But, even if no fault could be found with the salubrity of all the surgical wards, they would still remain unworthy of the Royal Infirmary, and the erection of a new medical hospital, in association for an indefinite time with two surgical hospitals of an earlier period, would injure the prestige of the Infirmary. Further, with the new Infirmary in process of erection on the existing site, necessitating the demolition of all the buildings, Edinburgh would be without a hospital for at least three years, thus depriving the sick poor of the means of treatment and interfering with medical education. "When the confined, smoky condition of the present site," he added, "is contrasted with the airy, cheerful and salubrious site now within reach, it is difficult to imagine what possible objection there can be to removal." Professor James Spence, whose work was conducted in the New Surgical Hospital, refuted some of Syme's statements and quoted, in support of his contention, a series of successful major operations performed by the surgeons attached to it in 1860-62, before the sanitary and constructional improvements had been carried out. Of twenty-five amputations through the thigh for disease only two died, and of five performed through the leg, all recovered; of twenty-one excisions of the elbow, all recovered, and seven lithotomies were also successful; and of twelve strangulated herniæ, only two died. These were results which he considered would contrast favourably with those of many model hospitals. Whatever decision might be reached regarding rebuilding of the surgical hospital he hoped no change of site would be made.

In consequence of Syme's strong protest, two questions arose: Was the whole Infirmary to be rebuilt on the existing site, or on the alternative site? These questions along with the comparative cost were remitted to the architect. As the position occupied by George Watson's Hospital was eventually selected, it is unnecessary to present in detail the different plans for the erection of the Infirmary on the old property. It will suffice to record that, in order to find an area adequate for a complete hospital, Mr Bryce proposed that the Infirmary Corporation should acquire the High School Yards and the ground extending northwards from it as far as the Cowgate; or, alternatively, should purchase an area on St John's Hill situated east of the Pleasance, making it accessible by spanning that roadway with one or two iron bridges. On the other hand, if a preference should be given to the Lauriston site he considered it would be necessary to purchase not only George Watson's Hospital and grounds, but, in addition, the Wharton property. In concluding his report Mr Bryce submitted that either was well adapted for erecting an Infirmary in the middle of a large town and that, while Watson's site was superior on account of the extent of ground available, the other had an advantage in its proximity to the medical school and to the poorer districts of the city.

The opinion of the Committee of the Court of Contributors was divided on both these big questions when the subject came before the adjourned meeting of the Court on 19th March 1869. Moreover, during the six months prior to that date public opinion had undoubtedly been influenced by Professor Syme's change of views which had been circulated in a letter to the contributors. Syme then moved the two following resolutions : 1. That the New Infirmary shall afford accommodation for surgical as well as medical patients: 2. That the New Infirmary shall be built on the grounds of George Watson's Hospital. An amendment was presented by Mr Millar of Sheardale and seconded by James Spence to the effect that, having considered the report of the committee, the Court resolve that the present site be retained and the whole question of the rebuilding of the hospital be remitted to the managers with full powers. On a vote being taken, 144 were in favour of James Syme's motion and 50 voted for the amendment.

Thus terminated the Battle of the Sites and, for the second time in the history of the Infirmary, negotiations were commenced between the managers and the governors of George Watson's Hospital. Widespread interest in the struggle had been aroused not only in the public Press but amongst all classes of the community. Syme's *volte face* was in later years chronicled in verse in the following lines written by a well-known Fellow of the Royal College of Surgeons of Edinburgh :[1]—

. . . . . .

So 'twas Hamish Syme spoke it in a letter—
If you want a site there is not a better ;
For ta air and licht are they not a treasure,
An' ta price of all is just at your pleasure.

Here ta patients wull, long pefore they leave us,
Be as strong as kye on ta great Ben Nevis ;
For it's here they cure children's diseases
Only by ta pure air an southlan' breezes.[2]

Goot day to you, sir, and what is it you've spoken ?
Had we not your word, Hamish, which you've broken ?
So you spurn ta place for your occupations,
Where your great forbears did all their operations.

Looking back over a period of sixty-eight years with the experience that these years have given, no one today will

[1] " How ta New Infirmary Arose," by J. S. in *Lays of the Colleges*, 1886.

[2] The Royal Edinburgh Hospital for Sick Children, in 1869, stood in proximity to the south-west corner of the grounds of George Watson's Hospital.

regret that Syme had the courage of his convictions and succeeded in impressing his views upon the majority of the contributors. Yet he could hardly have foreseen that, within less than half that period of time, even the new site in Lauriston Place would prove too small for the inevitable extensions of the Royal Infirmary. Within a month of the date of the fateful meeting of the contributors, Syme had an apoplectic seizure which necessitated his resignation of the chair of clinical surgery and his position as surgeon to the hospital. For several months he was able to attend to a little professional work, but he died on 26th June 1870, aged seventy years, and was interred in the family vault at St John's Episcopal Church, Princes Street.

Syme spent the evening of his life in his beautiful home of Millbank in the Grange district of the city amongst the flowers which he loved, his matchless orchids, his heaths and azaleas. " Sensitive, strong-willed, shy, bent upon reaching reality and the best in everything " he had struggled in his early years with imperfect means and family disaster. Short in stature but well-formed, with a finely modelled forehead, expressive eyes and strong well-shaped hands, he was invariably neatly dressed, and his checked neckerchief tied as a bow was a characteristic feature of his apparel. The times in which he lived were not always peaceful in the medical profession. There were giants in those days, but very combative and quarrelsome giants, and he not infrequently found himself engaged in controversies which sometimes terminated in estrangement with men who were formerly his friends. " He was keen in the pursuit of his science, single-minded and earnest in the discharge of surgical duty and influential for good in an immeasurable way." [1]

An agreement having been reached regarding the site, an offer was made for the building and grounds of George Watson's Hospital ; but although accepted by the governors the suggestion met with opposition on two occasions from a minority of

[1] *Horæ Subsecivæ*, by John Brown, M.D. First Series, vol. iii, p. 360, *et seq.* London : A. & C. Black, 1897.

the members of the Edinburgh Merchant Company when brought before them for confirmation. An Interdict from the Court of Session was sought but this was refused.[1] The contiguous Wharton property on the west side of the grounds of George Watson's Hospital, along with the houses in Wharton Place facing Lauriston Place, was also acquired, the whole area comprising eleven acres.[2]

In view of the decision to build the Infirmary on a new site, the Bill, previously introduced into Parliament to legalise the purchase of the ground and houses facing the University, was withdrawn and a second Parliamentary Bill was prepared and introduced in December 1869. It contained *inter alia* the following important sections :—1. Confirmation of the agreement between the Company of Merchants of the City, the governors of George Watson's Hospital and the Infirmary Corporation for the sale of the property in Lauriston : 2. Power to the Infirmary Corporation to dispose of the lands and buildings now belonging to and occupied by them, in whole or in part, either by sale or in consideration of annual payments : 3. Powers to the Infirmary Corporation to repay those persons who had previously subscribed for the erection of a new hospital on the old site and who dissented in the application of their contributions to the new proposal :[3] 4. Authority to the Infirmary Corporation to appropriate and apply towards the purchase of lands and buildings, monies now in their hands, whether accumulated capital or annual proceeds.[4] The Bill passed through both Houses without opposition and received the Royal Assent on 20th June, as the Edinburgh Royal Infirmary Act, 1870.[5] An interesting point arose at that time as to whether subscribers to the building fund could be regarded as contributors, within the meaning of the statutes, and therefore

[1] *The Company of Merchants of the City of Edinburgh and its Schools, 1694-1920*, by John Harrison : the Merchants' Hall, Edinburgh, 1920.

[2] The governors obtained a new site for George Watson's College by purchasing from the Merchant Maidens' Trust the Merchant Maidens' Hospital which stood on the west side of Lauriston Lane, facing the Meadows.

[3] Only eighteen dissentients finally sought repayment, entailing the return of £224.

[4] See Sections 11, 12, 14 and 15 of the Edinburgh Royal Infirmary Act, 1870. Appendix VII.

[5] Chapter XII, p. 216.

be privileged to vote at the General Court of Contributors. Counsel's opinion on the matter was thus expressed :—" If the money subscribed to the building fund is paid to the amount of £5 the subscribers will be members of the General Court of Contributors and entitled to vote at the meetings of the Corporation. Although the money is supplied to a special object it is none the less a contribution to the Infirmary. So long as the money, however, is held by the committee of the building fund, it is not yet handed over to the Infirmary and so the subscribers cannot vote till that is done, as they are not yet members of the General Court." [1]

On 13th October 1870, the Foundation Stone of the New Royal Infirmary was laid with full Masonic honours by H.R.H. Albert Edward, Prince of Wales, Patron of the Freemasons of Scotland, in the presence of H.R.H. the Princess of Wales and a large and distinguished company. The visit of Royalty, combined with the national character of the event which brought the Prince to Edinburgh, aroused widespread interest throughout Scotland and in the capital. There was a general suspension of business in the city, and the main streets decorated and beflagged were lined by troops along the route of the procession. Over 4000 Freemasons representing 170 of the Lodges in Scotland, under the leadership of the Grand Master, the Earl of Dalhousie, assembled in Charlotte Square and marched by way of Princes Street and the Mound to the rendezvous in Lauriston. The scene of the Ceremony was set in the north-east corner of the grounds of the Hospital where the stone was laid by the Prince with correct Masonic ritual—with plumb and level, square and mallet ; and finally, the contents of the cornucopia, the horn of plenty, and of the vases containing the oil and wine were poured upon the stone, in a cavity in which were placed plans of the hospital, current coins of the realm, a copy of Oliver and Boyd's Almanac for the year 1870 and Black's Guide to Edinburgh.[2]

When a commencement was made with the construction of the new Infirmary the disposal of the old buildings of

[1] Minutes, Royal Infirmary, 22nd March and 24th May 1869.

[2] No trace of the Foundation Stone now exists.

necessity became a matter for careful consideration. The University, being then desirous of obtaining more accommodation for the several departments of Medicine, expressed the wish to acquire the property in Infirmary Street, so the Senatus opened negotiations with the Board of Management. Valuations of the whole area, made independently by each of the parties, estimated the value of the property at £20,705. After subtracting the cost of the buildings used as the Lock and Fever Hospitals at the east end of the area next to the Pleasance, which the Infirmary would require for the treatment of fever patients after the new Infirmary was occupied, the west portion was revalued at £15,690 : to this sum there fell to be added £5335 which the managers had previously paid for the houses in South Bridge facing the University. The Senatus expressed their willingness to give £21,025 for this site on the understanding, however, that they would acquire the east portion, valued at £5015, when the Infirmary ceased to have further use for it.

The Committee of the Court of Contributors in their report of January 1871 took exception to this transaction on the ground that a considerably larger sum might be realised if the property were disposed of by public sale : they also expressed doubt as to whether the managers had the power to sell. The majority of the committee considered that it was both the right and the duty of the Court of Contributors to refuse their consent to the sale, but, at the adjourned meeting of the Court on 23rd January, the greater number of those present, without expressing either approval or disapproval of the transaction, remitted the whole matter to the new Board of Management for consideration.

It is unnecessary to record in detail the various phases of the further discussions.[1] Two Notes of Suspension and Interdict against the managers implementing their bargain with the Senatus were lodged in the Court of Session, an interim interdict being obtained in each instance. Both actions were defended by the managers who considered that they were

[1] Details of the proceedings are contained in the Annual Report of the Managers for the years 1869-70 and 1870-71.

bound to fulfil their agreement with the Senatus, and the cases were debated before the Lord Ordinary who declared the interim interdicts perpetual. The judgment of the Court of Session was communicated to the Senatus Academicus who generously absolved the managers from their bargain, and no further steps were taken at that time by the Infirmary Corporation to dispose of the property.

The whirligig of time, however, eventually placed the University in 1904 in possession of all that was then left of the old buildings of the Royal Infirmary. In the long interval between 1871 and the above date events occurred which had an important influence upon their future disposal. The Public Health (Scotland) Act, 1867, having given powers to Local Authorities to make provision for the treatment of infectious cases during periods of epidemics, the Town Council of Edinburgh, as the Local Authority, in 1871 prepared the Canongate Poorhouse for that purpose.[1] Further, as the managers of the Infirmary refused to admit cases of smallpox or cholera, premises in King's Stables Road and in part of the Poorhouse in Forrest Road were fitted up as temporary hospitals to meet any emergency that might arise, a wise procedure in view of the fact that another epidemic of cholera then threatened the city. But, in 1881, on the advice of Sir Henry Littlejohn, the medical officer of health, the Town Council took further steps for dealing with epidemics by purchasing from the managers of the Infirmary for £16,000 the two Surgical Hospitals with accommodation for 218 beds.[2] At the same time they bought the old Medical Hospital for £8500; and finally, in 1885, old Surgeons' Hall which, since the occupation of the New Infirmary, the managers had been using for the treatment of infectious fevers during ordinary seasons, passed into the hands of the Town Council for £4000.[3] Thus, through the disposal of the old property the Infirmary obtained a sum of £28,500.

At last the Local Authority had assumed the responsibility for the treatment of all cases of fever occurring in the city:

[1] Minute, Town Council, 29th March 1871.

[2] *Ibid.*, 11th March 1881. [3] *Ibid.*, 14th July 1885.

this old and much vexed question was then settled and the Infirmary was relieved of a burden which it had borne, not always patiently, for one hundred and fifty-seven years. The old Medical Hospital was demolished in 1884 and, on part of the site, the School Board erected one of its schools, still used as such by the Edinburgh Corporation Education Committee and on what was left of the ground the Corporation baths were built. For nearly twenty years the City Fever Hospital occupied this corner of Old Edinburgh till, in 1903, it was transferred to the fine situation at Colinton Mains on the southern outskirts of the city.

The way was now opened for placing in the hands of the University what remained of the old Infirmary buildings. Having failed to acquire the property in 1871, the University had turned elsewhere for a suitable position on which to accommodate the several departments of Medicine which could no longer be housed in the Old College. An extensive scheme was inaugurated in 1874, and properties in Park Place and Teviot Row were purchased in the vicinity of the site upon which the new Infirmary was under construction. There the New Medical School was erected, thus maintaining proximity between the school and the hospital, not in the manner formerly envisaged by the Joint-Committee of the Managers of the Infirmary and the Court of Contributors, sitting and deliberating in 1866 upon the site of the new hospital, but by the University following in the footsteps of the Royal Infirmary. In 1904 the University Court, being actively interested in acquiring more ground for the extension of two of the departments of science, opened negotiations with the Town Council for the purchase of the buildings vacated by the Fever Hospital, and were fortunate in obtaining them for the sum of £15,000. The old High School whose walls had once echoed to the youthful voices of Sir Charles Bell and Lord Cockburn, of Henry Brougham and Francis Horner, of Sir Walter Scott and Francis Jeffrey was thus rededicated to educational purposes ; and, in the autumn of 1905—with its external walls left unaltered—was ready for the use of the Department of Engineering, continuing to serve that purpose till 1932, when the department was transferred to the King's Buildings on the eastern slope of the Blackford Hill. The High School was then refitted for the Department of Geography. In 1906, the Department of Natural Philosophy was installed in what had once been the New Surgical Hospital, and old Surgeons' Hall became the Headquarters of the University Officers' Training Corps.

The future story of this historic area of the city has still to be told and, whatever the story may be, the fact remains that for more than three and a half centuries this part of old Edinburgh has continued uninterruptedly to minister to the educational needs of successive generations of youthful citizens. It has more than fulfilled the purpose desired by the Town Council of 1561 that the property once owned by the Black Friars and confiscated at the Reformation " should be applyit to mair proffitable and godlie ussis sic as for sustenying of the trew ministeris of Goddis word, founding and biging of hospitalis for the pure and Collegis for leirnyng and upbring of the youth and sic other godlie warkis." [1]

[1] See Chapter VI, p. 78.

CHAPTER XIV

THE LAST DECADE IN THE OLD ROYAL INFIRMARY
1870 to 1879

JOSEPH LISTER AND THE REGIUS CHAIR OF CLINICAL SURGERY—MEDICAL EDUCATION OF WOMEN IN THE ROYAL INFIRMARY—PLANS FOR THE CONSTRUCTION OF THE NEW ROYAL INFIRMARY—THE OPENING CEREMONY.

WHEN James Syme resigned the chair of clinical surgery in the summer of 1869 Joseph Lister was elected his successor and, in a letter to the managers of the Royal Infirmary dated 25th August, he wrote as follows :—" Having been appointed Professor of Clinical Surgery in the University of Edinburgh I beg to express the hope that you will provide me with the means of giving my lectures in connection with the Infirmary. It is hardly necessary to say that, if you honour me with your confidence, the interests of the patients committed to my charge will be the primary object of my attention." At the same meeting of the Board a letter was read from James Spence, professor of systematic surgery, whose term of office as an acting surgeon of the hospital was about to expire. In it he solicited an extension of his period of service as the charge of beds would enable him to make the teaching of the chair more in accordance with the system of instruction then recognised as desirable. An affirmative answer was given to both these applications, but, as the managers were considering a rearrangement of the whole surgical department, the allocation of the beds was not communicated to the two professors till 4th October.

At that date the Old and the New Surgical Hospitals contained 190 beds available amongst five surgeons, the three acting or ordinary surgeons and the two professors of surgery. Of the 77 beds in the Old Surgical Hospital 50 were allotted to Joseph Lister and 20 to the third or junior surgeon : the remaining 7 beds in two reserved wards were retained for the use of the whole surgical staff and were only to be occupied with the consent of the managers. In the New Surgical Hospital 113 beds were allocated in the following way :— 50 to the senior acting surgeon, 35 to the second surgeon and the remaining 28 to James Spence. Thus with 50 beds Lister commenced his work as surgeon in the old High School building in which his predecessor in the chair had laboured for thirty-six years.

Lister had many friends in the city who gave him a cordial welcome ; he was not a stranger to Edinburgh because, in the autumn of 1853, on the completion of his medical studies at University College, London, he had travelled north to the Scottish capital. His intention had been to stay for one month ; but the month was prolonged to six months and the six months to nearly seven years, so unrivalled were the opportunities offered him for work in the school of medicine and in the Royal Infirmary : as supplementary clerk and house surgeon with Syme ; as an extra-academical lecturer in surgery at High School Yards ; as assistant surgeon to the hospital in 1856—in which year he married James Syme's daughter—the long period terminating in the spring of 1860 with his appointment to the regius chair of surgery in the University of Glasgow. Throughout the whole of that time he had worked indefatigably, investigating the phenomena of the early stages of inflammation and the microscopical changes associated with the coagulation of the blood, his mind constantly dwelling on the problem of the origin of inflammation in wounds and of those distressing complications which were the source of the shocking mortality in hospitals after operation and injury.

During his absence of nine years in Glasgow the staff of the Royal Infirmary had undergone several changes : a few of his former colleagues remained to receive him, but a number had left and their places were occupied by less familiar faces. Hughes Bennett, Thomas Laycock and Sir James Young Simpson were still clinical professors and his colleagues on the Senatus.[1] None of the ordinary physicians of 1860 remained: of these, William Tennant Gairdner had been appointed professor of medicine at Glasgow where he and Lister had been colleagues in the University. The three physicians were Daniel Rutherford Haldane, George W. Balfour and Thomas Grainger Stewart, while Claud Muirhead and Thomas Richard Fraser had just been appointed to the newly created assistant physicianships. William Walker was still ophthalmic surgeon but Douglas Argyll Robertson had been elected in 1862 to assist him in the eye department. James Matthews Duncan, who became Lister's life-long friend, was acting as an extra-physician for the diseases peculiar to women. Of the former surgical staff, John Struthers had gone to Aberdeen as professor of anatomy, but James Spence as professor of surgery and James Donaldson Gillespie, as the senior acting surgeon, remained. The two junior acting surgeons were Patrick Heron Watson and Thomas Annandale, the latter afterwards Lister's successor in the clinical chair, and the two assistant surgeons, recently appointed, were Joseph Bell and John Duncan.

The years of Lister's professorship in Glasgow had been pregnant with the discovery of a great scientific truth: Louis Pasteur, as the result of careful observation and experiment had demonstrated conclusively, in 1864, that fermentation and putrefaction were vital phenomena due to the action of micro-organisms everywhere present in the atmosphere. He thus laid the foundation of the Germ Theory on which Lister proceeded to build his conception of the antiseptic or anti-putrefactive treatment of wounds, the essential basis of which was the destruction of the minute organisms that had already obtained access to the wound, and their subsequent exclusion during the process of healing. He effected a complete revolution in surgical practice and by so doing he destroyed the active factors in the causation of putrefaction and of those frequently occurring and often fatal complications, pyæmia,

[1] Douglas Maclagan elected professor of forensic medicine in 1862 and William Rutherford Sanders appointed to the chair of pathology in 1869 were also clinical professors in the Royal Infirmary at this date.

erysipelas and hospital gangrene. Writing in 1867 regarding the state of his wards in Glasgow Royal Infirmary, following his early efforts to banish the deplorable conditions which were then the rule and not the exception in hospital practice, he said : " Since the antiseptic treatment has been brought into full operation, and wounds and abscesses no longer poison the atmosphere with putrid exhalations, my wards, though in other respects under precisely the same circumstances as before, have completely changed their character ; so that during the last nine months not a single instance of pyæmia, hospital gangrene or erysipelas has occurred in them." [1] The following impressions of one of his students in Edinburgh are thus recorded :—

> I can well remember with what excitement we crowded into the operating theatre in the Old Infirmary, young lads of 17 and 18, fired by the rumours of what we had heard of dashing operations—disarticulations of the hip in ten seconds with oceans of blood and marvels of dexterity—to be met by a modest, shy, retiring figure with lisping utterance, and with nothing before him except a dozen glass bulbs filled with beef-tea, urine, and milk, on the aseptic qualities of which he discoursed in a quiet unobtrusive way. I must confess that it all came as a shock of disappointment. It was all too like the chemical lecture through which we had yawned in the morning, and we could not but feel that we were being defrauded. No doubt we were only silly boys, but what could you expect ? We had had no previous experience to guide us, we had not seen epidemics of pyæmia decimating whole wards, and it was thus impossible for us to grasp the magnitude and importance of his discoveries. Even when it did come to operations, the comparison with the other surgeons of the day was not flattering. There was no dash or brilliancy, but slow methodical plodding, the immediate results covered by carbolic putty and obscured by clouds of antiseptic spray, while as to the immediate results, though we heard that they were wonderful, we knew too little to appreciate at their true value their import or magnitude.[2]

In the old Surgical Hospital in the High School Yards Lister, on his return to Edinburgh, continued his beneficent work improving and simplifying the technic of his antiseptic

[1] *British Medical Journal*, 1867, vol. ii, p. 246.

[2] *Edinburgh Medical Journal*, vol. ix, 1912. " Some Memories of Old Harveians," by C. W. MacGillivray, M.D.

methods; and, after six years, he was able to record that during that period hospital gangrene had been banished from his wards, only one case on which he had operated had developed pyæmia, and erysipelas had been a very rare occurrence. Owing to the great demand made on his beds he had felt justified in accommodating as many as seventy patients by means of extra beds and "shake-downs," so that there were rarely as few patients in the wards as the hospital regulations permitted, while the annual cleaning of the wards, previously a necessary procedure in the Infirmary, was postponed during an interval of three years.[1] Moreover, surgery was no longer being confined to the major operations of the pre-Listerian days. Although attempts had been made from time to time to extend the boundaries of the surgeon's endeavour, sometimes with success but as a rule with uncertain results, the field soon became definitely extended and no part of the human body was regarded as outside the province of the surgeon. But Lister did more than bring security to the practice of surgery; he laid the foundation of hygiene and preventive medicine.

Notwithstanding the successful results which he obtained and which spoke for themselves, Lister did not escape the opposition and hostile criticism of some of his colleagues in Edinburgh; but nowhere was this feeling so pronounced as in London. Consequently, in 1877, when the chair of clinical surgery at King's College, London, became vacant through the death of Sir William Fergusson, Lister accepted the invitation extended to him. He was convinced that he still had a mission to perform and that "the importance of converting the greatest centre of learning and education in England justified almost any sacrifice." So, after twenty-four years' residence in Scotland, he left the Royal Infirmary which he loved, his large classes of enthusiastic students and his many friends and colleagues in the northern city. Preparatory to his departure in the autumn he wrote to the Board of Management on 1st August: "As my attendance at the Infirmary must for the future be at the best very irregular I beg now to

[1] *British Medical Journal*, 1875, vol. ii, p. 769.

resign the position of surgeon which I hold from you, and at the same time to express my sense of the forbearance and kindness on your part which have accompanied my tenure of office." Lister took with him to London four men to form the nucleus of his staff at King's College Hospital, William Watson Cheyne as his house surgeon and John Stewart as his clerk, along with two still unqualified students of medicine, William Henry Dobie and James Altham, as dressers.

Edinburgh, conscious of its loss, bade farewell to a dignified and charming personality, to a man gentle and unassuming, always courteous and kind; never disheartened, or with his serenity disturbed by temporary failures, but, " with faultless patience his unyielding will " pressed on by steady determination and perseverance to the goal he had set before him. He died on 12th February 1912. A general desire was expressed that he should be interred in Westminster Abbey, but, in fulfilment of his wish that he should be buried by the side of his wife, his remains were laid in West Hampstead Cemetery after a great public funeral service in the Abbey. There, a marble medallion placed in the north transept recalls the features and the name of Lord Lister.

The lively discussions and controversies, the actions in the Court of Session, and the keen public interest which characterised the early struggle for the admission of women to the study of medicine in the University of Edinburgh, on the same terms and under the same conditions as male students, are now matters of ancient history. It has been told elsewhere in considerable detail;[1] but the Royal Infirmary, then the only hospital in the city capable of giving the women the clinical instruction necessary for qualification, provided during the 'seventies of last century a stage on which some of the early encounters took place.

In the person of Miss Sophia Jex-Blake, a young English lady born in Hastings in 1840, the movement had a protagonist who was not deterred by serious opposition or by initial failure. In the spring of 1869, previously foiled in her attempt to

[1] *The Life of Sophia Jex-Blake*, by Margaret Todd, M.D. Macmillan & Co., London 1918.

gain entry to the Harvard Medical School at Cambridge, Massachusetts, she came to Edinburgh to explore the possibilities of obtaining instruction in its University. It was not her first experience of gauging public feeling in the city on this question, because in 1862, when attending the University classes for the Higher Education of Women held in Shandwick Place, she had, along with Miss Elizabeth Garrett, already tested opinion as to the prospects of obtaining a university degree in medicine. And now, in 1869, notwithstanding a reception more hostile than friendly, she reopened a campaign which, if it did not realise all her expectations, at least met with a certain degree of success.

In the spring of that year the University Court were not prepared to make temporary arrangements in the interests of one lady, or to adjudicate finally on the question of the admission of women, and accordingly recalled the favourable resolution previously passed by the Senatus. In her second attempt during the summer she appealed on behalf of herself and her fellow students for instruction in separate classes. The Senatus Academicus having then decided by a majority to admit women to the study of medicine in the University, resolved that they should receive instruction in classes confined entirely to them, but only from such professors as were willing to teach them, or from extra-academical lecturers whose courses were recognised by the University as qualifying for the degree in medicine. The University Court approved the decision of the Senate which, on 29th October 1869, was homologated by the General Council. Thus in theory, if not in actual practice, admission was gained to classes within the University.

The privilege then conceded had its repercussions in the Infirmary, as clinical instruction was essential for a complete medical education. In the hospital the gradual development of the movement may be appropriately, if briefly, considered in the three phases which distinguished it: the first short, initial period from 1870-73, the second phase consequent upon the powers granted to the Scottish Universities by the Universities (Scotland) Act, 1889, to confer medical degrees on women, and the third and final phase, in 1916-17, when during the War women were admitted to all the classes in the University in conditions similar to those open to graduation for men.

Careful perusal of the minutes of the Infirmary, however, reveal that, prior to the advent of Miss Jex-Blake, two fortuitous applications—both unsuccessful—had been made by women to obtain instruction in the wards of the hospital. In 1854, Miss Emily Blackwell, a naturalised American and a pioneer in the feminist movement, asked permission to visit the female wards during her temporary residence in Edinburgh, a request which was refused by the Board on the advice of the medical managers' committee.[1] Again, in 1862 the managers received a letter in the following terms from Miss Elizabeth Garrett : [2]—

> I purpose studying medicine with a view to practising as a physican to women and children. As any theoretic instruction I may be able to obtain will be comparatively useless unless I can, at the same time, share the facilities offered to other students for the practical study of disease, I beg respectfully to request your permission to visit the female wards of the infirmary with any of the physicians and surgeons of the hospital who may invite me to do so.

After consultation with the medical officers this proposal was also rejected as it was considered " inexpedient to grant her request in the circumstances of the hospital." What these circumstances were is not recorded.

In the autumn of 1870, following upon the decision of the University Court above related, Sophia Jex-Blake and her seven companions desiring clinical instruction knocked at the portals of the Royal Infirmary ; but their request met with a definite yet courteous refusal.[3] The hospital with the crest bearing the motto " Patet omnibus " remained closed to this small but determined band of women students. But in spite of this rebuff

[1] Minute, Royal Infirmary, 12th June 1854. Miss Emily Blackwell and her sister Elizabeth afterwards opened a Medical School for Women in New York.

[2] Minutes, Royal Infirmary, 16th and 23rd June 1862. Miss Garrett, by marriage Mrs Garrett Anderson, qualified to practise medicine in 1865 by obtaining the licence of the Society of Apothecaries. She became lecturer in medicine and Dean of the London School of Medicine for Women. She was the mother of Dr Louisa Garrett Anderson, C.B.E.

[3] Minute, Royal Infirmary, 31st October 1870.

the struggle was maintained for two years before a final settlement was reached. During that period both professional and public opinion was divided on the question of recognising their claims. A petition signed by 1326 women in favour of the admission of their sex was presented to the managers, but another, with 1200 female signatures, expressed the opposite opinion : further evidence of the public interest in the question was seen in the large attendance at the annual meeting of the Court of Contributors in January 1871, when 443 votes were recorded in the ballot for election of six representatives to the Board of Management, certain of the candidates being in favour of, others adverse to, the admission of women students.

Sixteen of the nineteen members of the medical and surgical staff of the hospital opposed the movement. But the main issue in the controversy, in the event of entry being granted, centred in the question of the instruction of women in separate or mixed classes. The former would involve a considerable reduction in the number of beds—already insufficient—available for the teaching of male students, as the regulations were such that a qualifying course of clinical instruction must be given in a general hospital containing not less than eighty beds. Consequently by withdrawing eighty beds for this special purpose, the efficiency of the Infirmary as a teaching centre for a large number of male students would be greatly impaired. If, on the other hand, both sexes were taught daily in the same wards, but at different hours, it would expose the patients to the risk of being used for teaching purposes twice daily, an unnecessary hardship which the managers were not prepared to countenance. Some of the staff held the opinion that the only solution of the difficulty would be found in the establishment of a separate hospital for women.

Amongst the lecturers in the extra-academical school who were giving the women systematic courses, the opposition to mixed classes was not unanimous. Thus at Surgeons' Square Peter David Handyside and Patrick Heron Watson taught respectively anatomy and surgery to men and women together, and George William Balfour had admitted both sexes to his class of systematic medicine. Heron Watson and Balfour, both members of the staff of the Infirmary, signified their willingness to open their wards to the women students. But the staff as a whole were obdurate and for many months the door remained closed in spite of the continuous pressure from without. It finally yielded, however, on 23rd December 1872, when, on the motion of Professor David Masson, a member of the Board and a zealous supporter of the claims of the women, it was agreed " that the Managers of the Infirmary admit the Females already matriculated in the University and enrolled on the Students' Register of Scotland, to receive clinical instruction at a separate hour from that at which Male Students are admitted into the hospital, and in a stated number of wards, containing not less than 80 beds, to which Female Students must confine their visits." This was accepted as a temporary measure carrying no underlying implication that the privilege would be extended *in perpetuo*. Accordingly arrangements were made with George W. Balfour and Patrick Heron Watson, the former to teach clinical medicine on three days in the week, the latter reserving the hour of eleven to noon on Sunday for surgical instruction. When, later, objection was taken to his selection of the hour of Divine Service, Heron Watson substituted nine o'clock on Sunday morning and, being a busy man, refused any further modification of his plans.[1]

Although entry to the Infirmary had at last been obtained, the restrictions imposed were of such a nature as to make it extremely doubtful if the women were obtaining the instruction laid down by the regulations as qualifying for the examinations licensing them to practise. No opportunities were being given to them to attend the *post-mortem* room, to see major surgical operations, or to act as clerks and dressers, nor was there any attendance on clinical lectures. They therefore petitioned the managers to be allowed to occupy the gallery of the operating theatre and, thus secluded, to attain the second of these objectives. But the request was refused, Sir Robert Christison, always a strenuous opponent of the women's movement, carrying his amendment to the motion at a meeting of the Board.[2] Complaints were made that Heron Watson's ward

[1] Minute, Royal Infirmary, 3rd March 1873. [2] *Ibid.*, 8th December 1873.

visits on Sunday were not being strictly reserved for the one sex, as his male clerks and dressers attended for the purpose of dressing the wounds of the patients, thus establishing a mixed class, contrary to the intention of the managers and to the expressed wish of the contributors ; but on this point Heron Watson was not prepared to yield. Thus terminated the first phase which, although it settled the principle of the admission of women to the Infirmary, must have given but a qualified measure of satisfaction, in view of the incomplete course of training which it implied.

Nearly twenty years were to elapse before the stage of the Royal Infirmary was set for the second phase of the drama. During the interval considerable progress had been made in the recognition of the claims of women for equality of treatment and, throughout the whole of that period, Miss Jex-Blake continued in the van of the movement. Transferring the scene of her operations to London she was successful in founding a separate school of medicine for women with an efficient staff of lecturers and, in 1877, the Royal Free Hospital opened its doors for clinical instruction. The Medical Act, 1876—the Russell-Gurney Enabling Act—extended the powers of the licensing bodies to grant qualifications for registration to all persons, irrespective of sex, and in 1878 the Senate of the University of London resolved to admit women to medical examination and degree. In the following year, having previously graduated M.D. Berne, and armed with a legal title to practise in Great Britain as a Licentiate of the King's and Queen's College of Physicians in Ireland, Miss Jex-Blake returned to Edinburgh where she opened her dispensary, the nucleus of the future Edinburgh Hospital for Women and Children. In 1886, the Royal Colleges of Physicians and Surgeons of Edinburgh having resolved to admit women to the examination for the joint qualification, the Edinburgh School of Medicine for Women was created by her, and Leith Hospital, founded in 1848, opened its wards for the clinical instruction of women students.

When the Universities (Scotland) Act, 1889, granted powers to the Commissioners to enable each of the four

Scottish Universities to admit women to graduation in one or more faculties and to provide for their instruction, the second phase commenced, the managers of the Royal Infirmary, in July 1890, receiving from the recently established Association for the Medical Education of Women an application for their instruction within the hospital. Thus the former controversy was reopened proceeding along lines very similar to those of twenty years previously. Some of the old campaigners had passed away, but a few still remained to fight another battle. The same arguments were again employed, such as the objection to mixed classes, and the reduction in numbers of clinical cases available for the male students—of whom 2044 had in that year matriculated in medicine in the University—if eighty beds should be allocated for the instruction of twelve female students. But the conditions had changed in twenty years : the principle of admitting women to the Infirmary had already been accepted, and the licensing bodies had recognised their right to sit the examinations and to receive qualifications ; moreover, the large new Infirmary offered facilities which the old Infirmary had been unable to provide, and the visiting medical and surgical staff had increased in numbers. Both public and professional opinion on this much vexed question was undergoing a salutary change.

The managers, who were then considering further extensions of the hospital and were desirous of enlisting the sympathy and financial support of all shades of public opinion, recommended, on 2nd February 1891, that the women should be admitted and taught in separate classes, an exception, however, being made in the case of certain of the special subjects, should the teachers in these subjects decide in favour of mixed classes. But opposition continued to be offered by some of the die-hards of the medical and surgical staff and by the faculty of medicine, and progress was withheld till the following summer. In the intervening months adverse opinion had certainly weakened and at a conference of the managers and the staff held on 11th July 1892 it was evident that the tide had turned in favour of the women, and, when the winter session opened in October, arrangements had been completed for their instruction. The objection to mixed classes, a barrier which at one time seemed insurmountable, had been overcome by negotiating special arrangements. Two wards were reserved for surgical and medical instruction in separate classes and placed in the charge of the senior assistant physician and senior assistant surgeon, and the women were appointed clerks and dressers. Special clinics were held by the assistant physicians for separate instruction on medical out-patients ; and facilities were provided in the wards for diseases of women, in the female Lock ward and at *post-mortem* examinations. Mixed classes, on the other hand, were held in the departments for diseases of the eye, the ear and throat and diseases of the skin.[1]

In the meantime Ordinance No. 18—General No. 9 of the Commissioners, regulating the graduation of women and providing for their instruction in the faculty of medicine and other faculties of the Universities of Scotland, had been approved by Order in Council on 28th June 1892, and in 1894 the University of Edinburgh resolved to admit women to graduation in medicine. The ordinance made provision for their instruction in any of the subjects taught within the University, either by admitting them to the ordinary classes or by instituting classes conducted by the professors and lecturers in the several subjects : " provided always that the University Court shall not institute classes where men and women shall be taught together except after consultation with the Senatus, and provided also that no professor whose commission is dated before the approval of this Ordinance by Her Majesty in Council shall be required, without his consent, to conduct classes to which women are admitted."

During the years of the Great War and in the shadow of the world's crisis the whole situation became materially altered and the third phase unexpectedly supervened. The question of the medical education of women was no longer one involving the provision of instruction in the interests of a

[1] In August 1893, in preparation for the winter session an increased number of beds for the instruction of women was obtained in ward 27, the cost of maintaining them being defrayed by the Scottish Association for the Medical Education of Women.

comparatively small group of female students. Actuated by patriotic motives the women responded in large numbers to their country's call to service and many of them commenced the study of medicine. The subjoined table reveals at a glance how their decision became at once reflected in the rapid increase in the matriculation figures at Edinburgh.

Matriculated Students in the Faculty of Medicine at Edinburgh during the Years of the War.

Academical Year.	Men.	Women.	Total Students.
1913-14	1304	78	1382
1914-15	962	106	1068
1915-16	771	157	918
1916-17	709	240	949
1917-18	823	324	1147
1918-19	1310	373	1683
1919-20	1555	413	1968
1920-21	1550	417	1967
1921-22	1457	381	1838

In the session 1915-16, sixty-six women had commenced the study of medicine in the Edinburgh School of Medicine for Women, and the Dean of the School in 1916 approached both the managers of the Infirmary and the University Court relative to arrangements for coping with the instruction of the increasing number of female students. In July of that year the Court resolved to make provision within the University to teach them, so far as was possible on the same footing as men, and appealed to the Board of Management of the Infirmary to assist them. Within the hospital the conditions were otherwise than favourable, but definite action on the part of the Board was unavoidable. The medical and surgical staff were considerably depleted, a number being on foreign service, while many of those at home were not only engaged in the work of the Infirmary but were on duty in the military hospitals in the neighbourhood of the city. Moreover, the restrictions, introduced in 1892, limiting the women to certain wards and, in some instances to separate classes, were still extant so that in all these circumstances the action of the managers was considerably hampered in their endeavour to meet the new situation.

In July 1917, however, an Agreement was concluded between them and the University Court, introducing several changes, which, in the conditions prevailing, were to be regarded as only provisional and of a temporary character.[1] The clinical instruction of women in medicine and surgery was no longer to remain in the hands of two members of the staff and be confined to the two wards previously reserved for that purpose, but all the clinical teachers—academical and extra-academical—were to teach them in rotation. The former regulations regarding separate classes were to some extent relaxed and while the two sexes continued to be taught separately in the bedside clinics in medicine and surgery and, for the first time in the department for diseases of the skin, the clinical lectures in medicine and skin diseases were to be given in conjoint classes, but were to remain separate in surgery. The teaching of gynæcology was to maintain its separate character both in clinics and lectures, while all the instruction in the ophthalmic and aural departments continued to be given to mixed classes.

In the post-war years restrictions and reservations with but one particular exception have gradually disappeared. In 1927 the physicians obtained the sanction of the managers to have mixed male and female instruction in the wards,[2] but it was not till nine years later that a similar step was taken in the teaching of clinical surgery, when mixed classes were taught both at the bedside and in the clinical lecture theatre.[3] The struggle for the recognition of equal opportunities for both sexes in their medical education had thus been prolonged over a period of sixty-six years.

Throughout the whole of the decade 1870-79 the attention of those immediately concerned with the erection of the new Infirmary was directed mainly to the preparation of the plans

[1] Supplementary Agreement between the Edinburgh University Court and the Managers of the Royal Infirmary of Edinburgh, 31st July 1917.

[2] Minute, Royal Infirmary, 28th July 1927.

[3] *Ibid.*, 22nd June 1936.

and to the all-important question of finance necessarily associated with its construction. The Committee of the Court of Contributors in their report to the General Court for the year 1869-70 did not take a very favourable view of the financial position, when considered in its relation to the immediate future. Along with a deficiency in annual income of £786 during 1870 was the further fact that part of the Capital Stock of the Corporation would in all probability be apportioned to the building of the new Infirmary, a step legalised by the recent Edinburgh Royal Infirmary Act; the committee thus envisaged a considerable reduction in the future annual revenue of the hospital. The building fund to date raised by public subscription was £75,000, but from this a considerable proportion had to be deducted to meet expenditure already incurred. Thus, £5256 had been spent in advertising the appeal, in expenses connected with the Parliamentary Bill and in meeting the liabilities incidental to the preparation of plans for the extension of the Infirmary on the existing site. Moreover, £56,330 had already been spent on the acquisition of the new sites, of which £43,000 had been paid for George Watson's Hospital and grounds and £13,330 for certain contiguous areas on the west side of Watson's property. A sum of £61,586, therefore, required to be deducted from the total subscriptions, leaving £13,414 available for the purpose of erecting the new hospital. To this, however, had to be added £21,025, which the University was willing to pay for the buildings of the Old Infirmary—a sum which eventually became £28,500 when the property was purchased by the Town Council in 1885 [1]—and a further sum of £50,000 which the managers were prepared to withdraw from the Capital Stock; [2] calculated on this basis, £84,439 were available for the erection of the new Infirmary, a very insufficient sum on which to commence the construction of the large hospital that was contemplated. In the light of the proposed deduction from Capital it was not surprising that

[1] Chapter XIII, p. 236.

[2] The ultimate sum expended on the sites purchased totalled £62,438; the Capital Stock applied to building became £71,000.

some anxiety was expressed concerning the future maintenance of the Infirmary.

Early in 1872 the architect presented his plans and estimates for a hospital containing 750 beds, computing that the probable cost in round numbers and exclusive of site would amount to £270,000, which, with architect's fees, incidental expenses and furnishing, would eventually reach a total of not less than £300,000. These estimates, however, had been prepared on the understanding that provision was to be made for a large number of beds to accommodate patients during epidemics of fever. The managers had not entirely forgotten the experience of some of their predecessors: the heavy expenses incurred by the Infirmary, the embarrassments due to overcrowding and the increased labours of the medical staff in dealing with large numbers of cases of infection, to which more than one physician had fallen a victim, still lingered in the memory of some of the members of the Board. Moreover, the Public Health (Scotland) Act, 1867, had enacted that Local Authorities should provide temporary hospitals during epidemics of fever and assess the community for their maintenance. Consequently, a hospital containing the large number of beds proposed by the architect would not be necessary.

Accordingly, fresh plans were prepared for a hospital designed for 500 beds in the first instance, of which 276 were to be medical and 224 surgical, and instructions were given that the estimates should not exceed £150,000, this being regarded by the finance committee as the probable limit of the building fund at the date of the completion of the Infirmary. The competitive offers presented by the several contractors varied somewhat, being either just above or just below £170,000, and the addition of certain incidental expenses would probably raise this figure to £185,000. The difference between the estimates submitted and those suggested by the finance committee was due to a recent large rise in wages and in the cost of material. As it was essential that a commencement should be made with the construction of the Infirmary without further delay, arrangements were made to build the medical house in the first instance and to utilise Watson's Hospital for the administrative and domestic departments. The estimated cost of this part of the scheme was £100,000 for which the managers hoped to have at their disposal a sum of £104,303.

It was not till 1874 that a commencement was made with the erection of the surgical house, the delay having been due to the fact that the building fund was not deemed sufficient to meet the additional outlay which this entailed. As the managers were contemplating the withdrawal of a further considerable sum from the Capital Stock for this purpose, legal opinion was sought as to the correctness of this step. Counsel expressed the view that the Infirmary Act of 1870 had given powers to apply, for the purpose of building, only such sums as were already held by the Infirmary Corporation and he therefore considered that it would be wiser to obtain further Parliamentary sanction to utilise more recent legacies and donations for a similar object. Accordingly the necessary action was taken, a Bill was passed through Parliament and the building of the surgical house was begun.

During the period of construction of the new hospital the Infirmary was particularly fortunate in the number of large legacies it received, specially welcome when so many commitments required to be met. Among the bequests was one of £40,000 from Mr Thomas Grindlay, Edinburgh, another of £17,500 from Mr Thomas White, £13,630 from Mr Buchanan of Dura, £13,000 from Mr David Nisbet, an architect in the city, and £6000 from Mr James Lambert, Alloa. All these gifts with many others are permanently recorded on the mural tablets placed in the corridors of the Infirmary.

The new hospital was erected in the effective and picturesque Scottish Baronial style, a model favoured by Mr David Bryce who was one of its foremost exponents. As he died in 1876 he did not see the completion of his scheme which was finished by his nephew. The medical and surgical houses, constituting two distinct groups of buildings, were constructed on the pavilion system so as to permit of the free access of the maximum amount of air and light. Each pavilion consisted of a basement floor, three main floors containing the wards, and an attic floor. The four pavilions of the medical house standing close to the Meadows were linked together by a long corridor, superimposed upon which was an open balcony connecting the wards on the second floor. The surgical house occupied the higher section of the area next to Lauriston Place. It comprised six pavilions, four facing Lauriston, the remaining two looking towards the medical house. The main entrance and hall and the principal staircase of the hospital were placed in the centre of the surgical house and surmounted by the clock tower.

The administrative departments were situated in the old reconstructed George Watson's Hospital standing between the surgical and medical houses. These included the residency, the quarters of the house physicians and surgeons, the kitchen, the apothecary's shop, the house of the Lady Superintendent of Nurses, the Nurses' Home, and the panelled chapel in which the boys of Watson's Hospital had worshipped. The two houses were connected by a corridor and balcony. The boiler-house, laundry, linenry, carpenter's shop and pathological department were in the north-west corner of the grounds and the house of the Superintendent stood intermediate between the two hospitals, close to the east boundary of the property formed by the Middle Meadow Walk. Such was the general plan of the new Royal Infirmary, worthy of the city and of the architect who designed it.

As the building operations had progressed so satisfactorily it was confidently expected that the new Infirmary would be ready for occupation during 1879. But the furnishing of the hospital, not hitherto included in any of the previous estimates of expenditure, remained to be considered, and the managers decided to appeal to the public for funds for this special purpose. The response was at once most substantial and gratifying. It was estimated that approximately £17,000 would be necessary, and the money was collected mainly from the citizens. In this connection permission was sought by a lady and her daughter resident in the city to raise a fund amongst the ladies of Edinburgh sufficient to furnish one of the largest wards in the hospital. The proposal was gratefully accepted by the Board and £552 were subscribed. Other sections of the community also interested themselves in the same object: the Edinburgh Business Women contributed £320; a sum of £534 was collected by contributions from 6000 domestic servants with which two wards were furnished; the medical practitioners in the city contributed £341; the Royal College of Physicians gave a donation of £630 for the equipment of two wards; and the sister College of Surgeons sent £210 towards the fund.

The Building Accounts were finally closed on 30th September 1884, and the subjoined table gives at a glance the total expenditure connected with the erection of the new Infirmary.

Sum expended on erection of Buildings	£254,762	13	1
Cost of Sites	62,438	10	5
Expenses of Acts of Parliament	2,015	4	6
Architect's Commission, Salaries to Clerks of Works	11,694	15	9
Laying Foundation Stone, Public Burdens, Insurance	3,436	18	11
Interest paid on Building Fund Debt to 30th September 1879	1,367	8	6
Furnishing of the Hospital	16,110	15	6
	£351,826	6	8

When the accounts were paid on the completion of the new Infirmary the managers found that they were faced with a large deficit on the building fund to the amount of £50,885, a sum, however, which was gradually repaid in annual instalments and the debt finally liquidated in 1895. The subscriptions to the building fund had only reached the sum of £88,648, the greater part of the money utilised in the construction of the hospital being obtained by transferring a sum of £200,557, obtained in part from the General Fund of the Infirmary and in part from legacies.

With the decision made to open the new hospital on 29th October 1879, the public ceremony was staged in the open space between the surgical and medical houses. In the absence of Royalty, through unavoidable engagements, the

Right Hon. the Lord Provost, Mr Thomas Jamieson Boyd, afterwards knighted by Queen Victoria in 1881 on the occasion of the Great Volunteer Review in the Queen's Park, performed the ceremony. In the circumstances no more appropriate choice could have been made as it was largely due to his enterprise and untiring efforts that the building fund had been successfully raised: after his death in 1902 his bust executed in marble was placed in the entrance hall of the Infirmary. The general interest aroused in the opening event was shown in the vast number of persons who took advantage of the privilege of inspecting the hospital, nearly 40,000 passing through the buildings during the afternoon and evening when the wards and corridors were illuminated. Two days later the patients, to the number of 240, were conveyed in cabs and other conveyances from the old to the new Infirmary, and in the evening the whole of the staff occupied their new quarters.

One final scene was set in the old Royal Infirmary, haunted by so many memories of a great and imperishable past, memories which continue to cling to such of the venerable buildings as still stand on the old site and which, during so many decades, ministered to the needs of thousands of the sick and injured poor. In the dimly-lighted operating theatre behind the old High School, in which Syme and Lister had so successfully laboured, the medical and surgical residents gathered round the operating table and in solemn cadence sang thcir parting song, " Auld Lang Sync."

CHAPTER XV

THE NEW ROYAL INFIRMARY, 1880-1889

INFIRMARY VISITED BY ROYALTY—DISTRIBUTION AND ALLOCATION OF BEDS—CHANGES IN THE PERSONNEL, THE OFFICIALS AND THE HONORARY VISITING STAFF—ELECTION OF THE STEWARD—APPOINTMENT OF JOINT TREASURER AND CLERK—FINANCES OF THE INFIRMARY—TWO NEW SPECIAL DEPARTMENTS, DISEASES OF THE EAR AND THROAT AND OF THE SKIN.

WITH the completion of the hospital and the successful transference of " the family " and patients from the old to the new buildings, the Royal Infirmary took a fresh lease of life. Standing on a wide expanse of ground, eleven acres in extent, sloping gently downwards from Lauriston Place to the Meadows, with its southern exposure and freedom from any encircling barrier of lofty tenements, the hospital as a group of buildings was a pleasing architectural addition to the city. Soon after its occupation Her Most Gracious Majesty Queen Victoria honoured the Infirmary with a visit. She was then in residence at the Palace of Holyroodhouse in connection with the great Review of Scottish Volunteers held in August 1881, since known as " the Wet " Review on account of the continuous, torrential rainfall which converted the parade ground into a sea of mud. In commemoration of this visit a surgical and a medical ward were named respectively the " Victoria " and the " Albert." In August 1884 the Prince and Princess of Wales also inspected the hospital, naming one ward " Albert Edward " and another " Alexandra."

Although the general design and layout of the several pavilions have already been sketched, a more detailed description of the accommodation and of the resources of the hospital is essential : only with this knowledge can a correct impression be gained of its enormous expansion during the next fifty years, a period in which the Infirmary has become the largest voluntary hospital in Great Britain. The architect had been instructed to prepare plans for a hospital capable of containing 500 beds, but the actual number provided was 555, of which 279 were in the surgical and 276 in the medical hospital.[1] While the majority of the surgical wards contained 16 beds, all the medical wards, twelve in number, had 23 beds. A liberal floor space was allowed so that in future years when the necessity arose, as it very soon did, beds could be added without inconvenience. A somewhat greater proportion was assigned to male than to female patients.

It would be incorrect, however, to assume that all the beds were immediately available for patients. The managers were not in a position to meet the cost of maintaining the full complement, as it was still necessary to provide in part of the old Infirmary an establishment for the treatment of cases of infectious fevers during ordinary seasons (p. 255). This made a demand upon the funds which precluded the use of the whole of the accommodation in the hospital in Lauriston Place: consequently, four wards were at first held in reserve, two surgical—32 beds—and two medical—46 beds—or 78 in all, thus reducing the number available to 477 beds, rather more than those in daily use in the old Infirmary prior to its evacuation.

In these circumstances no increase was at first made in the personnel of the honorary medical and surgical staff which remained, as in the old hospital, twenty-four in number, eleven Fellows of the Royal College of Physicians and thirteen of the Royal College of Surgeons.[2] Of the former group five were professors of clinical medicine, one being in charge of beds for the treatment of diseases of women; three were ordinary physicians; two, assistant physicians; and one was extra-physician for diseases of women. The surgical staff was constituted as follows: the two professors of surgery, three ordinary acting surgeons, one extra acting surgeon without

[1] A certain number of cots is included in these figures.

[2] These figures do not include the consulting physicians and surgeons. The names of individual members of the staff will be found in Appendix II. The pathologist to the Infirmary, being in receipt of a salary, was not a member of the honorary staff and is not included in these figures.

beds, three assistant surgeons, two ophthalmic surgeons, one surgeon for the treatment of ovarian disease and one dental surgeon. Specialism in medicine, therefore, which during the next half century was to exercise so profound an influence upon the expansion of the Infirmary, was still in its infancy: the subjects then regarded as deserving of special study were comparatively few in number, and the beds set apart for the treatment of such cases formed a small proportion of the total bed accommodation.

The distribution and allocation of the 555 beds are seen in the subjoined table.

Table showing the Number, Distribution and Allocation of the Beds in the New Royal Infirmary, October 1879.

Total Beds.	Distribution.	Allocation.		
555	195 General Surgery *	2 Professors of Surgery	87	
		3 Surgeons-in-Ordinary	102	
		1 Casualty Ward	6	
				195
	208 General Medicine	4 Professors of Medicine	104	
		3 Physicians-in-Ordinary	104	
				208
		In the Surgical House		
	74 Special Subjects	Diseases of the Eye	20	
		Venereal Diseases (female)	16	
		Ovarian Diseases (surgical treatment)	4	
		Incidental Delirium	12	
		In the Medical House		
		Diseases of Women	22	
				74
	78 Reserve Beds	In Surgical House	32	
		In Medical House	46	
				78
555				555

* The 32 beds reserved in the Surgical House were originally earmarked for General Surgery, so that the total number of beds assigned to general surgical diseases in the new Infirmary was 227.

A glance in retrospect at this stage will reveal how the growing importance of surgery was increasing the demand for more accommodation. With the introduction of chloroform anæsthesia by Simpson in 1847, surgical operations became more numerous, and as Lister's antiseptic principles in the treatment of wounds were more generally adopted, ensuring greater safety and more success in their performance, the field of surgery became considerably extended. When the new Infirmary was opened, forty-five years had elapsed since James Syme, on his appointment to the chair of clinical surgery in 1833, had become a member of the staff: at that date, 103 beds were allocated to general surgery. With the election of Joseph Lister as his successor in the chair in 1869, the number of surgical beds was increased to 190; and, with the occupation of the new Infirmary, ten years later, 227 beds were earmarked for a similar purpose, although only 195 were at first in daily use. In 1936 as many as 392 beds had been assigned for the treatment of general surgical cases, and the surgeons were seven instead of five in number as in 1879.

*Table showing the Increase in the Percentage of Surgical Cases undergoing Operation following the Introduction of the Listerian Principles of Wound Treatment with its Influence on the Range of Surgery.**

Royal Infirmary of Edinburgh—Regius Chair of Clinical Surgery.

Year.	Surgeon.	Number of Beds.	Cases in Surgical Beds.	Operations Performed.	Percentage of Operation Cases.	Percentage Mortality of Operations.
1850-51	I. James Syme	43	486	75	15·4	2·6
1865	II. James Syme	72	...	210	...	7·1
1871	III. Joseph Lister	50+	239	88	37·0	11·3
1907 (9 months, April-December)	IV. Thomas Annandale	70	715	402	56·5	5·7
1935	V. John Fraser †	58	1103	913	82·7	7·6

* *The Scottish Medical and Surgical Journal*, vol. xi. (July to December) 1902. "Fifty Years' Surgery in the Royal Infirmary, Edinburgh," by E. Scott Carmichael, F.R.C.S. Edin.

† Through the courtesy of Professor Sir John Fraser, K.C.V.O., Regius Chair of Clinical Surgery.

Prior to the period of Lister the range of surgery was restricted: amputations of limbs, excisions of joints, the removal of simple and malignant tumours, operations for stone in the bladder and occasionally for the cure of aneurism formed a fair proportion of the operations performed. But, of the total, a very considerable number would be placed today in the category of minor surgical procedures. Operations on the abdomen and brain were conspicuous by their absence in the statistical figures in groups I, II and III in the Table. On the other hand, groups IV and V include a large percentage of abdominal operations, a number often of a serious nature for which immediate operation was undertaken in the hope of saving the lives of the patients. Consequently the percentage mortality in groups IV and V is adversely influenced by the inclusion of these grave cases.

At first there was very little increase in the membership of " the family " which came into residence in the new and more spacious buildings. Few additions were made to the nursing staff which, under the supervision of Miss Pringle and three assistant superintendents, numbered 101—65 nurses and 36 probationers.[1] The female domestic staff employed in the kitchen, laundry, linenry and wards were about sixty in number. The male staff in residence included those in the boiler-house and the two porters, who occupied the lodges at the main and east gates, the chief porter combining the duties proper to his office with those of gardener. Of the two dispensers the assistant, whose services might be in demand during the night, required to live in the hospital. In addition there were eleven resident physicians and surgeons. In anticipation of a considerable increase in the work and responsibilities connected with the catering department, hitherto in the hands of the housekeeper, the managers prior to entry to the new Infirmary appointed an official, the Steward, electing Mr John Macpherson to the post.[2] Receiving a salary of £100, with free house, coal and gas, he resided in the Infirmary and was responsible for the supply of provisions, stores and coals. He held the appointment for forty years and was succeeded in 1920 by Mr Andrew Whyte, the present Steward, who is not required to live in the

[1] Nurses were drafted for periods of training to the Fever House as required.

[2] Minutes, Royal Infirmary, 7th July and 4th August 1879. The Steward and the Assistant Dispenser had residential quarters in the basement of the south-east surgical pavilion.

hospital. " The family " then numbered somewhat less than two hundred : today the nursing staff alone is more than double that number.

During the first decade in the new Infirmary changes were made in the personnel of the officials responsible for the administration and internal economy of the hospital. Early in 1879 Mr Alexander McDougall had resigned the office of Treasurer.[1] Appointed Apothecary in 1839, Treasurer-Superintendent in 1846, and Treasurer in 1871, when the dual office was abandoned on the election of Deputy Surgeon-General C. H. Fasson as the first Superintendent, Mr McDougall thus served the Infirmary for forty years, during the whole of which period he proved a loyal and valuable servant to the Institution. The vacant Treasurership, with a salary of £300 per annum, was filled by the election of Mr Alexander Ellison Ross, S.S.C., who was at the same time granted permission to retain the post of secretary to the Society of Solicitors to the Supreme Courts.[2] But his tenure of office as Treasurer was brief, as he resigned in December 1880 on his appointment as Treasurer of the Free Church. At the same meeting of the Board of Management Mr James Spence Trainer, who since 1878 had acted as Cashier, was elected his successor to commence his work on 1st January 1881.

It was during his years of service that the dual offices of Treasurer and Clerk to the Corporation were combined. In May 1883 Mr Peter Bell, then eighty-one years of age, tendered his resignation as clerk on the ground that infirmities of age unfitted him for the further discharge of his duties. Appointed House Clerk in 1843 and Clerk to the Corporation in the following year, when Mr James Hope resigned, he had given forty years of continuous service to the hospital. Reluctant though the managers were to part with one who had so long and faithfully served them, they had no alternative but to accept his resignation, and in doing so continued his salary as a retiring allowance during the

[1] Chapter XII, p. 205.
[2] Minute, Royal Infirmary, 3rd March 1879.

remainder of his life.[1] Mr Bell died in 1884. Mr Trainer was appointed in 1883 to the conjoined offices of Treasurer and Clerk at a salary of £250 and, in order to help him in his work, Mr J. M. Buckmaster, a clerk in the Treasurer's department, was made his assistant at a salary of £100.[2]

In 1887, Miss Pringle, the Lady Superintendent of Nurses, having accepted a similar appointment of responsibility at St Thomas's Hospital, London, tendered her resignation to the Board. Appointed in 1874, with a thorough knowledge of the Nightingale system of training, she had given thirteen years of service to the Infirmary and, in minuting their appreciation of her work, the managers stated that the high character and efficiency of the staff of nurses and the general excellence of the domestic staff were due to her management.[3] The vacancy then created was filled by the election of Miss Frances Elizabeth Spencer who ten years earlier had joined the staff as junior Assistant Superintendent of Nurses.[4]

At this juncture changes also occurred amongst the members of the active honorary staff of physicians and surgeons. Of these a few now made their final exit: death claimed two or three, for others the hour of retirement had struck. In 1882, George William Balfour retired: born in the manse of Sorn in Ayrshire, one of the Balfours of Pilrig—the family into which Robert Whytt, the eighteenth-century physician, had married—he was the uncle of Robert Louis Stevenson. Spending most of his boyhood in the manse of Colinton where his father had become minister of the parish, George Balfour took the Licence of the Royal College of Surgeons of Edinburgh, graduated M.D. at St Andrews in 1845 and commenced practice in the villages of Corstorphine and Cramond. But eventually attracted to the city he became a Fellow of the Royal College of Physicians, lectured on medicine and was appointed to the staff of the Infirmary in 1867. Concentrating on clinical study he early achieved great

[1] Minutes, Royal Infirmary, 29th May and 11th June 1883.

[2] Mr Buckmaster died on 26th May 1891, and funeral expenses and one year's salary were granted to his widow.

[3] Miss Pringle died on 29th February 1920.

[4] Minutes, Royal Infirmary, 20th and 27th June 1887.

success as a physician and teacher, and the women whose cause he espoused in the early days of the movement for medical education were very fortunate in their champion.[1] As a widely recognised authority on diseases of the heart his writings on the subject were regarded as medical classics, and for several years after his retirement from the Infirmary he was a busy consultant. George Balfour died at Colinton, in 1903, at the age of eighty. With the retirement of Andrew Douglas Maclagan in 1885—he was knighted in the following year—the hospital lost the services of one who had been a member of both the medical and surgical staff. Graduating doctor of medicine at Edinburgh in 1833 and, in the same year, admitted a Fellow of the Royal College of Surgeons, he was appointed assistant surgeon to the Infirmary in 1842 and acting surgeon in 1848. But his tenure of this post was brief: medicine made the stronger appeal and, resigning in 1850, he began a course of lectures on materia medica in the extra-academical school and practised as a physician. But in 1862 he was appointed to the chair of forensic medicine " where he taught the lawyer Medicine and the physician Law." Admitted a Fellow of the Royal College of Physicians in 1864, he became eligible as a professor of medicine to take charge of clinical wards in the Infirmary. Sir Douglas became president of both the Royal Colleges and thus shared with his father, David Maclagan, and with him only, the unique experience of occupying both the presidential chairs.[2] This kindly, courteous, courtly knight occupied a position all his own in the medical profession of Edinburgh. He was the life of its social gatherings, the poet-laureate of its dining clubs, charming his fellow-guests with his own compositions sung in the purest tenor. He resigned the chair in 1896 and died in April 1900, aged eighty-seven years.

Patrick Heron Watson—knighted in 1903—was born on 5th January 1832 and, like his colleague George Balfour, was a son of the manse. A graduate of Edinburgh in 1853, he

[1] Chapter XIV, p. 247.

[2] Sir Douglas Maclagan was president of the Royal College of Surgeons in 1859 and of the Royal College of Physicians in 1884.

was house surgeon with James Spence in the summer of 1854 and one of the group of seven in the "Residency" along with Joseph Lister who held a similar appointment under James Syme. Joining the Army Medical Service in December of the same year, Heron Watson proceeded to the Crimea as surgeon. Appointed junior assistant surgeon to the Royal Infirmary in 1860, to fill the vacancy caused by Lister's appointment to the chair of surgery in the University of Glasgow, he commenced his long service to the hospital. On the termination of his period of acting surgeon in 1878, his application for extension as such was refused, but the position of extra-acting surgeon was given to him with the charge of fifteen beds, "this service being limited to the occupancy of the present building"; but he remained as extra-acting surgeon in the new Infirmary without the charge of beds till 1886. A skilful and bold surgeon, "as an operator no one could touch him. He had the elegance and rapidity of pre-anæsthetic days when speed was the great desideratum, while in the range of his operations he was a generation before his time: he had excised the larynx and the spleen and had performed hysterectomy when such operations had hardly been thought of by others." An impressive and dignified personality, nothing ruffled his composure, no sudden, unexpected emergency interrupted the even tenour of his surgical procedure. He was equally successful as a physician and his prescriptions and directions to his patients were characterised by their neat and faultless caligraphy. Sir Patrick was Honorary Surgeon in Scotland to two Sovereigns and he was twice elected president of the Royal College of Surgeons of Edinburgh. Joseph Bell, the great-grandson of Benjamin Bell, the eighteenth-century surgeon in Edinburgh, left the hospital in the same year as Heron Watson. House surgeon with James Syme, 1859-61, and house physician with William Tennant Gairdner, Bell was appointed assistant surgeon to the Infirmary in October 1865 to fill a vacancy in the junior staff, Thomas Annandale being elected as his colleague in the same year to a similar post. Becoming acting surgeon in 1871 Bell at once established himself as a favourite clinical teacher. He cultivated the habit of rapid observation, training himself to take note of details which to others might appear as unimportant trifles and this, coupled with the gift of accurate deduction, made him a remarkable diagnostician. To a larger public beyond the walls of the Infirmary he was recreated in the person of one of the most popular characters of detective fiction, the "Sherlock Holmes" in the writings of his former pupil Sir Arthur Conan Doyle. After leaving the Infirmary he became the first surgeon to be attached to the Royal Edinburgh Hospital for Sick Children.

In the light of the present-day income and expenditure, a statement of the financial position of the Infirmary at the close of the year 1879-80 must necessarily be one of considerable interest as establishing further evidence, if such be necessary, of the great expansion of the hospital and the many obligations incurred during the years that have since elapsed. On 1st October 1880—the end of the first financial year in the new Infirmary—the Ordinary Stock and Funds at the credit of the Corporation were represented by a sum of £131,164; but to this must be added certain further sums earmarked for special purposes—a balance at the credit of the Convalescent House at Corstorphine, another balance at the credit of the Furnishing Fund of the new hospital, and the special fund for the New Nursing Department—which together made a total sum of £133,225. From this it was necessary, however, to deduct £50,752, standing at the debit of the Building Fund Account, thus leaving £82,473 in the Stock and Funds of the Corporation at that date. But there remained a prospective asset of £30,000, the value attached to the old buildings in Infirmary Street, so that a potential sum of £112,473 then stood at the credit of the Infirmary.[1]

The Ordinary Income during the first year of occupation was £21,540—an increase of £2841 over that of the previous year—while the Ordinary Expenditure was £27,818, being an excess over Income of £6278: this excess of expenditure over

[1] The sum finally obtained from the sale of the old property was £28,500. Chapter XIII.

income was nearly double that incurred during the last year in the old Infirmary. The Extraordinary Income derived from donations and legacies above £100 in value amounted to £18,255 : after deducting from this the excess of expenditure for the year 1879-80 there remained for transference to Capital Account the sum of £11,977. The factors mainly responsible for the increased expenditure were the maintenance of the separate establishment in the old Infirmary implying a sum of £2000, and the larger outlay on wages, coal and light in the new Infirmary, involving a sum of £2930 in excess of what had been previously expended on these items. It was at once obvious that some economy in coal would require to be effected and an alteration made in the arrangements for heating the buildings, the necessity for which was further emphasised during the specially severe winter of 1880-81. As many as 477 fire-places had been originally introduced, more than double the number in the old Infirmary, yet the temperature of the wards proved very unsatisfactory. The removal from the wards of a number of the open fire-places, a step which later permitted of the addition of more beds, and the introduction of a system of steam heating at a comparatively small cost, not only reduced the expenditure on coal but greatly improved the comfort of the inmates.

The annual average cost of the upkeep of an occupied bed was then calculated to be £60 and, with a view to supplementing the funds of the Infirmary, the recommendation was made that individuals or groups of individuals should undertake to maintain one or more by subscribing towards their endowment. The bed thus endowed would henceforth be named after the donor by attaching a plate inscribed with his or her name to the wall at its head. For the purpose of endowment the annual sum of £50 or £60 was considered sufficient or, alternatively, a capital sum of £1000 to be paid into the funds of the hospital. The first benefactors to whom the Infirmary was indebted for this form of maintenance were "The Scholars of Merchiston Castle School" who endowed and named a bed, while the second by Miss Downie of Appin, Argyll, was called the "Appin Bed." Both these gifts were made in 1881 and the beds were placed in two of the surgical wards. The practice, thus started, has been continued through succeeding years and today 255 beds and cots are maintained by special donations and bequests. But with the ever increasing cost of maintenance, calculated in 1936 at £175 per bed, at least £3000 are required for endowment, but £2000 for a bed or £1000 for a cot are accepted and the donor's name is attached.

In computing the annual average cost of occupied bed it should be clearly understood that the sum is calculated upon the total ordinary expenditure incurred in defraying the day to day expenses of all the departments of the hospital, an expenditure which includes such diverse items as the salaries of the officials in the various administrative departments and the antiseptics and surgical dressings provided for the numerous out-patients. The cost does not comprise, however, payments made on items of extraordinary expenditure such as structural improvements upon existing buildings or on the construction of extensions.

Shortly after the occupation of the new hospital the Infirmary was again most fortunate in the receipt of certain legacies of an exceptional character which, when added to the Capital Stock, provided for a considerable increase in annual revenue. In 1882-83 three legacies of the total value of £140,765 were received: the sum of £13,520 from Dr Thomas Hunter, Deputy Inspector General of Hospitals; £27,245 from Mr Thomas Laing of Linhouse in the County of Midlothian; and £100,000 from Dr Duncan Vertue, Edinburgh, formerly in the Honourable East India Company's Service.[1] In recognition of these munificent gifts wards were named the "Hunter," "Laing" and "Vertue" wards.

Year by year the number of patients seeking advice steadily increased: during 1879-80, 5315 were treated in the wards, five years later they numbered 7624 and, in the final year of the decade, 8606 were under treatment.[2] The managers, when considering the requests of the physicians and surgeons

[1] Dr Duncan Vertue's estate eventually yielded £115,000.
[2] The first and second figures include the cases of fever in the old Infirmary.

for additional facilities, were compelled at first "to hasten slowly," so long as they were hampered by the expenditure on the maintenance of the fever patients. Further, they had to decide whether such potential resources as were available in the hospital should be utilised on behalf of the special branches in medicine and surgery, then claiming recognition, or whether something more should be done to meet the requirements of general medicine and surgery. The time had undoubtedly arrived when, both in the interests of the patient and in those of medical education, the demands of specialism could not be neglected; and, so far as circumstances then permitted, the managers endeavoured to act equitably in the interests of all the parties concerned.

In 1883-84 two special out-patient departments were established, one for diseases of the ear and throat and the other for diseases of the skin, but in neither case was any provision made for indoor cases till 1891. In March 1883 Peter McBride was appointed aural surgeon in charge of the ear and throat department and, in the spring of the following year, William Allan Jamieson was elected extra-physician for diseases of the skin. Both were lecturers in their respective subjects in the extra-academical school of medicine, so that the creation of clinical departments in the Infirmary gave due recognition to the status of both these specialties. Otology and laryngology had been struggling for some years to overcome the indifference with which they were regarded by the general hospitals and teaching schools in which, with very few exceptions, they had no *locus standi*, patients seeking advice for ear and throat complaints being relegated to the care of the junior surgeons and physicians. The pioneer work of Peter McBride placed the specialty on a firm foundation and, during twenty years of service in the Infirmary, he built up a large and important department from very small beginnings in a cramped and meagrely equipped out-patient room, communicating with the first-floor corridor of the surgical house.

As far back as 1848 special instruction had been given in diseases of the skin by John Hughes Bennett and later by Thomas Laycock who, as professors of medicine, taught in the clinical wards of the Infirmary. But no specialist in dermatology was attached to the hospital till the appointment of Allan Jamieson in 1884, in charge of an out-patient department. He established regular clinics which attracted an ever-increasing number of students, and the crowded benches of the large lecture theatre on Saturday mornings testified to the popularity of his practical demonstrations on "skins." When, a few years after his appointment, he applied for additional beds his request was refused, all the physicians on the staff expressing their dissent on the ground that his clinics had already proved hurtful to clinical teaching in the medical wards ![1] But two years later, in 1891, 12 beds were allocated to the two new departments, being equally divided between Peter McBride and Allan Jamieson in a male and female ward on the second floor of the surgical house, communicating with the north side of the main corridor.[2] Although no official ceremony marked this event the opportunity was taken by the resident physicians and surgeons to celebrate the occasion unofficially, utilising the wards as their sleeping quarters on the night prior to their occupancy by the patients, their presence being discovered in the early hours of the morning by an astonished night superintendent making her rounds of the hospital.

Further facilities were also extended to those services already regarded as deserving of special recognition : thus beds were added to the accommodation that had been provided for cases of incidental delirium in order to isolate those patients who became noisy and obstreperous in the general wards and a source of annoyance to their neighbours. A male Lock Ward of 16 beds was also opened and, in 1885, 20 additional beds were given to the extra-physicians for the diseases of women. For this latter purpose two rooms, each fitted with 10 beds, were prepared in the basements of the two central medical pavilions, access to them being obtained from the wards on the first floor immediately above them by constructing a covered-in spiral staircase outside one of the

[1] Minute, Royal Infirmary, May 1889.

[2] One of these wards is now fitted up as the X-ray Diagnostic Theatre, the other as the operating theatre connected with the fourth surgical charge.

two terminal circular turrets in each of these pavilions.[1] The rooms were used as sleeping quarters by the patients who were convalescing, as they spent their day and had their meals in the wards to which they had been originally admitted. Thus all the beds previously allocated to the gynæcologists were set free for cases of a graver and more urgent character. These basement rooms became familiarly known as the "Duck Ponds," and the origin of this requires some explanation.[2] The beds reserved for the treatment of diseases of women under one of the extra-physicians were situated on the third floor of the eastermost of the medical pavilions, and the convalescents, in order to reach their sleeping-quarters in the basement of the adjacent pavilion, had each evening to make a long trek. They descended two flights of stairs, passed along the connecting corridor on the first floor and entered the ward immediately above their allotted basement room: traversing this ward they finally disappeared down the circular staircase. This nightly procession of women waddling through the ward in single file, loosely clad, their feet shod with heelless slippers and preceded by their leader, a porter assigned to the duty, so tickled the sense of humour of the Sister in charge of the ward that she aptly described them as the ducks; hence the term "Duck Ponds." Under the Clinical Teaching Agreement between the University Court and the managers of the Royal Infirmary in 1913, the basement rooms in all the medical pavilions were fitted up and used for the instruction of students and they continued to be known collectively as the Duck Ponds.

In 1887, further five beds were given to Douglas Argyll Robertson for ophthalmic cases. In response to repeated requests by Thomas Keith for more facilities, 12 additional beds in the surgical hospital were assigned to him, between 1884 and 1887, to enable him to cope with the increasing number of cases requiring ovariotomy. Keith graduated at the University in 1848, was surgeons' clerk with James Syme

[1] None of the basements in the pavilions of the Infirmary are underground and all are provided with windows.

[2] The writer is indebted to Dr William Fordyce, M.D., Consulting Gynæcologist to the Royal Infirmary, for the explanation of the term.

in 1849-50 and, a few years later, joined the Royal College of Surgeons. Although established in general practice in Edinburgh with his brother George, he identified himself with obstetrics and gynæcology and, in 1862, three years before Lister treated his first case of compound fracture by antiseptic methods, Keith commenced his first series of operations of ovariotomy. His success in this special branch of abdominal surgery was attained by scrupulous attention to cleanliness in every detail. Having applied to the managers for facilities in the hospital, he was appointed, in 1870, extra-surgeon for the treatment of ovarian diseases and was given a small room of four beds in the old Infirmary, a room previously used for clerks and students suffering from infectious fevers. In accepting the accommodation he expressed the hope that he would obtain "something better when the new hospital opened." [1] He never enjoyed robust health: tall and spare, almost cadaverous in appearance, with his long hair and pointed beard, his clothes hanging somewhat loosely on his stooping shoulders, his figure was familiar in the streets of the city. When, in 1885, additional beds were allotted to him, his son Skene Keith was appointed special assistant to the surgeon for treatment of ovarian diseases. But in 1888 father and son left Edinburgh to continue their work in London and both the appointments expired. In accepting Thomas Keith's resignation the managers placed on record their sense of the importance and value of his work and of his skill and success in the Infirmary.

After the Town Council, in July 1885, had become responsible for the care of all cases of infectious fevers in the area, the managers proceeded to erect close to the west boundary of the property a small brick building on an open space between the surgical and medical houses: as an isolation and observation hospital it provided fourteen beds for patients suffering from erysipelas and for others whose symptoms suggested the possible onset of an infectious fever. "The Cottage," as it was sometimes called, still stands the first of several new buildings erected in the grounds of the

[1] Minute, Royal Infirmary, 7th November 1870.

Infirmary; but for many years it has ceased to be used for its original purpose. In 1920, it was fitted up as a small clinical research laboratory under the charge of Jonathan Campbell Meakins, the Christison professor of therapeutics; and in the summer of 1929, when no longer required for that purpose, it was re-equipped to accommodate the classrooms connected with the Preliminary Training School for Nurses.

The claims of general surgery and medicine, however, were not altogether neglected as, in 1883, the two wards originally held in reserve in the surgical house were opened. This did not add appreciably to the sum total of surgical beds as a smaller ward, previously used for surgical patients, was placed on the reserve list. At the same time the casualty ward on the first floor, near the entrance to the surgical house and which had not been employed to any extent, was handed over to the professor of clinical surgery, the reason assigned being that "as the lifts are now in operation there is now no necessity for a casualty ward!"[1] In the medical house one of the reserve wards was opened in 1885 for female patients, and James Ormiston Affleck—afterwards Sir James—was appointed in charge as fourth physician-in-ordinary. But the restrictions originally placed upon the number of beds assigned to the large surgical and medical wards were gradually removed and more beds were attached to each, the "side rooms" being also utilised for this purpose. Consequently, as the result of the several changes above enumerated, the managers were able to announce in their annual report, presented in January 1888, that 670 beds and 30 cots provided accommodation for 700 patients. Thus the new Infirmary in the first ten years of its existence had very rapidly expanded and increased its usefulness without the necessity—with the exception of "the Cottage"—of adding to the number of its original pavilions, proof of the care and foresight with which the architect had planned his scheme of the hospital. But the next decade was to witness a further remarkable expansion, so insistent became the demands of specialism.

[1] Minute, Royal Infirmary, March 1883.

CHAPTER XVI

THE NEW ROYAL INFIRMARY

THE EXTENSION SCHEME, 1890-1904

THE NEED OF HOSPITAL EXTENSION—THE CENTRAL HOME FOR NURSES—PURCHASE OF THE CHILDREN'S HOSPITAL AND THE JUNIOR SCHOOL OF GEORGE WATSON'S COLLEGE—THE NEW LAUNDRY—THE DIAMOND JUBILEE PAVILION—THE EYE, EAR AND THROAT PAVILIONS—THE NEW SURGICAL OUT-PATIENT DEPARTMENT—THE MEDICAL ELECTRICAL DEPARTMENT.

THE last decade of the nineteenth century witnessed the commencement of a remarkable era of expansion. It is an arresting and significant fact that, eleven years after the opening of the new Infirmary designed to accommodate 555 patients, it was necessary not only to build on the open spaces surrounding the original pavilions but to acquire fresh acres for a similar purpose. Since its foundation, in 1729, the Infirmary had never failed to respond to the demands of contemporary progress in Medicine and to give manifest proof of continued vitality and power of adaptability. The growth of the hospital had not been confined to the period of adolescence but, constantly reacting to stimulus from without, had persisted through middle life and even into the period which might legitimately be regarded as that of a respectable old age. Extension indeed has been the normal feature of the life-history of the Infirmary which thus retains both the appearance and the vigour of perpetual youth.

During the 'eighties, as related in the previous chapter, it had been possible to multiply the number of beds by utilising the potential capacity of expansion possessed by each ward, but the time had arrived when more accommodation could no longer be obtained in that way. The population in the areas from which the Infirmary drew the majority of its patients was steadily growing and, during the ten years in which the hospital had been in Lauriston Place, the number under treatment in the wards showed an increase of 80 per cent.; and figures were also produced to show that, during one month alone, 217 patients had been refused admission owing to the lack of the necessary accommodation. Moreover, the resources of the hospital as an integral part of the medical school were being severely taxed, and the small proportion of beds available for the clinical instruction of large numbers of students was a ground of serious complaint. The recent decision of the Board of Management to admit women to the hospital for a similar purpose only aggravated the prospective difficulties.[1]

The number of students commencing the study of medicine at Edinburgh at that period may be accurately described as phenomenal: the maximum reached in 1889-90 surpassed all previous records, nor have they since been exceeded even in the peak year of the post-war influx in 1919-20. Three periods may be quoted in illustration: in the academical year 1875-76, 896 students matriculated in the faculty of medicine of the University, in 1885-86 the numbers had risen to 1873 and, in 1889-90, 2044 enrolled. The curriculum of study for qualification in Medicine then covered an obligatory period of four years, voluntarily extended to five years by a certain proportion of candidates; and, although residence in Edinburgh was not required throughout the whole course of study, the majority undoubtedly selected to remain. While figures are not available to permit of a correct estimate of the actual proportion attending the hospital at any one time, those who were students of medicine during the 'eighties will retain a vivid recollection of the overcrowded state of the clinics in the wards in the charge of the clinical professors. At that period students in the extra-academical school preparing for the Triple Qualification of the three Scottish Medical Corporations were another factor to be reckoned with and, though barely fifty were then receiving clinical instruction in any one year, they nevertheless helped to swell the attendance in the Infirmary.

In the winter of 1885-86 the medical faculty had petitioned the Board of Management to provide additional beds not only

[1] Chapter XIV, p. 250.

to accommodate more female patients—many of whom had to be refused admission—but to give better facilities for the instruction of those students attending the University clinics in medicine. The figures quoted in the letter from the faculty are instructive as throwing some light upon the number of students in the medical hospital : " during the quinquennium, 1875-80, those attending the classes in clinical medicine in the winter session ranged from 92 to 188, but, during the succeeding quinquennium, they varied from 217 to 274 with every prospect of a further increase in the immediate future. Moreover, owing to the excessive numbers many are denied the opportunity of acting as clinical clerks in the wards." [1]

With all these facts before them the managers had no option save to give serious consideration to a new scheme of extension. But in the meantime another matter of urgent necessity claimed their attention. The time had undoubtedly arrived when a Central Home for the nursing staff seemed eminently desirable in place of the scattered quarters provided in dormitories in the attic floors of several of the pavilions of the hospital. Segregation of the nurses in a separate building, centrally placed, would offer a reasonable chance of procuring quieter surroundings and suitable accommodation for recreation, both conducive to maintaining a better standard of health. During the first ten years of occupation of the new Infirmary twenty-three nurses had been added to the staff and all the available rooms were being utilised. The proportion of nurses to patients was in the ratio of one to five, which was less than that in the principal hospitals in London where the ratio varied from one to 2.5 to one to 3 patients. Moreover, the number of surgical operations performed in the Infirmary during the same period had risen from 665 in the first year to 1811 in the last year of the decade, these figures excluding the operations in the ophthalmic wards. This entailed extra attention and threw a considerable strain upon the resources of the nursing department. Further, the large extension of

[1] Minute, Royal Infirmary, 9th November 1885. At that date the managers were unable to accede to the request for additional beds.

the hospital then in contemplation would necessitate an addition of 50 nurses, thus increasing the numbers of the whole establishment to 214, including the lady superintendents, the nurses and probationers.

Prior to the transference of the hospital to Lauriston Place a Special Fund for the New Nursing Department had been accumulating from voluntary subscriptions, but the immediate difficulty concerned the site on which the Central Home should be placed. The only suitable area appeared to be the open space between the medical and surgical houses on the west side of the corridor and balcony connecting these two groups of buildings and adjacent to the administrative department. With the final selection of this situation the preparation of the plans was placed in the hands of Mr Sydney Mitchell, the architect, whose firm became responsible for the execution of the whole extension scheme of that period. The Home, built of red brick—known in future as " the Red Home "—was designed in the form of a quadrangle and restricted in height to two floors so as to interfere as little as possible with the access of light and air to the adjacent buildings. The foundations were laid in July 1890 and the building was ready for occupation in the spring of 1892. Although originally estimated at a cost of £13,000 and providing 60 bedrooms, the completed structure involved an expenditure of £18,972 with the provision, however, of 121 rooms, a separate bedroom being allotted to each nurse : a large recreation room and accommodation for nurses on the sick-list were also included. Access to the Home from the adjacent administrative department, in which was the nurses' dining-room, was obtained by means of a conservatory, and sufficient space remained available for a small garden to which a tennis court was afterwards added. Some of the vacated dormitories in the attic floors were used as sleeping-quarters for members of the domestic staff.

On the eve of the opening of the Red Home the Infirmary had to mourn the loss of its first Superintendent, Deputy Surgeon-General Charles H. Fasson who, during the twenty years in which he held the post, had amply justified the decision of the managers to introduce a resident official with disciplinary powers.[1] He had seen the old system of nursing give place to the new and he had been largely instrumental in reorganising the department: he had carried through the difficult and responsible task of transferring the establishment from Infirmary Street to Lauriston Place and had rendered valuable assistance in the negotiations between the Town Council and the Infirmary when the municipal authorities finally accepted the care of all persons suffering from infectious fevers in the city. He had recognised the necessity of providing a Central Home for Nurses, " watched over its erection and died much lamented on the eve of its completion," as the mural tablet at its entrance bears testimony. Fasson combined firmness of purpose with unvarying courtesy to, and consideration for, others.

In the following year another important office became vacant, that of Treasurer and Clerk, through the death of Mr James S. Trainer in November 1893, after fifteen years of service to the hospital. He had been the first to fill the conjoint post of Treasurer and Clerk instituted in 1883 upon the retirement of Mr Peter Bell.[2] In his capacity as Treasurer, Mr Trainer had been very successful in advocating the claims of the Infirmary for greater financial assistance throughout the wide area of the Scottish counties from which many persons had received the benefits of treatment in the hospital. The vacancy thus created was filled by the promotion of Mr William Strathie Caw who had been in the service of the hospital for thirteen years, during six of which he had acted as Cashier.

The decision having been reached to proceed with the extension scheme which had in view accommodation for approximately 200 patients and the provision of a new laundry, the managers, in February 1891, appointed an Extension Committee under the sub-convenership of Professor John Rankine—afterwards Sir John. It was quite obvious that for these purposes the Infirmary must extend its boundaries. With the north, east and south sides of the property definitely closed to any extension, new ground could only be obtained on the

[1] Chapter XII, p. 206.
[2] Chapter XV, p. 265.

west side. A glance at the Plan facing page 232, illustrating the area bought in 1869 for the erection of the new Infirmary, shows a narrow roadway called Lauriston Lane extending from Lauriston Place to give access at its lower or southern end to the Royal Edinburgh Hospital for Sick Children standing between the foot of the Lane and the Meadows. The purchase of the houses on the west side of the Lane and of the Children's Hospital was an essential part of the scheme of expansion.

In 1891, two of the buildings near the upper end of the Lane had already become the property of the Infirmary, one being leased to the Incorporated Edinburgh Dental Hospital and School, the other to the Royal College of Physicians of Edinburgh as premises for its research Laboratory, founded in 1887 (Plan, p. 280). The Dental Hospital had held a lease of its house since 1889, paying the managers an annual rent of £65 and agreeing to provide gratuitous dental service to the patients in the Infirmary who required such treatment. Foreseeing that it would become necessary to vacate these premises the directors of the Dental Hospital purchased, in 1892, for £4000, number 31 Chambers Street which, prior to the town-planning scheme in that district, had been one of the houses in Brown Square. The College of Physicians, who were paying £80 of rent, proceeded to negotiate for property in the immediate neighbourhood of Lauriston Lane but in 1895 bought for a sum of £7350 the old parochial buildings at the corner of Bristo Place and Forrest Road, the site still occupied by the Research Laboratory.

Lower down the Lane were two houses, numbered 11 and 12, occupied by the Juvenile or Junior School of George Watson's College for Boys, and at the foot of the Lane, number 13, was the Hospital for Sick Children already referred to. Negotiations were commenced therefore between the managers of the Infirmary and the governing bodies of both these Institutions with a view to acquiring the two properties. The directors of the Children's Hospital, although willing to entertain the proposal, were unable to find a suitable site on which to build their new hospital ; consequently, the managers faced with a difficulty did not continue at this stage separate negotiations for the purchase of the School. No agreement having been reached an alternative scheme of extension was then considered. This embraced the acquisition of the remaining houses in the upper part of Lauriston Lane, along with others in Lauriston Place facing the main thoroughfare, and the open ground extending to the tenements on the east side of Archibald Place. It was proposed to erect on this somewhat restricted area a combined medical and surgical pavilion and, in addition, to build a surgical pavilion on the part of the existing property of the Infirmary immediately to the west of the surgical house. Consideration was given at the same time to the expediency of removing the laundry to the country.

As the original scheme was unquestionably the more attractive, offering a more spacious site with greater possibilities of sunshine, negotiations fortunately carried to a successful conclusion were reopened in 1892 between the several bodies concerned. The previous difficulty in obtaining a suitable locality for the new Children's Hospital had in the meantime been overcome, as the governors of the Trades' Maiden Hospital had expressed their willingness to sell their school buildings in Rillbank Terrace on the south side of the Meadows. The price suggested was £17,500 of which sum the managers of the Infirmary agreed to pay £12,500 and the directors of the Children's Hospital the remaining £5000. The offer then made by the governors of George Watson's College to dispose of the Juvenile School in Lauriston Lane for £12,000, with right of entry on 1st October 1893, was at the same time accepted by the managers, and the whole scheme received the approval of the Court of Contributors at a meeting specially summoned to consider it.[1] Thus, for the third time in the history of the Royal Infirmary, the managers, when desirous of enlarging the hospital, approached the Company of Merchants of the City to enable them to carry out their purpose.[2]

In 1893, preparations were made to issue an appeal to the public for a sum of £100,000 to meet the expenditure upon

[1] Minute, Royal Infirmary, 4th April 1892. [2] Chapters VI and XIII.

the site, accommodation for approximately 200 beds, the new laundry and certain necessary alterations in some of the departments of the Infirmary. Arrangements were also made to hold a public meeting in the Music Hall to inaugurate the scheme. But on the eve of launching the appeal came the news of the financial crisis in Australia with the failure of the banks, involving serious loss to many Scottish investors. The time therefore was regarded as unpropitious and, in the circumstances, it was deemed more prudent to postpone any further action. Although for two years the appeal remained in abeyance, subscriptions continued to be received and in 1895 £14,000 had been raised. In the same year prospects became considerably brighter with the receipt of the welcome news that the Infirmary would benefit, at Whitsunday, 1896, by two large bequests, both unhampered by any conditions—£50,000 from the Right Hon. George Philip, 14th Earl of Moray, and £25,000 from Mr Peter Waddell of Leith. The greater part of these sums having been devoted to the complete cancellation of the debt incurred by the hospital through recent borrowing, the remainder, amounting to £32,000, was added to the building fund account and plans were prepared for a slightly modified scheme of extension.

Commencement was made with the construction of the new laundry on the site of the Dental Hospital and the Laboratory of the College of Physicians, a decision only reached after some discussion as to the advisability of building it adjacent to the hospital. While some were in favour of its erection in the grounds of the Infirmary, others held the view that it would be more appropriately placed in the country or handed over to one of the public laundries in the city. That there should have been a difference of opinion on this point is not without interest at the present time, as the same question again occupied the attention of the Board of Management in connection with a more recent scheme of extension.[1] When the final decision was made not to depart from the oldstanding arrangement, Sir Henry Littlejohn, the medical officer of health, objected on the ground that the laundry in the neighbourhood of

[1] Minutes, Royal Infirmary, March, April, 1932.

Lauriston Place was contrary to the first principles of public health and should be placed in the country where the soiled bed and body linen could be washed under the best sanitary conditions and the occupants of the houses in the vicinity of the Infirmary would thus be relieved of a source of great annoyance.[1] But the managers, although appreciating Sir Henry's public spirit, saw no adequate reason to alter their decision. It was essential that the part of the laundry work requiring immediate attention should be carried out on the premises; further, two laundries were an undesirable arrangement entailing additional cost and labour: moreover, the necessary mechanical power had already been introduced and could not be transferred elsewhere. There was no legal objection to the existing site and no nuisance was anticipated, as every care had been taken in planning the new building to provide good ventilation. The laundry was therefore built and was ready for occupation early in 1898. In its construction a division was made into two separate departments, the one for the laundry of the patients, the other for that of the nursing and domestic staff. Accommodation for thirty-one laundry maids was also provided on the upper floors, along with a dining room and bathrooms, care being taken that these rooms should not be situated immediately above the washing and ironing departments.

Good fortune once more came to the assistance of the Infirmary at this critical time. During 1896 plans were in preparation for two new pavilions, one mainly for the treatment of diseases peculiar to women to be erected on the sites of the former Hospital for Children and on that of the Juvenile School and, between these and the laundry, the second and smaller pavilion to accommodate patients suffering from diseases of the eye. But at this time the citizens of Edinburgh, considering how they might commemorate the Diamond Jubilee of Her Majesty Queen Victoria, resolved to raise a fund, nine-tenths of which were to be devoted to the erection of the pavilion for women at the Royal Infirmary and one-tenth to the Queen Victoria Jubilee Institute for

[1] Minute, Royal Infirmary, 3rd August 1896.

Nurses. Thus the way was opened for a more complete realisation of the extension scheme, making it possible to include in it the construction of a third pavilion to provide a larger number of beds for patients with diseases of the ear and throat.

As the cost of the first pavilion was to be in part defrayed from this special fund, it was desirable that it should not only be known as the Diamond Jubilee Pavilion but that it should embody some architectural features to distinguish it from the other pavilions of the hospital. Although of greater length and more massive than its neighbours it was decided that the two terminal turrets on the south elevation should be made octagonal in shape instead of in the circular pattern which characterised those of the other buildings ; and, in addition, it was proposed to introduce a stone slab into the balustrade protecting the central balcony on the south front outside the ward on the second floor, this stone to bear the following inscription :—

> Dedicated to the glory of God and the healing of human suffering in commemoration of the sixtieth anniversary of the accession to the Throne of Her Most Gracious Majesty, Queen Victoria, the thank offering of many for great benefits bestowed upon the realm during her reign.

The distinction between the jubilee pavilion and the others was destined to be achieved in a much more striking fashion than that obtained by octagonal turrets and a commemoration stone. The new Infirmary for the most part had been constructed of grey stone excavated from the Hailes Quarry, on the western outskirts of the city situated between Slateford and Colinton, one of the several quarries around Edinburgh supplying stone for its buildings and for the paving of its streets. When informed by the architect that fresh excavations would be necessary at Hailes and that probably twelve months would elapse before sufficient stone was available for the construction of the pavilion, the managers decided that the best course to pursue was to use the red stone of the Corsehill and Corncockle quarries in Dumfriesshire and thus definitely distinguish the new pavilion from the others.[1] Force of circumstances, therefore, had compelled the erection of a building, the colouring of which was out of harmony with the rest of the Infirmary. On its completion the opening ceremony was performed by H.R.H. Princess Henry of Battenberg on 26th October 1900, the occasion being suitably commemorated on a mural tablet placed outside the entrance to the ward on the first floor of the pavilion.

The jubilee pavilion, like all the others, comprised a basement which contained the Baths Establishment, three main floors for wards, two reserved for the treatment of the diseases of women and the third as a male ward for ordinary medical cases, and in the attic storey separate rooms for nurses and servants. Each ward accommodated 26 patients, making a total of 78 in the pavilion. This arrangement remained in operation till 1922 when a third gynæcologist was appointed and the three wards, with the beds increased to 90, were devoted to the treatment of diseases of women. When this specialty first received recognition in the Royal Infirmary, on the appointment of James Young Simpson to the staff in 1850, the title of extra-physician for diseases peculiar to women was attached to the office. But just prior to the erection of the new pavilion, the managers, on the recommendation of the Fellows of the Royal College of Physicians, agreed to apply the designation of gynæcologist to those in charge of the department, the change being made in 1898 after it was agreed that Fellows of the Royal College of Surgeons should become eligible for these appointments.[2]

The financial assistance derived from the jubilee fund for the erection of the gynæcological pavilion, supplemented in 1898 by a handsome legacy of £38,822 from Mr James L. B. Yule, a citizen of Edinburgh, which the managers resolved to apply to the scheme, made it possible to proceed with the rest of the extension. Consequently, early in 1900, a commencement was made with the construction of the two smaller pavilions on the vacant ground between the Juvenile School

[1] Minutes, Royal Infirmary, 10th, 17th, 24th January 1898.

[2] Minute, Royal Infirmary, 20th December 1897.

and the laundry. Both were built of the grey stone from Hailes Quarry and were ready for occupation in 1903. The larger of the two appropriated for diseases of the eye gave accommodation for 44 beds and the smaller for diseases of the ear and throat made provision for 28 patients.[1] Each formed a complete unit providing in addition to the wards an out-patient and teaching department.[2] And so this extension scheme, initiated in 1891, had been steadfastly pursued to a successful termination after twelve years of varying fortune and in spite of frustrated hopes and delays from quite unexpected causes. Its completion terminated the labours of the committee which, under the sub-convenership of Professor John Rankine, had borne the burden and heat of the day. Sir John was Professor of Scots Law in the University of Edinburgh from 1888 to 1922, and a member of the Board of Management of the Infirmary continuously for thirty-three and a half years, 1889-1922, on which he represented alternately the Senatus Academicus and the Faculty of Advocates. His professional advice was of great value to the Law Committee of the Board on many occasions, he was its convener for twenty-seven years and, as sub-convener of the Extension Committee, he handled difficult situations with tact and circumspection.

In the subjoined table the receipts and expenditure in connection with the extension scheme are briefly recorded.

A. *Receipts.*

Donations	£34,966
Transferences from Extraordinary Account	41,601
Legacies applied to Building Fund	59,673
Interest, Rents, Income Tax returned, miscellaneous	6,401
Balance Royal Bank on account of Fund	1,642
	£144,286

[1] In 1926, two new wards were added to the ear and throat pavilion containing 31 beds, thus making 59 beds in the department.

[2] The large eye ward vacated in the Surgical House was not again occupied by patients till 1907 when it became, along with the new Ward 1, the enlarged department for diseases of the skin.

B. *Expenditure.*

Sites, Lauriston Lane Houses and Children's Hospital	31,886
New Laundry	16,320
Diamond Jubilee Pavilion	40,808
Eye, Ear and Throat Pavilions	48,818
Drainage, connecting corridors, grounds, etc. . .	6,441
	£144,286

Note.—The totals are expressed in round numbers, thus explaining the apparent error in calculating the total amounts. The sum received from the Jubilee Fund, included under donations, was £17,638. The Red Home for Nurses was a separate scheme and is therefore not included in the statement.

The large scheme of extension was not the only project with which the managers were then concerned. Although the Infirmary buildings were of comparatively recent date and in the 'nineties might reasonably be regarded as modern, the rapid advances in science compelled the introduction of improvements which could not be withheld. In 1897, it was deemed highly expedient to replace the old system of lighting with gas by a complete installation of electric illumination. This necessitated wiring of all the pavilions and the substitution of the original 2690 gas burners with the requisite number of electric lamps, entailing an expenditure of £5500. At the same time the opportunity was taken to introduce the system of telephonic communication throughout the hospital which, ten years later in an amended form, was placed under the control of the National Telephone Company. A new boiler-house and plant for heating of the most approved type were introduced, and a taller chimney erected to obviate the smoke-nuisance complained of by the neighbours. A kitchen to meet the needs of the enlarged hospital was also necessary, a reconstruction which incidentally terminated the long series of Kitchen Concerts, popularly known as the " K.C.," and conducted annually by the resident physicians and surgeons.[1] When it became obvious that the life of these concerts would be threatened by the inevitable

[1] Minute, Royal Infirmary, 26th October 1896, " permission granted to the Residents to hold the K.C. on 18th December." Minute, 23rd August 1897, " request to hold the K.C. declined."

changes in the kitchen that were forecasted, the decision was made to found the Edinburgh Royal Infirmary Residents' Club to carry on the traditional reunion of past and present residents by holding an annual dinner in Edinburgh.[1] But perhaps the most important and certainly the most costly improvement then carried out was the new system of plumbing and drainage, as that originally introduced had become obsolete. This extensive work commenced in 1900-01, but not completed till 1908, involved an extraordinary expenditure of £34,000.

Reorganisation of the Surgical Out-patient Department was first considered in 1895, if the term department can be appropriately applied to the arrangements then in operation in the Infirmary for the attendance upon the surgical out-patients. In the early days of the new hospital, a reception room at the entrance to the surgical house provided accommodation for the preliminary examination of casualties and for such minor treatment as was deemed necessary, if the injury or ailment did not require treatment in the wards. But during the recognised visiting hours of the surgeons the majority of the out-patients proceeded to the wards of the surgeon on duty for the day, where they were examined and treated in accommodation which left much to be desired. The system was not satisfactory either in the interests of the patients or of the students of medicine, who were denied opportunities of obtaining useful experience in the treatment of the lesser surgical ailments which constitute a considerable part of daily professional work.

The alterations in the out-patient department included the provision of a large waiting-room obtained by reconstructing what had been the original casualty ward on the first floor of the north-east surgical pavilion, the ward handed over in 1883 to the professor of clinical surgery as part of his surgical charge when the lifts in the hospital first came into operation.[2] In addition, a series of small rooms was converted into "dressing rooms" for the treatment of wounds, and the whole department was supervised each day by the assistant surgeon attached

[1] The first dinner of the Club was held on 3rd May 1895. [2] Chapter xv, p. 276.

to the surgeon on duty. Such an arrangement, although effecting some improvement, could scarcely give complete satisfaction ; consequently, in 1904, a large committee of the managers were appointed to discuss with the staff a new plan for the conduct of the department. Following their deliberations a small theatre was built for the treatment of patients and the instruction of students, a casualty ward was again attached to the department and more dressing-room accommodation was provided. Three resident house surgeons were appointed, along with the requisite number of nurses and porters. The care of the out-patients was entrusted to the two junior assistant surgeons alternately for periods of six months at a time, while the clinical teaching was carried out by the assistant surgeon attached to the surgeon on duty for the day. This arrangement permitted of a more prompt and efficient service. Some years later (1921) the whole service of the department, examination, treatment and clinical teaching, was placed in the hands of the two junior assistant surgeons ; and, as recently as 1936, a casualty ward of six beds was opened for the temporary accommodation of patients whose condition was not deemed of such a nature as to require admission to the general wards ; and for patients operated upon by the surgeons in charge, when their immediate return home was not considered advisable.

Specialisation, however, continued to make still further demands upon the resources of the Infirmary. The employment of electricity as an aid in the diagnosis and treatment of disease and injury was becoming of increasing importance and, after the installation of the electric current throughout the hospital, the establishment of a Medical Electrical Department could not be delayed. The period coincided also with two remarkable discoveries which were soon to revolutionise medical practice in two particular directions. In 1895, Professor Röntgen had discovered that certain radioactive electrical waves, invisible to the eye—named the X-rays—could penetrate opaque substances impervious to ordinary light and affect sensitive photographic plates. In the following year Henri Becquerel announced that the emission of similar radio-active rays was produced from the metal uranium, and, in 1898, the investigations of Monsieur and Madame Curie led to the discovery of other substances with precisely similar properties, with varying degrees of penetration, amongst which was the element to which they gave the name of Radium.

The arrangement and equipment of the Medical Electrical Department were intrusted to Robert Milne Murray who, in November 1896, was appointed Medical Electrician to the Infirmary. As physician to the Edinburgh Royal Maternity and Simpson Memorial Hospital and as lecturer in midwifery and gynæcology in the extra-academical school he had mapped out his professional career as a specialist in these two branches of medicine ; and in accepting this new office he made the proviso that his chances of election to the post of assistant gynæcologist to the Infirmary, when such became vacant, should not be jeopardised. A man with many interests, a lover of the Arts, with a fine appreciative sense of the value of old prints, a musician, a chemist, mineralogist and geologist, Milne Murray had added the study of electricity to his other pursuits, and his intimate knowledge of the subject as a science and in its application to medicine eminently fitted him to take charge of the new department.[1] Dawson Fyers Duckworth Turner, lecturer in physics at Surgeons' Hall, was at the same time appointed assistant medical electrician. He early recognised the importance of the X-rays in their application to medicine and the possibilities inherent in radium as a remedial agent and, having purchased a small quantity of that element, he generously placed it at the disposal of the Infirmary.

The very limited accommodation available for the electrical department was found beneath the operating theatre of the professor of clinical surgery. The old splint room and the plumber's workshop were ingeniously converted into four small rooms, two of which were used as examination rooms and for the calibration of the electrical instruments, while the

[1] Robert Milne Murray was elected assistant gynæcologist to the Infirmary in 1901 ; he died in 1904 at the early age of 49 years.

X-ray diagnostic room—the only use then made of the Röntgen rays—and the photographic development room were placed in the basement beneath, reached by an ill-lit and precipitous staircase. The necessary equipment and apparatus were installed for the modest sum of £500; and these cramped and dingy quarters were made the temporary home of a young department which was to become, a few years later, of increasing usefulness and importance as an aid in the diagnosis and treatment of disease and injury. Better accommodation was soon a matter of urgency and, in 1903-04, the whole of the basement of the south-east surgical pavilion in which were the residential quarters of the Steward and the Dispenser, was reconstructed and adapted for its new purpose.[1] There the work was carried on for twenty-two years, often under difficulties as it continued to increase, till the new Radiological Department, built and equipped at a cost of nearly £50,000, was opened in 1926.

The events narrated in this and the previous chapter carry the story of the Infirmary to the close of the first quarter of a century of its life in Lauriston Place. The occasion seems suitable to review very briefly the course of events during those twenty-five years, and the appended table will show at a glance its remarkable capability of expansion and its extended sphere of usefulness.

Number of Beds and Patients Treated.	1879-80.	1903-04.
Beds in the Infirmary	555	850
Patients treated in the wards	5,315	11,125
Average daily number in wards	469	810
Highest number on one day	525	852
Out-patients treated	15,000	33,412
Ordinary Income	£21,541	£33,814
Ordinary Expenditure	£27,818	£49,808

Then as now, ordinary expenditure exceeded ordinary income.

[1] After this date these two officials no longer lived in the Infirmary.

Through the kindness of a friend of the hospital the two scriptural texts which for so many years had been inscribed on the front elevation of the old Infirmary were carved upon the stone above the main doorway of the new, "I was a stranger and ye took me in," "I was sick and ye visited me"; and between these two inscriptions was engraved the Pelican, part of the crest of the Royal Infirmary and beneath it the motto, "Patet Omnibus." In addition, two dates are recorded, 1730 : 1879. The first has no special significance in the history of the Infirmary and, in all probability, should be 1729, the year of the foundation of the hospital; 1879 commemorates the year of the opening of the present building.

CHAPTER XVII

THE ROYAL INFIRMARY IN THE TWENTIETH CENTURY—THE YEARS BEFORE THE WAR 1900-1914

APPOINTMENTS OF OFFICIALS, THE SUPERINTENDENT AND THE LADY SUPERINTENDENT—INTRODUCTION OF THE AGE-LIMIT OF SERVICE OF THE MEDICAL AND SURGICAL STAFF—THE CLINICAL TEACHING AGREEMENTS OF 1913 AND 1929 — CHANGES IN THE MEDICAL AND SURGICAL STAFF.

THE passing of the years brought changes in due course in the personnel of the Infirmary and, very early in the century, death or retirement on account of age released certain of the officials of the hospital from their labours. Following the death of Surgeon-General Fasson in 1892,[1] a successor as Superintendent had been found in Surgeon-Major-General Stewart A. Lithgow, C.B., D.S.O., M.D., Army Medical Service, then stationed at Portsmouth as Principal Medical Officer to the Southern District. He had joined the army in 1855 as surgeon with the 75th Regiment and, during thirty-eight years many of them spent on active service at the Cape, in India during the Mutiny and in Egypt, he had held both at home and abroad several administrative posts which had qualified him for his new appointment. But his tenure of the office of Superintendent was brief: he died when on leave in the autumn of 1899, without seeing the completion of the large extension scheme which had occupied so much of his attention and time during the eight years of residence in the Infirmary. Colonel William P. Warburton, C.S.I., M.D., who had recently retired from the Indian Medical Service, was selected as his successor. Like his predecessor he was a graduate of Edinburgh, one with very considerable administrative experience gained in India as Medical Officer to the Native State of Kapurthala and in the more responsible

[1] Chapter XVI, p. 280.

position of Inspector-General of the Civil Hospitals of the North-West Provinces and Oudh, when he controlled both financial and medical arrangements. He retired from his post in the Infirmary in July 1911, but his days of leisure were few in number as he died in the month of October. During his predecessor's tenure of office a rise in the price of foodstuffs and an enforced increase in the salaries and wages bill of the Infirmary had raised the average cost of occupied bed to £71 per annum, as it had been found necessary to augment both the nursing and domestic staff in order to provide more opportunities for rest and recreation. Notwithstanding this rise in expenditure Warburton was able before the end of his period of office to reduce the annual cost of occupied bed to £60, an evidence of his faculty of combining economy with efficiency in administration. Colonel Warburton was succeeded in the post of Superintendent by Lieut.-Colonel Sir Joseph Fayrer, Bt., Royal Army Medical Corps, Commandant of the Military Hospital, Hong Kong, from 1909 : he commenced his duties on 1st August 1911.

About the same time another important administrative post in the Infirmary fell vacant through the retirement in June 1907 of Miss Frances Elizabeth Spencer, the Lady Superintendent of Nurses, after thirty years in the service of the hospital. Coming to Edinburgh in 1877 as junior assistant superintendent she succeeded Miss Pringle ten years later, and a memorial tablet placed in the chapel of the Infirmary by the unanimous resolution of the managers commemorates her devotion to duty. She died on 15th April 1908, within less than twelve months of her retiral, being buried at Dollar where her grave is marked by a Celtic cross raised to her memory by her fellow-workers and the nurses whom she trained. Her post was filled by Miss Annie Warren Gill, C.B.E., R.R.C., Matron of the Royal Berkshire Hospital at Reading, after her return from South Africa in 1902. Her appointment as Lady Superintendent of Nurses in the Royal Infirmary meant a return to the scene of her former labours as she had been one of the assistant superintendents of nurses prior to 1900. On that date she was appointed matron of the Edinburgh and East of Scotland South African Hospital which left Edinburgh in March of the same year with David—Sir David—Wallace and Francis Darby Boyd, both members of the Infirmary staff, as the surgeon and physician in charge.

At varying intervals of time new rules and regulations were deemed necessary for the management of the hospital and, as those approved of and put into practice in 1881 had with a few modifications been in use for a number of years, the managers, in 1897 and again in 1903, considered it advisable to submit them to a thorough revision. The large extension of the Infirmary, completed early in the century, with the increase in the personnel in several departments, necessitated alterations in the rules, and the opportunity was taken to reconsider more particularly those concerned with the terms of service of the honorary physicians and surgeons. Since the Board of Management had first become responsible in the middle of the eighteenth century for the selection of members of the medical and surgical staff, the duration of their period of office had been extended more than once and, when the revision was undertaken in 1903, the rule governing their appointments, which had been approved by the Court of Contributors in January 1897, was as follows :—" The Physicians and Surgeons shall be appointed for five years with eligibility for reappointment at the discretion of the managers for a second and third term of similar duration. The whole term of office shall not exceed fifteen years." To this the following footnote was appended : " The terms Physicians and Surgeons include Professors having wards in the Infirmary, excepting under that portion of the Rule limiting the term of office to fifteen years." In other words, while all the members of the honorary staff were subject to election for five years and re-election at intervals of five years, the period of service of the professors was not to be terminated at the end of fifteen years, but was to continue during the tenure of their chairs. In 1900 an addition had been made to the above rule to the effect that " Power is reserved to depart from this limitation in the case of Physicians and Surgeons who have charge of wards devoted to special classes of disease, when, in the opinion of the managers, such departure would, for special reasons stated, be deemed expedient in the interests of the Infirmary."

The committee, to whom had been assigned the duty of again revising the rules in 1903, proposed to the Board that they should "fix an age-limit beyond which no one could hold office as Physician or Surgeon, and suggest sixty years as a suitable age." This motion was agreed to, "it being resolved, however, that the Rule shall not apply in the case of Physicians and Surgeons who are presently serving their second or third term of office, or to the Professors."[1] Although the introduction of an age-limit in the case of the medical and surgical staff was an entirely new departure in the history of the Infirmary, the possibility that such a measure might become necessary in the future had been brought to the notice of a previous Board of Management in 1886, when the question of delay in promotion of members of the surgical staff was under consideration. The suggested remedy was the introduction either of an age-limit applicable to the appointment and retirement of the surgeons, or the election of the assistant surgeons for a limited period of five years. On the motion of Dr—Sir John—Batty Tuke, a member of the Board, a committee was appointed to consider whether modification of the existing arrangements in the surgical department was desirable, there being at that time a vacancy in the staff of the assistant surgeons. Sir John in presenting a minority report contended that under the existing regulations if the vacancy was filled by the election of a candidate aged thirty years he could not be promoted surgeon till he had reached the age of fifty-six and, under the time-limit of fifteen years, he would not be due to retire till he was seventy-one years of age; again, when the next vacancy should occur and a candidate aged thirty was elected, he would be fifty-four when promoted and sixty-nine at the time of his retirement. It was essential for the success of the hospital and the reputation of the medical school that surgeons should hold appointments during the years when they would prove

[1] Minute, Royal Infirmary, 23rd March 1903.

most efficient as practitioners and teachers.[1] As the committee of the Board were of the opinion that the ordinary accidents of appointments to other schools, of retirements and of deaths amongst the staff would, in the future as in the past, prevent the position of surgeons being held by men too advanced in years, no further consideration was given to the question of age limitations, and the managers proceeded to the election of an assistant surgeon.

As the resolution of the managers to fix an age-limit had been adopted in 1903 without any previous consultation with the physicians and surgeons, it was only natural that the staff should desire the opportunity of expressing their views upon a change which would have such an important and far-reaching effect upon their future connection with the Infirmary. As the assistant physicians and surgeons were frequently appointed when they were considerably over thirty years of age, they did not as a rule obtain charge of wards till fairly late in life, so that the enforced retirement at the suggested age of sixty would greatly curtail their period of office as physicians and surgeons. Enquiry on the part of the staff revealed that, in eleven of the large hospitals in London, eight had a retiring age-limit at sixty-five, and two at sixty, while in one there was no limitation on an age basis. In three of the hospitals in London, where a time- and an age-limit coexisted, the former was fixed at twenty years, and in hospitals elsewhere in Great Britain twenty years were also the prescribed period. Moreover, if the age-limit of sixty was introduced in the Infirmary it would shorten the term of office of every member of the medical and surgical staff and, further, it would mean the coincident retirement at recurrent intervals of several members of the staff. Thus between the years 1912 and 1915 the hospital would lose the services of five physicians and, between 1912 and 1918, as many as ten—physicians and surgeons—would be obliged to retire. It was felt that the loss of so many senior men of experience would be detrimental to the interests of the Infirmary in its dual capacity as a hospital for the treatment of the sick and injured and as a teaching centre.

1 Minutes, Royal Infirmary, 12th April and 8th November 1886.

Upon the question of delay in promotion of the junior members of the staff to senior posts, emphasis was laid by the staff on the fact that this was in part attributable to the long term of service of five of the senior staff—three professors of clinical medicine and two professors of surgery—who would not be affected by the introduction of the age-limit, as the resolution of the Board agreed to on 23rd March 1903 exempted the professors from retirement at the age of sixty years. The staff suggested that the age-limit should be fixed at sixty-five years and, further, that an additional surgical charge should be created with a view to relieving the slow promotion in the surgical house. As the result of their conferences with the staff the managers, on 26th October 1903, altered the previous resolution and agreed " to fix an age-limit beyond which no one could hold office as Physician or Surgeon, and that the limit be sixty-five years of age " ; but the rule was not to be retrospective in the case of those physicians and surgeons serving their second or third term of office, nor apply to the professors then holding chairs.

Under Section 23 of the Edinburgh Royal Infirmary Act, 1870, the General Court of Contributors " may from time to time alter any of the Statutes of the Infirmary Corporation or make new Statutes in relation thereto. . . ." Consequently, the new rule was submitted to the Court at the annual meeting on 4th January 1904. It was agreed by a majority that in the public interest the age-limit of sixty-five enacted by the managers for the ordinary physicians and surgeons should be made applicable also to those physicians and surgeons who were professors in the University. But at the statutory adjourned meeting of the Court of Contributors a majority ruled that the approval of the new rule be delayed and that a special committee of the managers and of the Court should consider the whole question and report. The two contentious points were, should an age-limit of service be introduced and, if so, should it apply to the professors holding appointments as physicians and surgeons? In submitting their report at a special meeting of the Court on 14th November 1904, the special committee, although divided in their opinion, recommended by a majority that no age-limit should be adopted for members of the ordinary medical and surgical staff, and that, accordingly, the resolution agreed to by the Court, on 4th January, requiring professors to retire at sixty-five be rescinded. The approval of the committee's report was moved and seconded, but an amendment recommending that an age-limit be adopted for all physicians and surgeons, including the professors, and that the age-limit be sixty-five was carried by a majority and became the finding of the meeting. Obviously opinion was divided upon the question of establishing an age-limit for the professorial members of the staff of the Infirmary.

This rule, which took effect on 1st January 1905, still regulates the appointment of all the members of the honorary visiting staff, its full terms being as follows :—

> The Physicians and Surgeons shall be appointed for five years, with eligibility for re-appointment at the discretion of the managers for a second and third period of similar duration, but no Physician or Surgeon shall hold office after attaining the age of sixty-five years. The whole term of office shall not exceed fifteen years. Power is reserved to depart from the latter limitation in the case of Physicians and Surgeons who have charge of Wards devoted to special classes of disease, when, in the opinion of the Managers, such departure would, for special reasons stated, be deemed expedient in the interests of the Infirmary.
>
> The terms Physicians and Surgeons include Professors having Wards in the Infirmary, excepting under that portion of the Rule limiting the period of office to fifteen years.[1]

Thus the age-limit was imposed upon all members of the staff holding the office of physician or surgeon, whether professors in the University or not ; but, in the case of those who were not professors, the period of service was also curtailed by the time-limit of fifteen years, their tenure of office ceasing when either the age-limit or the time-limit was reached. In those days professors in the universities of Scotland held

[1] The new Rule, introduced on 1st January 1905, was not made retrospective in the case of professors then occupying their Chairs or of those physicians and surgeons who at that date had completed five years of service as such. It was not till 1918 that the Rule became applicable to every member of the staff.

their chairs *ad vitam aut culpam* as no compulsory age-limit for retirement was then in force. When the Universities (Scotland) Act, 1922, conferred powers upon the several Courts to make ordinances for the superannuation and pensioning of Principals and Professors, the University Court of the University of Edinburgh by an Ordinance approved by Order in Council, dated 25th July 1924, made provision for the retirement of the professors at the end of the academical year in which each attained the age of seventy years.[1] But those professors whose appointments were otherwise regulated through the position which they held as physicians and surgeons in a hospital were subject to the rules of retirement of the Institution in which they held office.

Although the professorial members of the honorary staff were exempted from that part of the rule which limited their period of service to fifteen years, it was the practice of the Board of Management for a number of years, when appointing the professors of medicine, surgery and midwifery to posts on the staff of the Infirmary, to elect them for a period of five years, re-electing them for further similar periods, subject to retiral on reaching the age-limit. This procedure continued to be carried out by the Board till 1929 when the revised Clinical Teaching Agreement between the managers and the University Court made provision for its discontinuance.[2]

The first professorial appointment to the Infirmary following the adoption of the age-limit occurred in 1908 when the death of Thomas Annandale, on 20th December 1907, created a vacancy in the regius chair of clinical surgery.

In 1877, Thomas Annandale had been appointed successor to Lister in the chair of clinical surgery. Born in Newcastle-on-Tyne in November 1838, where at the age of fifteen he had received his baptism in surgery in his father's practice, Annandale came to Edinburgh in 1856 to study medicine. After acting as house surgeon with James Syme during 1861-62 and as his assistant in the years that followed, he was promoted

[1] The retiring age of the Principals of the Scottish Universities was fixed at seventy-five years.

[2] Clinical Teaching Agreement, 1929, Article 7: also Article 3 of Appendix relative to the Regulations of the Board of Management.

to acting surgeon in the Infirmary in 1869. He was thus intimately linked with the older school of surgeons whose dexterity, rapidity of action, resourcefulness and courage were essentials of their craft, all of which qualities Annandale possessed. " Surgeons are born not made " was a favourite dictum of his which was certainly illustrated in his own person, and both as an operator and as a teacher of clinical surgery he followed closely the methods he had learnt from Syme. Of medium height, sprightly in his walk, neat in his dress, with his coloured necktie knotted in a loose bow after the fashion of his old master, he was a familiar figure in the streets of Edinburgh, saluted by the policemen on duty and by the " cabbies " on the ranks, for all of whom he had a cheery greeting. Himself the soul of punctuality he expected the same from his assistants who, in the early morning, not infrequently found him on his doorstep at 34 Charlotte Square ready to start for the nursing home two or three minutes before the pre-arranged hour. The vacancy in the regius chair was filled by the appointment of Francis Mitchell Caird. Having on his election resigned his appointment as ordinary surgeon to the hospital, he was placed by the managers in charge of two university wards for a period of five years with eligibility for reappointment subject to the condition regarding his retirement at sixty-five.[1]

When the question of delay in promotion of the junior members of the honorary staff had been under discussion, it will be recalled that the suggestion was made that an additional surgical charge should be created with a view to accelerating promotion. Prior to 1904 the surgical beds were distributed amongst five surgeons, the two professors of surgery and three ordinary surgeons, but in that year the managers had promoted to full surgeoncy—and incidentally to full physicianship—the senior assistant surgeon and assistant physician in charge of the two wards assigned for the clinical instruction of women students.[2] Thus an additional or fourth ordinary surgeon had been added to the staff. The creation of a fifth surgical charge

[1] Minutes, Royal Infirmary, 22nd June and 20th July 1908.

[2] Chapter xiv, p. 251.

followed shortly afterwards, the assistant surgeons again approaching the Board with a view to the appointment of another ordinary surgeon when the chair of clinical surgery should become vacant. It was proposed that the necessary beds should be obtained by taking one ward from the charge of the new professor and one from that of the senior ordinary surgeon, three wards having for many years constituted the charge of each of these two surgeons.

This proposal not unnaturally led to considerable discussion. Objections were raised by the ordinary surgeons who claimed that, in order to overtake the work involved, three wards—with an average of from 60 to 70 beds—were necessary, and that that number was imperative if the instruction of students was to be properly carried out. That the faculty of medicine of the University did not share this view is seen in a resolution of 3rd March 1906, quoted in the minutes of the Infirmary: "The Faculty are not prepared to say that the uniform provision of two-ward charges does not present certain advantages both from the point of view of affording a more efficient means of treating patients and also of affording increased facilities for clinical instruction." Moreover, reports from other hospitals disclosed that 40 beds were the average number allocated to surgeons and, in the Royal Infirmary itself, in the case of one of the surgeons with only 36 beds in his charge as many operations were performed in one year as in one of the three-ward charges. Although the additional surgeoncy would accelerate promotion for a limited period only, it would have the advantage of distributing the students more equally amongst the surgeons, and the sister in charge of two wards instead of three would certainly have her work lightened. The Board of Management by a majority decided that such charges should be discontinued and that a fifth ordinary surgeon should be appointed with two wards allocated to him.[1]

Shortly after the introduction of the age-limit of retirement for all members of the medical and surgical staff of the

[1] Minute, Royal Infirmary, 22nd June 1908.

Infirmary—a regulation which was to affect their period of service as physicians, surgeons and specialists—the problem of how to improve the system of clinical teaching then in operation in the hospital presented itself in a somewhat acute form. In 1908, the Government had appointed a Departmental Committee, with Lord Elgin as Chairman, to consider the claims of the Scottish Universities to receive increased grants from the Treasury ; and the committee, while taking evidence, had their attention drawn to the large number of students receiving their medical education at the Universities of Glasgow and Edinburgh and to the difficulty experienced in providing a sufficient number of patients for their clinical instruction.[1] At Glasgow the problem of supply had been considered and satisfactorily solved by an arrangement with the managers of the Royal Infirmary who had placed their wards, along with the medical and surgical staff, at the disposal of the University of Glasgow, thus supplementing the accommodation at the Western Infirmary in which the greater part of the clinical teaching of university students had hitherto been carried on.

At Edinburgh, where the available beds in the Royal Infirmary were relatively few in proportion to the large number of students attending the hospital, the problem was more difficult of solution. But the recent appointment of two of the ordinary surgeons as lecturers in clinical surgery in the University had effected an improvement in the surgical house by placing at the service of the University more beds and two additional teachers, thus augmenting the number of patients available for clinical instruction and for the purpose of the final professional examinations for the degrees in medicine and surgery. In the opinion of the Elgin Committee full use was not being made of all the resources of the Infirmary : the weakness of the system, long in practice, was not due so much to the lack of patients as to the need for an organisation which would permit more beds and all the members of the medical and surgical staff to be utilised for teaching and examining.

[1] Report of the Committee on Scottish Universities, with a memorandum by Professor G. Sims Woodhead, presented to both Houses of Parliament, 1910.

In the gradual evolution of the Edinburgh School of Medicine, which has been traced in earlier chapters, it will be recalled that within the Infirmary the physicians and surgeons became differentiated into two groups, the professorial or academical, and the ordinary physicians and surgeons or extra-academical group.[1] In their rôle as teachers in the hospital, the professors instructed and examined the university students who formed the great majority of those attending the Infirmary; the extra-academical group taught and examined the students of the School of Medicine of the Royal Colleges who were preparing for the diploma of the three Medical Corporations in Scotland, but, in addition, they also gave clinical instruction to such students of the University as selected to attend their clinics. Although they examined for the diploma, they took no part in the examination for the university degree, unless, as from time to time was the case, one or more of their number were appointed assessors or co-examiners with their professorial colleagues. The patients in their wards could not be used for purposes of examination save in these circumstances. Consequently the extra-academical teachers who were not at the same time university examiners were placed at some disadvantage, as students not unnaturally desired to obtain part of their instruction from those who were later to test their knowledge. Again, as there was no limitation placed upon the number attending the clinics the distribution of the students throughout the wards was frequently unequal, those of the professors and of the more popular extra-academical teachers being overcrowded while others were sparsely attended; moreover, the large clinic lost some of its value from the absence of personal contact between teacher and taught and overcrowding was detrimental to the comfort of the patients.

The appointment of two ordinary surgeons as university lecturers had been attended with considerable success, leading to a more equable distribution of the students in the clinics and, with the lecturers as examiners, to improvement in the examinations, more patients becoming available for that purpose.

[1] Chapters VIII-IX.

The Elgin Committee, therefore, advocated not only an extension of this system but also the inclusion as university teachers of the assistant physicians and assistant surgeons and, to some extent also of the clinical tutors, so as to increase the numbers of the clinical teaching staff of the hospital. The Memorandum prepared by Professor G. Sims Woodhead and appended to the Elgin Report became the basis of the Clinical Teaching Agreement signed on 20th and 23rd June 1913 by the managers of the Royal Infirmary and the University Court, after consultation with the faculty of medicine and with the physicians and surgeons of the hospital.

Briefly stated, the principle underlying the Agreement was a fusion between the academical and extra-academical groups *quâ* teaching in the Infirmary and, while both should share in the instruction of university students, the latter were to retain their right to teach the students in the School of the Royal Colleges both within and outside the hospital. The Agreement therefore provided for a more equal distribution of students throughout the wards with some limitation in the size of the clinics and with their subdivision into senior and junior students, while the younger members of the staff of the hospital were to participate in the clinical instruction; further, in order to give better facilities for conducting the professional examinations for the degree of the University, the ordinary physicians and surgeons became co-examiners along with their professorial colleagues.

During their term of office on the staff of the Infirmary the ordinary physicians and surgeons were to be designated senior lecturers in the University, the assistant physicians and surgeons as lecturers, and the tutors as university clinical assistants. Hitherto appointments had been made to the honorary staff by candidates applying directly to the whole Board of Management in whose hands lay the selection of the most suitable candidate. But, in future, nominations for an appointment were to be placed in the hands of a Selection Committee of the Board consisting of seven members :—the two University representatives on the Board, one each of the representatives of the Royal College of Physicians and the Royal College of Surgeons, and three other members selected from the Board, this committee nominating two candidates for the post of assistant physician or assistant surgeon in order that the Board might select one for the appointment. When a vacancy occurred in the office of ordinary physician or surgeon the same Selection Committee was to nominate one of the assistant physicians or surgeons for appointment by the Board, it being understood and agreed that the senior assistant physician or surgeon should be nominated, unless in the opinion of the committee there were special reasons why they should not be nominated. Clinical Boards comprising the professors and the senior lecturers were also set up to become responsible for the arrangements regarding clinical teaching and for its direction and supervision. Special arrangements were also made for the payment of all the teachers coming within the scheme, with the receipt of honoraria from the University in respect of the instruction given to university students, the senior lecturers, in addition, receiving a proportion of the net amount of the fees paid into a separate clinical account in the University Fee Fund.

Arrangements along very similar lines, and incorporated in the Agreement, were made in one of the special departments of the Infirmary, that reserved for the treatment of the diseases of women, or clinical gynæcology ; this was in future to be dissociated—*quâ* teaching—from its old relation with clinical medicine, and to become a separate department of the hospital. The junior of the two gynæcologists on the staff who was an extra-academical teacher was appointed a university lecturer and examiner and the two assistant gynæcologists were also made university lecturers. The method and the terms of their appointment as members of the staff of the Infirmary were on identical lines with those of the physicians and surgeons through nomination of the Selection Committee : honoraria were agreed upon as remuneration for their services as teachers, and a Clinical Gynæcological Board exercised a general supervision over the arrangements connected with the instruction of the students.

In the preparation of the new scheme of clinical teaching in the Infirmary, on the lines just described, the University Court were contemplating a further change which would involve a break in the old association between the hospital and two of the long established chairs in the medical faculty, the occupants of which for many years had been professors of clinical medicine. More than a century and a half had elapsed since " the managers of the Infirmary granted liberty to the Professors of Medicine to give clinical lectures on the Cases of the Patients " and, during the long interval since the days of John Rutherford and his three colleagues, a number of new chairs had been added to the faculty and some of their occupants had acted for a time as clinical professors. But as the duties of the systematic chairs became more arduous and their occupants were less able to devote their time to the calls of the Infirmary, in due course they ceased to act as physicians ; so that in 1912 when the Clinical Teaching Agreement was under consideration, the professors of pathology and materia medica, along with the professor of medicine or practice of physic, alone remained on the staff of the Infirmary as three professors of clinical medicine.

The resignation of William Smith Greenfield in the summer of 1912 from the chair of pathology, to which he had been appointed in 1881, paved the way for dissociating that chair from clinical teaching ; and, in order that the University might retain its connection with the Infirmary, the Court proposed to found a chair of clinical medicine. With that end in view they expressed the hope that the managers would allocate to the new professor the wards previously in charge of the professor of pathology.[1] At the same time the Court contemplated a change of a similar nature when the chair of materia medica should in due course become vacant, with the expectation that the wards thus vacated would be allocated to a professor or professors of the University. In order that the Board of Management might be consulted prior to the appointment of these professors, a Joint-Committee of seven members was to be appointed, consisting of three chosen by

[1] Minute, Royal Infirmary, 5th August 1912.

the University Court and of three managers of the Royal Infirmary selected by the Board, with the Principal of the University as chairman : the Joint-Committee would then nominate two persons of whom the Court would elect one as the professor, this procedure to remain in effect as vacancies occurred in these chairs in the future.

When the appropriate Ordinance had been prepared by the Court and approved by Order in Council on 24th June 1913, the Joint-Committee proceeded to nominate two persons to the chair of clinical medicine and, in the following October, the University Court elected William Russell, one of the ordinary physicians to the Infirmary, as the Moncrieff Arnott professor of clinical medicine.[1] Having resigned his appointment as ordinary physician, the managers placed him in charge of the equivalent number of beds previously in the care of the professor of pathology and thereafter promoted the senior assistant physician in the Infirmary to the charge of the beds which William Russell had vacated. The chair of pathology in the University was filled by the election of James Lorrain Smith, a graduate of Edinburgh in Arts and Medicine and professor of pathology at Manchester. Under the terms of the new agreement, he was appointed by the managers as consultant pathologist to the Infirmary on the understanding that when the office of pathologist to the hospital became vacant he would succeed to that post.

With the retirement of Sir Thomas Richard Fraser from the chair of materia medica in 1918, to which he had been elected in 1877 in succession to Sir Robert Christison, the second of the three long-established chairs in the faculty of medicine became dissociated from clinical teaching in the Infirmary, as had been foreshadowed in the Agreement of 1913 ; and the new occupant of the chair, relieved of this obligation, was free to devote his time to scientific research and to the other duties connected with his professorship.

Sir Thomas R. Fraser during the long period of forty years

[1] The chair of clinical medicine was thus named to perpetuate the memory of James Moncrieff Arnott, a graduate in medicine of the University, and of his daughter Jane Moncrieff Arnott, benefactors of the University.

as a physician to the Infirmary became one of the outstanding personalities of the Edinburgh School of Medicine. Possessing in a remarkable degree the qualities essential for success as a scientific investigator—the greatest accuracy and care in observation and an inexhaustible patience and persistence—he soon established a reputation through his work on the pharmacological action of such poisons as the Old Calabar bean, on *Strophanthus hispidus*, the African arrow poison with its use in medicine as an alternative to digitalis, and on the snake poisons and their antidotes. As a lecturer he had a happy gift of varying the monotonous descriptions of a series of salts and powders by introducing an illuminating and often humorous account of their actions and uses. But his alert mind found other outlets than the laboratory and classroom. As dean of the faculty of medicine, a member of the University Court, a representative on the General Medical Council, a member of the Council and president of the Royal College of Physicians of Edinburgh and president of the Indian Plague Commission, he had opportunities of exercising his faculties in other directions. Sir Thomas died on 4th January 1920 within a month of his seventy-ninth birthday.

A new chair was created by an Ordinance of the University Court with the object of promoting the subject of therapeutics and of enabling the holder to engage in clinical teaching. To commemorate the eminent services rendered to the science and art of medicine by the late Sir Robert Christison, Bt., the Christison chair of therapeutics was founded in 1918, to which Jonathan Campbell Meakins of Montreal was appointed in the following year as a whole-time professor ; and by arrangement with the managers of the Infirmary the beds previously in the charge of the professor of materia medica were allocated to him. Thus the University retained its old connection with the hospital, continuing to give instruction in the wards by three professors of clinical medicine, the professor of practice of physic, the Moncrieff Arnott professor of clinical medicine and the Christison professor of therapeutics.

In 1917 a Supplementary Agreement of a provisional and temporary character was concluded between both parties to amend the original Agreement in so far as to give facilities within the Infirmary for the education of the women students attending in large numbers during the war.[1] The opportunity was taken to insert a clause permitting of the termination of the old Agreement by mutual consent at any time, or, on 30th September in any year, after not less than nine months' notice in writing by either party.

The scheme embodied in the Agreement of 1913 was undoubtedly a step in the direction of removing one cause of weakness in the old system of clinical teaching : by making provision for utilising the services of a larger number of the honorary staff as teachers, the students were more equally distributed throughout the wards, the clinics became less overcrowded, and better facilities were obtained for the conduct of the final professional examinations in clinical medicine and surgery. If, through the fusion of the academical and extra-academical teachers, some of the former friendly and healthy competition had disappeared, nevertheless better use was being made of all the resources of the hospital and the position of the medical school as a whole was more firmly ensured against the growing competition of other schools in the country. But some years later it was considered advisable for various reasons to revise the terms of the existing Agreements, some of the clauses of which were no longer applicable, and, by the introduction of new clauses, to effect some much desired improvements.

Following many protracted conferences and discussions, the Board of Management, in March 1929, concluded two new Agreements on more or less identical lines, one with the University Court and the other with the Governing Board of the School of Medicine of the Royal Colleges, both becoming operative as from 1st October 1928. The new Agreement with the University brought within its scope all the departments of the hospital engaged in clinical teaching, both general and special : it continued the system of distribution of the students throughout the several wards, giving both university and extra-academical students, as far as reasonably possible, free choice

[1] Chapter XIV, p. 253.

of teacher, provided that the number did not exceed forty in each clinic unless with the special consent of the Board. It recognised the members of all the clinical departments in the Infirmary as members of the University Clinical Teaching Staff, but in the case of the ordinary physicians and surgeons it discontinued the use of the former term senior lecturers in the University : it entitled any member of the hospital staff to resign his university appointment on giving due notice, without prejudice to his Infirmary appointment ; and further, it provided for equality of status as between all the physicians and surgeons, including the professors, with precedence within the Infirmary in the order of seniority of their Infirmary appointments, unless otherwise determined by the Board. Moreover, the new Agreement continued the appointment of the Joint-Committee of seven persons to nominate two for the election of one by the University Court to future vacancies in the Moncrieff Arnott and Christison chairs ; and it perpetuated the Selection Committee, henceforth to be a Statutory Committee of the Board and named the Clinical Committee, for nomination to the Board of persons as assistant physicians, surgeons and specialists and for their promotion to senior appointments on the staff when vacancies occurred. The Agreement also widened the basis of the composition of the different Clinical Boards by introducing members of the assistant staff and it provided that the secretaries of the Clinical Medicine and Clinical Surgery Boards should be appointed by the University as members of the medical faculty. It revised the financial arrangements previously reached relative to remuneration for teaching and for the payment of the ordinary physicians and surgeons as coexaminers with the professors, and for such assistant physicians and surgeons as might act from time to time as principal examiners.

By a subsequent arrangement between the Board of Management and the University the professor of pathology was recognised as in charge of, and as the official head of, the pathological department of the Infirmary and responsible to the Board for its general supervision and direction, with the title of honorary pathologist. As the nature of the work of the bacteriological department of the hospital did not call for the same close supervision by the professor of bacteriology, the latter was appointed to the honorary staff of the hospital as honorary bacteriologist, continuing in his former position as official head of the department, the bacteriologist to the Infirmary consulting with him in matters of major importance.

The successful completion of the new Agreement of 1929 after prolonged negotiations, often of an intricate and delicate character, and the smoothness with which it continues to fulfil its purpose, owe much to the legal acumen, tact and persuasive powers of the late Right Honourable Charles D. Murray, then the representative on the Board of the Senators of the College of Justice and convener of the Special Committee appointed by the managers to confer with the University Court.

The chapter closes, as it opened, on a somewhat sombre note, again recording the loss to the hospital of many who had given to it years of valuable service. In the short pre-war period of the new century the ordinary accidents associated with routine retirements, with unexpected resignations for reasons of ill-health or other causes, and the vacancies caused by death, accounted for more than the average number of changes usually met with in the personnel of the medical and surgical staff in other periods of similar duration. No fewer than twenty-three members passed from the active list during the years 1900 to 1913; ten joined the consulting staff as they reached the statutory limit of their period of active service, eight resigned—six on account of ill-health and two voluntarily—and of the remainder, death claimed five.[1]

At a time when the Edinburgh School of Medicine was specially fortunate in its group of able teachers, Sir John Halliday Croom, as an extra-academical lecturer in midwifery, enjoyed a popularity which was the more remarkable as his short course of lectures did not qualify for the degree in medicine.[2] He took infinite pains in their preparation and

[1] In 1900 the active honorary staff numbered forty; in 1913 the staff had increased to forty-six.

[2] This course of lectures covered a period of three months, the qualifying course being six months.

no medical student considered his education complete without attendance at his class. Tall, erect, and immaculately dressed, his forceful personality held his audience ; and his presentation of the subject, enriched by a strong sense of humour and a felicitous choice of illustration culled from an abundant store of facts, made an indelible impression upon his listeners, teaching them as no text-book could ever do. His retirement from the staff of the Infirmary in 1901 did not terminate his active career as, in 1905, he was elected to the chair of midwifery in the University on the retirement of Sir Alexander Russell Simpson, thus continuing to give to further generations of students the fruits of a ripe and extended experience.[1] In 1909 John Chiene resigned the chair of surgery to which he had been elected in 1882 as successor to James Spence, and with his retiral from the Infirmary he severed a long association of thirty-eight years. A faithful and ardent disciple of Lister he taught and practised the antiseptic treatment in the early days of its introduction, and he fought Lister's battle in the wards of the hospital after he left Edinburgh for London. Beneath a somewhat rugged exterior Chiene had a very human and sympathetic interest in his fellow-men and his students will long remember his many acts of kindness. He early recognised the importance of giving facilities for research to the young graduate and, on his appointment to the chair of surgery, established in his department the first bacteriological laboratory in the University.[2] The year 1912 saw the retirement from the Infirmary of Sir Byrom Bramwell, a graduate of the University in 1869, and one of the numerous Englishmen who, from time to time, have brought distinction to Edinburgh in Medicine, Science and Arts. After spending ten years in North Shields and Newcastle-upon-Tyne he recrossed the Border to return to the city in which he had spent his student days. Commencing at once to teach medicine in the extra-academical school he joined the staff of the Infirmary in 1882 as pathologist, the first step to his future appointment

[1] Sir J. Halliday Croom died on 27th September 1923, aged seventy-six years.

[2] Professor John Chiene, C.B., died 29th May 1923, aged eighty years.

as assistant physician and to his goal as physician. His commanding presence and impressive manner, his clear and concise delivery, arrested the attention of his students and, from his accumulated knowledge of clinical facts gained from years of exact observation, he expounded the essential features of the disease from which the patient before them suffered and on which he had based his diagnosis. A voluminous writer, covering a large field of medicine, he embodied his personal experience of diseases of the nervous and circulatory systems in several volumes which, widely read, enhanced his reputation and that of the school in which he was an ornament. But perhaps he is best remembered by his Wednesday " Duck Pond " clinics. They were models of what clinical instruction ought to be, and many old students of Edinburgh must retain vivid recollections of the masterly way in which on these occasions he presented and illustrated the essentials of medicine.[1]

One member of the consulting staff of the Infirmary calls for notice at this time. When Douglas Argyll Robertson died in 1909, while on a visit to India, ophthalmology lost one of its most eminent exponents, a man with a world-wide reputation, and the medical profession in Edinburgh mourned the death of him who for twenty-nine years, from 1867 to 1896, had been a distinguished member of the staff of the hospital and a lecturer in diseases of the eye. A dignified figure in his grey frock coat and top hat, his tall and athletic frame, his handsome features and air of distinction, combined with a genial and old-world courtesy of manner, made him conspicuous in any assembly.

With the passing of the Victorian era, the silk hat and the frock and morning coat, so long recognised as the correct dress of that period, have disappeared and, with the advent of the twentieth century, physicians and surgeons have lost something of the dignity and impressiveness of their fathers. Save on special occasions, the lounge suit and the soft Homburg hat, or one of its many variations in neo-Georgian times, have replaced the once familiar professional costume. The motor

[1] Sir Byrom Bramwell died on 27th April 1931, aged eighty-three years.

car has been substituted for the smart brougham and the high swung C-spring carriage with its pair of horses and, with the coming of the automobile, the slower and more stately means of progression has been displaced. If there be moments of regret at the disappearance of those dignified figures and the more leisurely means of transport, there is undoubtedly the gain in personal comfort and in the time- and life-saving powers—sometimes, alas ! life-destroying—of the modern motor car. *Autres Temps, Autres Mœurs !*

CHAPTER XVIII

THE WAR AND ITS AFTERMATH—1914-1920

THE CALL TO SERVICE—ACCOMMODATION FOR SAILORS AND SOLDIERS —GIFTS IN KIND FROM HOME AND OVERSEAS—THE FINANCIAL POSITION OF THE HOSPITAL—AN APPEAL AND THE RESPONSE.

THE abnormal conditions suddenly created by the national crisis at the beginning of August 1914 threatened to dislocate the uniform routine of the Infirmary as members of the various departments responded to the call of military service. Although a considerable strain was thus thrown upon those who remained to carry on the work, the general efficiency of the hospital was not impaired nor was the comfort of the patients neglected either during the four anxious years of the war or in those that immediately followed its conclusion. The responsibilities falling upon the shoulders of the managers were enormously increased when faced with the task of rearrangement and of filling the temporary vacancies ; but in this they were assisted by the willing cooperation and readiness of all to undertake such additional duties as were necessary.

The Superintendent, Lieut.-Colonel Sir Joseph Fayrer, Bt., at once took over the command of the 2nd Scottish General Hospital at Craigleith, the Territorial Army Hospital serving the area. His post at the Infirmary was temporarily filled by Robert McKenzie Johnston, a former member of the honorary staff and of the Board of Management ; but in October 1915, William S. Caw, the Treasurer and Clerk, while continuing as such, was appointed Acting Superintendent till Sir Joseph Fayrer should be relieved of his military duties.[1] With his intimate knowledge of the affairs of the hospital Mr Caw's services in this office proved of the utmost value. An unexpected number of vacancies occurred amongst the nursing staff, but Miss Gill the Lady Superintendent, previously

[1] Sir Joseph Fayrer returned to duty at the Infirmary in February 1919.

appointed Principal Matron of the Hospital at Craigleith, was able to remain on duty in the Infirmary and to reorganise the nursing department. Two of the assistant superintendents of nurses and ten sisters were called up for military service. By arrangement with the War Office thirty trained nurses had been placed at its disposal in the event of hostilities but, in 1914-15, as many as sixty-one were enlisted. In the ensuing years large numbers, after completing their training, left the Infirmary to join the Army Nursing Service and therefore were not available to fill the vacancies normally occurring in the staff. Moreover, during the first year of the war arrangements required to be made to give more than one hundred members of the Voluntary Aid Detachments short courses of training preparatory to their entering the military hospitals. Evidence of the desire of many young women to assist their country as nurses was furnished in 1915-16 when more than one thousand applied for entry to the Preliminary Training School, a number unprecedented in any one year in the history of the Infirmary. A serious drain was also made upon the several administrative departments when officials and employés to the number of seventy-nine—dispensers, clerks, tradesmen and porters—were transferred to military duties.

The medical and surgical staff of the Infirmary were depleted at the outbreak of war, as those holding commissions in the Naval Reserve and in the Territorial Army left the hospital for national service elsewhere ; while a large number holding commissions in the Royal Army Medical Corps, Territorial Force, formed the Staff of the 2nd Scottish General Hospital to which they had been appointed some years previously as *à la suite* officers. For them, military duties were superadded to their routine civil occupations : the civilian population still required attention, and clinical teaching in the Infirmary made even greater demands than formerly with the growing need of meeting the call of the Navy and Army for medical, surgical and specialist officers. In 1915-16 as many as fourteen members of the honorary staff were absent overseas. Before the end of August 1914, twelve of the twenty house physicians and house surgeons had resigned their appointments and volunteered, and very soon the whole of the work in this department of the hospital was being undertaken by students in their final year of study. But the work of the hospital was carried on without interruption in spite of many difficulties. With the exception of Denis Cotterill, appointed junior assistant surgeon in 1913, all the members of the honorary staff who had been on national service eventually returned to duty at the Infirmary. At the outbreak of war he offered his services and, in November 1914, was attached to the Red Cross Hospital at Rouen. In January 1918 he was transferred to the 50th Casualty Clearing Station at Bohain where he died after the Armistice, falling a victim to the severe influenzal epidemic which was then raging. His early death removed from the staff a young surgeon of great promise.

Notwithstanding the arrangements made by the Admiralty and War Office for the provision of hospital accommodation in the area for sick and wounded sailors and soldiers in the event of war, it was inevitable, especially with the proximity of Rosyth as a naval base, that additional means would require to be found to meet any sudden emergency that might arise either at sea or on land. Consequently, when the managers of the Infirmary were approached in August 1914 by the naval and military authorities, they at once responded to the appeal to place at their disposal two wards in the Infirmary, afterwards increased to three, or approximately one hundred beds, the majority being surgical. True to its traditions the hospital once again opened its doors to those who were serving their country, as it had done in the early days of its history. In common with the decision reached by the Boards of Management of the larger hospitals in London and elsewhere, the managers, in view of the national emergency, at first suspended the practice of exacting payment for the maintenance of sailors and soldiers; but after October 1915, and following the example of the other hospitals, they reversed their previous decision and accepted the Government's allowances. With the prolongation of the war and the large number of men admitted for treatment, it was hardly justifiable to meet from the voluntary subscriptions of the public the extra cost thus entailed. Payment was therefore made at the rate of four shillings per head per day: in 1756, fourpence per day or twenty-eight pence per week had been offered, with the fourpence deducted by the military authorities from the soldier's pay, and, in 1915-16, four shillings per day or twenty-eight shillings per week! In the spring of 1918 the rate of payment was increased to four shillings and ninepence, and an allowance of sixpence per day was granted for each unoccupied bed placed at the disposal of the military authorities, both of these concessions taking effect as from 1st October 1917.[1]

During the year 1915-16, 270 men from the Navy and 633 from the Expeditionary Force received treatment in the wards: of the former, 68 sailors were admitted after the naval engagement off Jutland on 31st May 1916, and on 17th June the Infirmary had the honour of a visit from H.M. the King, accompanied by Vice-Admiral Sir David Beatty. In the same year the sum of £6915 from the Government was credited to the receipts of the Infirmary and, in 1917-18, the amount received from the same source was £10,128: as arrangements had then been made for the treatment of disabled ex-sailors and soldiers, as pensioners under the Ministry of Pensions Scheme, the above sum included £2700 for their maintenance. After the establishment of the various Women's Auxiliary Corps members who were sick or injured were treated in the ordinary civilian wards.[2]

Although during the war years additional beds were made available in the Infirmary, the reserve surgical ward being requisitioned for wounded sailors and soldiers, yet the returns of the total number of patients, civilian and military, during the period of hostilities showed that fewer patients were treated in the hospital than in the immediate pre- and post-war years. The explanation is probably to be found in the more prolonged stay in hospital of the military casualties, the nature of the injuries received by men of the Expeditionary Force and by

[1] Minute, Royal Infirmary, 11th March 1918.

[2] Minute, 23rd September 1918, states that women members of the Royal Air Force if requiring hospital treatment will be received in the Infirmary at a maintenance charge of 4s. 9d. per head, per day.

those in naval action, being such as to require a longer course of treatment. A further number of beds remained unoccupied, reserved on behalf of the War Office in case of some sudden emergency. Therefore the "turn over" of patients was not so rapid as in time of peace. The accompanying table, to which has been added the number of patients treated in the several out-patient departments, illustrates the position :—

Year to 30th September.	Indoor Patients.	Average Duration of Days in Hospital.		Outdoor Patients.
		Medical.	Surgical.	
1914-15	13,102	32·5	20·1	36,639
1915-16	12,399	35·2	22·2	37,649
1916-17	12,022	34·1	23·5	33,924
1917-18	12,481	26·7	29·1	38,064
1918-19	12,550	29·5	22·1	43,478
1919-20	13,320	30·2	16·6	48,117

A remarkable feature in the daily life of the Infirmary during the years of conflict was the many acceptable gifts in kind received not only from generous donors in the home country but from friends of the hospital in distant parts of the Empire ; and so numerous were these donations that they materially lessened the annual expenditure on maintenance. In the early part of the eighteenth century Scotsmen resident in the Colonial possessions had come to the assistance of the Royal Infirmary with gifts of money to swell the building fund of the old hospital ; and in the twentieth century new generations in the British Dominions beyond the seas, not forgetful of the needs of the old country, sought to help with gifts in kind. The Canadian Red Cross Society supplied hospital clothing and surgical dressings ; from the West Indies the Jamaica Agricultural Society and the planters of Trinidad sent oranges and grape fruit, and from Montserrat came guava jelly. Through the Agent General in London, Queensland gifted thousands of pounds weight of beef and mutton along with fruits, flour, bacon, honey and butter, and with the aid of the Patriotic Fund of the Brisbane *Courier*, sugar and cornflour were supplied in large quantities ; Sydney sent similar consignments of beef and mutton, along with 1489 rabbits. From the home country the King presented game and fruit to his sailors and soldiers. The National Egg Collecting Scheme was responsible for the supply of 3875 dozen of fresh eggs and great quantities of game, fruit and flowers, a similar service being rendered by the various branches of the British Red Cross Society in Scotland and by the Edinburgh and District Ladies' Egg Collecting Committee. Last but not least were the vegetables and potatoes produced by the labours of the many allotment holders in the district, a voluntary offering to the sick and injured.

In spite of the relief from Government assistance and the many gifts in kind, the financial position of the Infirmary was still a cause of anxiety as the prices of provisions and coals continued to rise. In 1914-15 the annual ordinary expenditure was £60,944, while the average cost of occupied bed was £67 : in 1918-19 the corresponding items totalled £102,549 and £115. For the first time in the history of the Infirmary ordinary annual expenditure had reached six, and the cost of occupied bed, three figures. But in spite of the many claims upon the sympathy and liberality of the people during the years of war, it is remarkable that the ordinary annual income did not diminish but actually showed year by year an increase. The voluntary contributions which in 1914-15 amounted to £31,260 had in 1918-19 risen to £41,984 ;[1] and yet, notwithstanding every effort to maintain a strict economy, the adverse balance became larger each year increasing from £24,470 in the first to £31,927 in the last year of the war. A striking feature of the special effort to give the Infirmary the maximum of assistance was the encouraging response from the employés in the various public works and business establishments in the city and from the miners in the coal and shale areas, all the more gratifying in view of the difficult financial position.

The economic strain was prolonged into the post-war period. The aftermath of heavy taxation, high prices and

[1] In 1914-15 the total ordinary income was £46,474 ; in 1918-19 it was £70,622.

unemployment, with the consequent shrinkage in resources, brought increasing diminution in the margin of surplus which the public had available for charity. Some more active step required to be taken to restore the finances of the hospital and to make provision for long over-due improvements. It was obvious from the report prepared by the Superintendent in November 1919, that cleaning, painting and repairs, of necessity postponed during the war, could not be indefinitely delayed. But more than cleaning and painting were necessary; once again the kitchen, the laundry and the boiler-house proved insufficient for the greater demands made upon them, while additional accommodation for nurses and a new medical electrical department were imperative. Accordingly, at the annual meeting of the Court of Contributors in January 1920, the managers announced their intention of issuing a special appeal.

On 27th March a public meeting, over which Lord Provost Chesser presided, was held in the City Chambers, when an appeal was launched to raise a capital sum of £250,000, with the object of improving the condition of the existing fabric and of providing the necessary extensions; and an additional sum of £50,000 was asked for in support of the annual income. The appeal letters were signed by the Lord Provost and Sheriff Gerard L. Crole, the convener of the finance committee of the Board, and a further personal letter from the Lord Provost was addressed to the numerous Sports Clubs, by whom a widespread response was made. Public interest was aroused in all classes of the community, and eight months later a sum of £60,383 had been raised by subscriptions. Although falling very short of what was desired, the funds of the Infirmary benefited still further from other sources. The City of Edinburgh Branch of the British Red Cross Society made the valuable contribution of £15,000, specially earmarked for the new radiological department; the St Andrew's Society of Hong Kong sent £11,000; the 10th Service Battalion of the Black Watch, 42nd Royal Highlanders, gave £1600 towards the endowment of a bed, and as many as thirteen beds were endowed as war memorials by friends and relatives of those who fell in the war. In the distribution of the National Relief Fund in 1921, £16,097 were received by the Royal Infirmary. Altogether a sum approaching £125,000 was contributed to the maintenance and extension funds of the Infirmary through the post-war appeal. Thus a situation which seemed to threaten for a time the very existence of the voluntary system was relieved by the generous response of those whose belief in the future of the Royal Infirmary remained unaltered.

CHAPTER XIX

THE IMMEDIATE POST-WAR YEARS
1920-1928

VISIT OF ROYALTY—A FURTHER PERIOD OF EXTENSION—THE CLINICAL MEDICINE LABORATORY — THE NEW RADIOLOGICAL DEPARTMENT—LECTURESHIP IN RADIOLOGY—BEECHMOUNT—DENTAL DEPARTMENT—VENEREAL DISEASES DEPARTMENT AND LECTURESHIP—TUBERCULOSIS, PSYCHIATRY, TROPICAL DISEASES—SOCIAL SERVICE DEPARTMENT—DIETETIC DEPARTMENT—ASTLEY AINSLIE INSTITUTION—RETIREMENT OF OFFICIALS.

IN the summer of 1920, with conditions gradually becoming normal, the Infirmary received an unexpected visit from King George and Queen Mary, accompanied by their daughter, Princess Mary. The visit was of a purely informal character and was not part of the official programme which included the ceremony of the laying of the Foundation Stone by His Majesty of the Department of Chemistry, the first of the new science buildings of the University at " The King's Buildings," and the laureation of Queen Mary as an Honorary Doctor of Laws. After inspecting a surgical and a medical ward Their Majesties graciously responded to the invitation of the resident physicians and surgeons to inscribe their names upon the old dining-room table in the "Residency." On an oval area on the central leaf beneath the date 5th July 1920, are clearly carved in the wood the signatures, George R.I., Mary R. and Mary, a permanent record of a delightful visit which will not readily fade from the memory of those who were privileged to be present.

The dining table used by the resident medical and surgical officers, " bearing the means of sustenance of the present, and the names of the past, residents," while from time to time enlarged as their number increased with the expansion of the hospital, new leaves being substituted for the old as the names accumulated, is one of the " vestigia " of historic interest in the Infirmary. For more than sixty years each resident has carved his name upon its surface, but unfortunately time, assisted by repeated scrubbings, has rendered undecipherable many of the names inscribed in the days when the table, along with the horse-hair sofa and chairs, stood in the small and somewhat dingy dining room of the old Infirmary built out from the south side of the medical hospital : its windows faced the line of the Flodden Wall and the houses in Drummond Street beyond, while conspicuous in the foreground was an ancient cherry tree which blossomed annually but was reputed never to have borne a crop of fruit.[1]

The report on the internal condition of the Infirmary prepared by the Superintendent—to which reference has been made in the previous chapter—constituted the basis of the appeal to the public launched in the spring of 1920 : it not only placed emphasis upon the wear and tear of the existing fabric and the urgent necessity for immediate attention, but, in addition, the report stressed the need for enlargement of some of the departments and for the provision of new buildings. An essential and frequently recurring item in hospital expenditure which is apt to be overlooked by those interested in the welfare of such an institution as the Royal Infirmary, but who are not concerned in its management, is the large outlay on cleaning, painting and repairs to maintain the buildings in a proper state of preservation. This expenditure, like that more frequently exacted by the progressive developments in the science and practice of medicine, must be met from time to time if a hospital is to keep its reputation as a modern House of Healing ; and, in illustration of the cost entailed in preserving the fabric of the Infirmary, it is necessary to cite only one item, the sum of £35,000 estimated after the war as requisite for the repainting of all the pavilions and administrative buildings.

Less than twenty-five years had passed since a new system of lighting and heating had been introduced and the scheme

[1] "The Edinburgh Royal Infirmary Old Residents' Club," by Alexander James, M.D., *Scottish Medical and Surgical Journal*, 1898, p. 136. The earliest names carved on the oldest leaf are those of residents between 1870 and 1879.

of drainage entirely remodelled, when it was again considered imperative to instal new plant for steam heating and for an improved hot-water service throughout the hospital, the cost of which was estimated at £16,000. Extension of the kitchen, in order to give greater facilities for independent cooking arrangements for the nurses, who numbered from 320 to 350, was also very desirable: each day thirty-one different types of meals were prepared and nearly 1400 persons in the hospital were provided with food, so that it was not surprising that some delay occurred in the preparation of the daily dinner. When so much important work required attention the managers were fortunate in obtaining the services of Mr Thomas W. Turnbull appointed as the new Clerk of Works in February 1920.[1] His promotion as architect in June 1929 was a well-merited recognition of his ability and skill in hospital design and construction, all the extensions subsequent to his appointment as clerk of works being built according to his plans.

The period immediately following the occupation of the new Infirmary in 1879 had been one of continuous progress in medical science, and the hospital, accepting its responsibilities, had responded to the best of its ability to the many calls made upon its finances. But, with the advent of the twentieth century, scientific research had disclosed fresh avenues of approach to the study of man's body in health and in illness: experimental methods of investigation in the laboratory were becoming of greater assistance to the physician and surgeon in their work in the wards, supplementing both clinical observation at the bedside and the knowledge gained by the examination of the patient's body after death. The new physiology and the study of the chemistry of the body in the living were teaching the clinician not only the chemical processes controlling its normal functions, but the means of detecting very early departures from the normal, before pathological changes in the structure of the body were recognisable. Hence the diagnosis of disease in its incipient stages and its appropriate early treatment were becoming

[1] In 1924 the title of Clerk of Works was changed to that of Master of Works.

greatly assisted and the practice of medicine placed on a less empirical basis than formerly. But biochemistry was not the only recent avenue of exploration : clinical medicine and surgery were still further reinforced by the progress made in the science of physics : the greatly extended employment of the X-rays with the more accurate interpretation of the nature of the changes which they revealed were facilitating diagnosis, while their therapeutic value, along with that of radium, was enhanced as a more exact knowledge of their specific action upon the tissue cells was ascertained. Further, the experience gained in the treatment of war injuries had contributed to a fuller appreciation of the value of heat, light, massage and graduated exercises as remedial measures, rendering necessary the provision of more commodious premises and a larger staff of remunerated experts. The time had also arrived when more attention was being paid to the care of the patient after his or her discharge from hospital during the important period of convalescence : consequently, appropriate departments and a "follow-up" system permitting of closer contact with the patient in his own home were becoming indispensable. To meet these increasing demands expansion of the Infirmary at a very early date was essential : although the ordinary revenue in 1920, in response to the special appeal made in the month of March, was much larger than that of the previous year, it still failed to meet the ordinary expenditure which, exceeding all former records, had reached the sum of £130,668.

Amongst the new departments established within the Infirmary in the post-war period, one of the most important was the clinical medicine or biochemical laboratory as an integral part of the scientific equipment of the hospital ; but before proceeding to describe the building and what led to its foundation, reference may appropriately be made to an earlier attempt to bring experimental physiological investigation into closer association with the clinical work of the physician in the wards. It is necessary therefore to revert to the year 1910, when, through the influence of George

Alexander Gibson, one of the physicians-in-ordinary from 1900-1913, with a wide reputation as a specialist in diseases of the heart, a small laboratory was opened for their special study. Through the generosity of an anonymous donor a Clinical Research Trust was founded, the income from which was to be devoted to the investigation of cardiac disease. Recent observations had revealed the importance to be attached to the condition of the muscles of the heart, their capacity for maintaining the circulation of the blood, even when disease of the valves was present, and their power of recuperation, being the real proofs of cardiac efficiency. The introduction of the electrocardiograph, an instrument of great precision, had provided the means of accurately studying and testing the action of these muscles both in health and disease. Accordingly, accommodation was obtained for a small laboratory, and a room previously occupied by one of the indoor porters of the hospital was fitted up with the necessary apparatus, electrical supply being installed and placed under the charge of Harry Rainy, one of the assistant physicians. The laboratory was opened on 1st October 1910 by the late Sir Clifford Allbutt and, for a number of years, valuable work was carried on in premises which certainly could not boast of the advantages of the more modern laboratory.[1]

Ten years elapsed before the next step was taken to develop coordinated work between the clinician and the physiologist. In 1920, on the suggestion of the medical and surgical staff, the managers resolved to utilise as a biochemical laboratory the small building erected in 1885 as an isolation and observation ward, when the Town Council of Edinburgh became responsible for the treatment of all cases of infectious fevers occurring in the city.[2] The cost of converting the building for its new purpose, estimated at £875, was met partly by the Infirmary and in part by the University Court, the latter also undertaking to meet the expenditure upon the fittings and equipment. Regulations for the conduct of the laboratory were drawn up and approved by both bodies,

[1] When the new Clinical Medicine Laboratory was opened in 1928, the electrocardiographic apparatus was transferred to it.

[2] Chapter xv, p. 276.

an advisory committee was appointed and the Christison professor of therapeutics, Jonathan Campbell Meakins, was placed in charge.[1] The function of the new laboratory was twofold : to give opportunities for research to the professor and his assistants in the department of therapeutics, and to furnish reports to the medical staff of the hospital on behalf of the patients under their care in the wards. The reporting work which was of a highly technical character increased to such an extent during the first twelve months that an addition to the staff of the laboratory became necessary, the advisory committee recommending the appointment of a whole-time thoroughly trained biochemist.[2]

Such were the small beginnings of a scheme of collaboration which was shortly to develop on a considerably larger scale. During the summer of 1923 the medical faculty of the University had been contemplating a rearrangement of the departments of medicine and surgery and, with that in view, the Court had sought the cooperation and financial assistance of the Rockefeller Foundation in New York. The proposals put forward had been favourably received by that body, so that in the month of December the University Court learnt that there was no longer any doubt as to the realisation of their plans which included a biochemical or clinical laboratory. For this purpose the Rockefeller Foundation was prepared to make a contribution to the University of a sum of £35,000, of which £33,000 would defray in part the cost of the construction of the building, while the remaining £2000 would assist in its initial equipment, provided always that the site was found upon the property of the Infirmary and that an assurance was obtained that the additional cost of the future maintenance of the laboratory was secured. The object which the Foundation had in view in the creation of the building was "the provision of higher teaching and research in the clinical subjects with especial reference to the development of a true university clinic under the direction of Professor Meakins."

[1] Minutes, Royal Infirmary, 1920 and 1921.
[2] Minute, Royal Infirmary, 7th August 1922.

After the terms of this offer had been communicated to the managers of the Royal Infirmary and a committee of the Board appointed to confer with the University Court, an agreement was reached in July 1924, the site selected and the preparation of the plans entrusted to Mr Turnbull, the master of works. The choice of site had presented considerable difficulty as few open spaces remained on the property of the Infirmary capable of furnishing an area suitable for a building of the size desired, while the ground recently chosen for the new radiological department had reduced still further the field of selection. Eventually, however, this was acquired by taking part of the garden on the south side of the Superintendent's House—which incidentally deprived him of his tennis court—the ground at the east entrance to the medical house, once occupied by the old carriage shed or the motor shed used by the staff, and by incorporating part of the east medical lecture theatre. In addition to the facilities offered by the laboratory, the scheme included the provision of two small wards for male and female patients, each containing six beds, for the observation and treatment of such patients as required particular clinical investigation and special dieting, for whom the general wards of the hospital were not so suitable: these patients remained either under the care of the members of the honorary staff recommending them, or were placed, if desired, in the hands of the physician in charge of the department of therapeutics.

Construction was commenced in June 1926, tenders having been accepted estimating the total cost at £27,366 which was considerably less than the sum assured by the Rockefeller Foundation. The laboratory was ready for occupation in 1928, but as Jonathan Meakins had resigned the chair of therapeutics in 1924 on his appointment as professor of medicine and director of the department of medicine at McGill University, Montreal, his successor in the Christison chair, David Murray Lyon, assumed the directorship. On its completion the laboratory became the property of the managers of the Infirmary who were responsible for the maintenance of the fabric and for the expenditure connected with cleaning and painting, heating and lighting, and for the necessary electrical power supply. The University Court, on the other hand, met the expenses of the staff required for teaching and research and the outlays upon equipment and chemical materials. The new building provided scope for work on a more extended scale than that carried out in the old laboratory, all the members of the medical and surgical staff having the privilege of using the accommodation provided for research. The routine reporting work on behalf of the patients in the Infirmary continued to increase in volume and year by year made greater demands upon its resources.

Coincident with this undertaking the managers had to face the more serious problem of the reorganisation of the Medical Electrical Department. Since its inauguration by their predecessors in its cramped and somewhat makeshift quarters in an obscure corner of the surgical house, this special branch of science in its application to medicine had become more and more essential to nearly every department of the hospital. The accommodation which had served, however imperfectly, to meet the requirements in 1896 had become hopelessly inadequate in 1920, notwithstanding more than one attempt to enlarge it and increase its efficiency. Nothing less than an entirely new building would serve the purpose and, at the earnest desire of the medical and surgical staff, the reforms, which had been discussed in 1914 but necessarily abandoned during the years of the war, were again given consideration; and, while plans were being prepared for the erection of a modern pavilion, temporary expedients were introduced and accommodation was found for the massage staff in the surgical out-patient department. In 1923 a special committee of the Board was appointed under the convenership of Sir James Hodsdon, K.B.E., to whose untiring industry, sound practical judgment and efficiency as convener, the Infirmary owes a lasting debt of gratitude.

A central situation was selected upon unoccupied ground between the surgical and medical houses on the east side of, and contiguous to, the long corridor and balcony connecting these two sections of the hospital, so that it might be made readily accessible to both houses. In the basement which contained the heavy electrical machinery, were the mechanics' work-shops, the stores and the safe for radium: the first floor accommodated the radiographic apparatus necessary for diagnosis and treatment, for X-ray screening, deep X-ray therapy and dental X-ray work along with the photographic and dark rooms for the development of films, and a large room for purposes of demonstration and teaching. The second floor constituted the department of massage and physical therapeutics, with a gymnasium and rooms for general electrical treatment, light and heat therapy and accommodation for the necessary staff. In planning the internal arrangement the committee had the valuable assistance of Robert Knox, radiologist to King's College Hospital, one of the foremost authorities on the subject in the country, who acted throughout as honorary expert adviser. The cost of construction including part of the fittings and equipment was £39,500, to which required to be added a further sum of £9087 for the installation of the X-ray plant, thus bringing the total expenditure to £48,587. This outlay was met in part by the gift of £15,000 from the City of Edinburgh Branch of the British Red Cross Society and in part from the balance of the money received in response to the special appeal to which more than one reference has been made.

The department, which offered unrivalled facilities for the purposes for which it was planned, was completed in the summer of 1926 and the official opening ceremony was performed on 9th October of the same year by H.R.H. the Duke of York who was accompanied by H.R.H. the Duchess of York.

The increased cost incurred in maintaining the new building with its larger and more highly paid staff was at once reflected in the figures disclosed in the accounts of the annual ordinary expenditure of the hospital. In 1922-24, prior to its opening, the upkeep, equipment and appliances in the old department cost £2346 and, in 1926, in which year the work in the new department was carried on for six months, a sum of £4071 was expended; but, in 1929, the outlay had been more than doubled, totalling a sum of £9027.[1] These figures supply striking proof, if such were needed, of the constantly increasing strain upon the finances of the Infirmary in meeting the demands of one department, nor do they include the extra-ordinary expenditure on new plant, a frequently recurring item.

From the first it was anticipated that the new department would require to be placed in charge of a whole-time medical officer and, further, that the growing importance of radiology as a branch of medicine would necessitate the provision of suitable facilities for the instruction of the student and graduate. For a number of years the work of the department had been carried on by three part-time officers ; but in 1925, Dawson F. D. Turner, who had latterly acted as extra-medical electrician for the treatment of patients requiring radium, retired and was placed on the consulting staff and, in the following year, William Hope Fowler and Archibald McKendrick on the completion of their period of service as medical electricians were made consulting radiologists. The way was thus open for a change in administration. Dawson Turner and Hope Fowler, like other devoted pioneers in the work of this young science, had not escaped the physical disabilities supervening upon repeated exposure to the röntgen rays before satisfactory precautionary measures had been rightly understood : Turner did not long survive his retirement, dying on Christmas Day, 1928.[2]

In a communication from the managers of the Infirmary to the University Court in June 1923, the suggestion was made that the Court should consider the institution of a lectureship in medical electrical therapeutics and radiology and that the lecturer should be the official appointed by the Board as radiologist to the Infirmary. The proposal was favourably received by the Court, but on the understanding that the University should have "an adequate voice" in the selection of the person whom the managers might appoint in charge of the department. When in the following year the Board

[1] In 1935-36 the ordinary expenditure in the department was £12,700. This item as well as those of 1926 and 1929 included the salaries of the staff.

[2] William Hope Fowler, C.V.O., died on 4th October 1933.

decided to recommend as medical officer, John Miller Woodburn Morison, then the head of the radiological department at the Manchester Royal Infirmary, the University Court concurred in the recommendation and appointed him lecturer in radiology as from 1st June 1925, agreeing to contribute £400 towards his salary on the condition that the equipment of the department should be available for the instruction of students without further charge on the University.[1] Subsequently, in 1926, the University Court established a diploma in radiology open to graduates in medicine and surgery of the University, and to candidates holding corresponding degrees or qualification of some other licensing body registrable with the General Medical Council in Great Britain, or of such other universities or medical schools recognised for the purpose by the University Court.

In the massage and physio-therapy department on the second floor of the radiological building an increasing number of patients came under treatment each year; and, in 1929, three years after the department was opened the new patients numbered 2200 and the return visits 50,000, with an average daily attendance of 200 patients.[2]

The increasing demand for the employment of radium in the treatment of cancer and other diseases led the managers towards the end of 1928 to give serious consideration to the establishment of a complete radiological institute under their management and direction. As the additional beds required for the care of these patients could not be readily obtained within the Infirmary itself, they decided to reconstruct and equip with the necessary plant the mansion house of "Beechmount"—property bequeathed to the Infirmary in 1926—situated on the southern slope of the high ground at Murrayfield on the western outskirts of the city. But the scheme as originally contemplated was not proceeded with when the Royal Infirmary, shortly afterwards, became recognised by the National Radium Commission as the

[1] Dr J. M. Woodburn Morison resigned the dual appointment in 1930 on his election as Director of the Radiological Department, the Cancer Hospital, Fulham.

[2] In 1936, new patients, 3680; return visits, 68,000; average daily attendance, 300.

National Radium Centre for Edinburgh and the South-Eastern Area of Scotland. Beechmount was, however, fitted up as an Auxiliary Hospital to accommodate approximately forty patients before and after receiving radium treatment in the Infirmary. But the story of the Infirmary as a National Radium Centre and the coordination and expansion of its work in the fight against malignant disease post-date the period covered by this narrative and must be left to a future historian to record.

From time to time the attention of the managers was drawn to the necessity of providing more adequate dental treatment for the patients admitted to the wards of the Infirmary. As far back as 1863 a dental surgeon had been appointed to the honorary staff, the position being held for twenty-five years by John Smith, a Fellow of the Royal College of Surgeons of Edinburgh and its president in 1883. After his resignation from the post in 1888 the staff of the Dental Hospital and School, which occupied premises from 1889 to 1893 in Lauriston Lane rented from the Infirmary, gave gratuitous dental service to the patients in the Royal Infirmary and, by arrangement with the managers, conducted short courses of instruction in dental surgery for the more advanced students of medicine. But the transference of the Dental Hospital to Chambers Street terminated this arrangement and a surgeon was again appointed to the Infirmary. Following representations made by the medical and surgical staff that more facilities should be provided, an assistant dental surgeon was added to the department. As this failed to satisfy the growing needs of the Institution additional appointments were made so that in 1927 as many as six dental surgeons had been appointed, thus providing a daily service.

Prior to the conclusion of the war the Local Government Board for Scotland [1] had prepared a scheme and drafted regulations for the care and treatment of those suffering from venereal disease, which, if carried into effect, would establish for the first time within the Infirmary a Venereal Diseases

[1] Afterwards the Department of Health for Scotland.

Department. Since the early days of the hospital this group of patients had been treated in beds specially set apart for the purpose, but the wards had not been assigned to the care of a specialist, having been allocated from time to time to different members of the surgical staff. The scheme projected an entirely new form of administration and, as the success of the measures proposed would depend in great part upon the active cooperation of the large general hospitals with the Local Authorities in the various areas, the managers of the Infirmary, on the suggestion of the Local Government Board, appointed a committee to confer with the Public Health Committee of the Town Council : following their deliberations a satisfactory working scheme was drawn up and the terms of the co-partnership were finally approved in December 1918.

Briefly, it embodied the provision within the Infirmary of the necessary accommodation and facilities, while each party to the agreement was responsible for the administration of its own particular part of the scheme. The selection of a clinical medical officer and assistant medical officer to take charge of the department was made by a Joint-Selection Committee of the Corporation of the City and the managers of the Royal Infirmary, the names of the candidates thus nominated being then submitted to the Corporation for election as clinical medical officers, and to the managers for election as members of the honorary staff of the Infirmary with all the rights and privileges of that position. Their duties as officers of the Corporation were under the direction, supervision and control of the medical officer of health of the city, and those in the Infirmary under the sole and entire control of the managers of that Institution. To complete the staff necessary for the work of the department two assistant clinical pathologists were appointed by the Board of Management. The financial expenses connected with the scheme were to a large extent met by the Corporation who paid the salaries of the clinical officers and pathologists, made allowances towards salaries and wages of nurses and attendants, for material used in the necessary examinations, and for part payment for board and lodging of such patients resident in the city who required indoor treatment within the hospital. The managers, however, reserved to themselves the right of treating, either as in-patients or out-patients, those residing outside the jurisdiction of the Corporation of Edinburgh, and of receiving payment for the same from the different Local Authorities concerned, with the right also to direct and control the whole internal arrangements of the department within the Infirmary.

On 22nd September 1919, the Board of Management accepted the recommendation made by the Joint-Selection Committee and appointed David Lees, D.S.O., a graduate of Edinburgh and the first elected clinical medical officer, to be a member of the honorary staff of the Infirmary and to conduct the work of the new department. David Lees, after active service in France during the early years of the war, had received special training in this group of diseases in the military hospitals at Newcastle and Glasgow and had been adviser to the Derbyshire County Council: with exceptional administrative ability he was eminently qualified to undertake the duties of the post assigned to him and to lay the foundation of the department.[1]

The creation of a lectureship in venereal diseases in the University, already contemplated, was not long delayed, and after the faculty of medicine and the Senatus had approved of the introduction of a course of obligatory instruction in the subject as part of the medical curriculum, the University Court agreed to the appointment of David Lees as lecturer from 1st January 1920, the Corporation of the city concurring in this decision.

Other departments, to which beds were not attached and which might be more appropriately termed sub-departments within the field of general medicine and surgery, were instituted at this time. In 1922, when Sir Robert William Philip, professor of tuberculosis in the University since 1917, completed his term of fifteen years as ordinary physician to the Infirmary, he was appointed by the managers physician consultant in

[1] David Lees died on 25th March 1934, aged fifty-four years.

tuberculosis, so that his colleagues on the staff might continue to have the benefit of his valuable opinion and long experience in diseases of the lungs. The title " consultant " was employed to designate an office intermediate between that of ordinary physician and consulting physician to the hospital, the position carrying with it certain regular duties, such as attendance at bi-weekly clinics to which patients were referred from the general wards for consultation.[1] Another appointment on similar lines was made in 1923 when George Matthew Robertson, professor of psychiatry in the University and superintendent of the Royal Edinburgh Hospital for Mental and Nervous Disorders was made physician consultant in psychiatry. As far back as 1902 a movement had been made to establish such a department in the Infirmary, but, although the honorary staff generally approved of the scheme, neither the finances of the hospital nor the necessary accommodation were available.[2] A few years later, in 1929, a position on the staff of the Infirmary was assigned to the lecturer in the diseases of tropical climates, Lieut.-Colonel Edward David Wilson Greig, C.I.E., I.M.S., retired. Since his appointment as lecturer in 1924 the systematic instruction in the course for the diploma in tropical medicine had been given in the University buildings, while the facilities for clinical teaching had been placed at his disposal by the physicians in the hospital. But accommodation in the University being no longer at his command, arrangements were made that in future the systematic teaching and research should be carried on in the clinical laboratory, as the Deed of Gift permitted of its use for higher teaching in medicine (p. 331) ; and in order that the lecturer might have an official status in the Infirmary, the managers appointed Colonel Greig physician consultant in the diseases of tropical climates.

For many years by the aid of the Convalescent House at Corstorphine the medical and surgical staff had been able to

[1] The term surgeon consultant had been employed in 1921 when the writer, on the termination of his period of service, was appointed as such in the Ear, Nose and Throat Department.

[2] Minutes, Royal Infirmary, January, March, July 1902.

maintain contact for a short period of time with a limited number of patients after their discharge from the wards, and with others again, if desired, through the assistance of the Ladies' Committee and Almoners of the Royal Infirmary Samaritan Society. This Society, founded in January 1879, the year in which the new Infirmary was opened in Lauriston Place, rendered valuable help in various ways to the specially necessitous cases by providing small weekly payments to families whose bread-winners, while in hospital or even after leaving the Institution, were unable to work ; it also supplied clothes, artificial limbs and other necessities and arranged for the provision of diets in particular cases. The Society thus formed a temporary link between certain of the recently discharged patients and the Infirmary, but no organised general "follow-up" system existed.

The years subsequent to the war, however, saw considerable expansion of the social service movement and a greater effort on the part of voluntary organisations to participate in various aspects of social welfare, necessitating a demand for trained workers in that field. In 1923, at the request of the University School of Social Service, the managers granted permission to the lady pupils to obtain practical training by visiting the necessitous medical out-patients in their homes and by giving them assistance on lines somewhat similar to those so long provided by the Samaritan Society. The success attending the movement led to the inauguration in 1924 of a social service scheme, the Society's almoners continuing to undertake on behalf of the in-patients the work they had formerly done, while a new Social Service Department with its own staff of three almoners became responsible for the care of the out-patients. Amongst the manifold activities of this department may be mentioned the provision of grants to patients requiring special diets, the supplying of insulin for diabetic patients, arrangements for the attendance of Queen's Nurses at their homes, and monetary help from the Public Assistance Authorities and in special cases from the various relief societies. The almoners also kept in touch with those receiving grants from certain funds administered by the Infirmary, such as the

Murray Keith Fund and the Stedman and Charles Black bequests. But the new service was of further material assistance by acting as a "follow-up" department both in town and country and in tracing patients when special lines of investigation were being carried out by members of the honorary staff of the hospital. As an illustration of the extent of its work during the year 1928-29, 1939 visits were paid by the almoners and interviews were held with 6209 individuals.

With the establishment of the Dietetic Department in April 1924 and the appointment of a whole-time Sister Dietitian, there was introduced another organisation contributing to the health of many former patients by instructing them as to the nutritional value of simple articles of diet and the importance of a proper scheme of meals. In numerous instances a better standard of health was thus preserved, making readmission to hospital unnecessary and leaving beds available for the treatment of cases of greater urgency. With diets planned in the department according to the physicians' prescriptions many patients were enabled to continue their work and several hundreds attended the department every week. In 1928 a diet-kitchen was opened in connection with the two small wards attached to the clinical laboratory (p. 332) and patients in these wards were served with specially cooked meals when a complicated diet was desired.[1]

An exceptional opportunity of continuing the supervision and treatment of patients, whose illness involved a prolonged convalescence, was presented to the Infirmary through the munificent bequest of the late David Ainslie of Costerton, Midlothian, a landowner and a successful stock exhibitor who died in 1900. In his Trust-Disposition and Settlement he directed his trustees, after the expiry of fifteen years, to apply the residue of his estate to "the purpose of creating, endowing and maintaining a hospital or institution to be called the Astley Ainslie Institution for the relief and behoof of the convalescents in the Royal Infirmary of Edinburgh. . . ."

[1] A School of Dietetics was founded in the Department in 1934 under the supervision and instruction of Sister Ruth Pybus. In 1936 the new patients seen at the Department numbered 1262 and the return visits numbered 14,056.

As the war, with the consequent restrictions on building, postponed the commencement of operations, it was not till 1921 that the Court of Session approved a Deed of Constitution and Trust, and a Board of twelve governors was formed, five of whom were appointed by the managers of the Infirmary from their own members, with Sheriff Gerard L. Crole, K.C., one of the representatives of the Infirmary, as the first chairman.

The site selected for the Astley Ainslie Institution was ideal for the purpose. The several properties purchased in the Grange district of Edinburgh, covering an area of nearly thirty-one acres, had a southern exposure with an uninterrupted view of the Blackford, Braid and Pentland Hills. Amongst the mansions and gardens acquired stood the house of Millbank, formerly the country home of James Syme, in which his daughter Agnes was married to Joseph Lister in 1856 and in which Syme spent the closing days of his life. Two of the existing mansion houses were preserved and adapted for the new service, but the work of the Institution was carried on mainly in a number of specially constructed pavilions. One of the two houses retained was opened in 1923 providing accommodation for thirty-five female patients, but, with the completion of the east and west pavilions in 1929, ninety beds became available and in that year 410 patients were treated during their convalescence.[1]

The policy adopted by the governors was twofold: to enable patients preparatory to undergoing a serious operation in the Infirmary to have a short period of rest and treatment; while the main object of the Institution was to make provision whereby the convalescent patients might be sufficiently restored to health and able to resume work without incurring the risk of an early relapse. It was not the intention of the governors to establish a home for incurables or for those debilitated by old age or suffering from a permanently disabling affection. No time-limit was laid down as to their duration

[1] In 1936 the beds numbered 169, and 744 patients were admitted. In 1932, when Millbank became available, it was found necessary to demolish the house and to construct a pavilion upon its site.

of stay, but so long as the patients continued to improve, with every prospect of recovery, accommodation and treatment were provided for them. Their earlier removal from the Infirmary was thus made possible and the pressure upon its beds correspondingly relieved. Hitherto investigation had been directed mainly to the study of the causation of disease, but in the Astley Ainslie Institution a new field was opened for research in the observation and examination of patients during a prolonged period of convalescence.[1]

Mr Gerard Lake Crole, Sheriff of the Lothians and Peebles, the first chairman of the Board of the Astley Ainslie Institution, was a very active manager of the Royal Infirmary for eighteen years, as a representative alternately of the Faculty of Advocates and the Court of Contributors. He died while still in office on 26th October 1927. As convener of several of its special committees he placed his business ability, legal knowledge and wide experience of affairs at the service of the hospital; and he specially identified himself with the arrangements made for coordinating clinical teaching in the Infirmary, with the special appeal of 1920, and with the subsequent extension movement. He was an ardent supporter of the inception of the League of Subscribers.

In this post-war period the Infirmary lost the services of some of its experienced senior officials. In May 1924, Sir Joseph Fayrer, the Superintendent, reached the age-limit of sixty-five years. Appointed in 1911, his period in office had been considerably encroached upon by his absence during the war as commandant of the 2nd Scottish General Hospital. In his position as administrator he exercised his authority with a geniality and charm of manner which gained him the willing help and cooperation of every member of the Institution with whom he was brought into contact.[2] From a particularly strong list of applicants the managers selected as his successor, Colonel George David St Clair Thom, C.B., C.M.G., C.B.E.,

1 "The Astley Ainslie Institution," by Alexander Miles, M.D., *University of Edinburgh Journal*, vol. iii, 1929-30.

2 Sir Joseph Fayrer died at Gullane, East Lothian, on 13th April 1937, aged seventy-eight years.

a graduate of Edinburgh in 1893. His experience in the Army Medical Service had extended over twenty-nine years and in the war he held responsible posts in the Dardanelles, in France and finally at Archangel, having been specially selected to reorganise the medical arrangements of the Allied Forces in North Russia. Strongly recommended on account of his administrative capacity, which was of a high order, Colonel Thom was eminently fitted for a post of responsibility and trust.[1] In 1925 Miss Annie Warren Gill, C.B.E., retired from the office of Lady Superintendent after eighteen years in that position which included the arduous period of the war. She was a member of several Associations concerned with the advancement of the profession of nursing, the status of which she was indefatigable in promoting.[2] The vacancy was filled by the appointment of Miss Ellen Frances Bladon, the senior assistant superintendent of nurses who, commencing her career as a probationer in the Infirmary, had passed through all the grades during twenty-eight years of residence in the hospital.[3]

When, in December 1893, the managers had promoted Mr William Strathie Caw from the post of cashier to fill the vacant office of Treasurer and Clerk they acted with a shrewd knowledge and intelligent appreciation of his ability to occupy that position, a selection which time and experience fully justified. Although reaching the age-limit for retirement in 1927, Mr Caw at the unanimous request of the Board of Management remained for a further two years. On his retirement in December 1929, the chairman, Harriet, Lady Findlay, in expressing the great regret of the Board at his departure after the long period of forty-nine years, thirteen in the Cashier's office and thirty-six as Treasurer and Clerk, voiced the feeling of every member when she said that, " although the personnel of the Board had changed many

[1] Colonel St Clair Thom died on 7th April 1935 during his final year as Superintendent, having been given one year of extension. The office was filled by the appointment of Lieut.-Colonel Alexander Dron Stewart, C.I.E., M.B., I.M.S.

[2] Miss Gill died on 2nd March 1930.

[3] Miss Bladon retired on 30th September 1931, and was succeeded by Miss Elizabeth Dunlop Smaill, O.B.E., R.R.C.

times during that long period, the fact that its tradition of willing service to, and happy relation with, the Institution remained unchanged, was in no small measure due to Mr Caw's personality and his coordinating influence in every branch of the work of the Infirmary." At the close of the meeting Mrs George Kerr, the senior member of the Board, presented him with a silver salver, the gift of the managers, as a mark of their respect and appreciation. The vacancy was filled in June 1929 by the appointment of Mr Henry Maw, secretary to the Clayton Hospital, Wakefield, the office being henceforth designated as that of Secretary and Treasurer. He commenced his duties on 1st January 1930.

CHAPTER XX

THE BICENTENARY YEAR—1929

THE COMMEMORATION SERVICE—THE BICENTENARY EXTENSION SCHEME—THE MATERNITY HOSPITAL AND THE NEW HOME FOR NURSES—RETROSPECT.

1729 to 1929—two centuries of time since the Royal Infirmary first opened its door in Robertson's Close; and the story of its simple origin, with its small beginnings, steady growth and expansion throughout these years, reaches the final chapter. Little requires to be added save to relate how the bicentenary anniversary was commemorated and made the occasion of an appeal to the public to contribute to the continued prosperity of the heritage handed down to them.

"As Men and Christians we have the strongest Inducements and even Obligations to this sort of Charity, as it is warmly recommended and injoyned in the Gospel as one of the greatest Christian Duties. . . ." In these words, written more than two hundred years ago, John Monro made the first appeal to the citizens of Edinburgh to help him to found an Infirmary. With the Christian spirit as the basis of the appeal for the relief of human suffering, it was meet and right that the bicentenary commemoration should take the form of a religious service; and for such a ceremony no more fitting shrine could have been chosen than the ancient and venerable pile of the Cathedral Church of St Giles in which, for a thousand years, generations had been wont to assemble and, in times of national mourning and thanksgiving, to raise their voices in prayer and praise. In 1926, within the same historic building the medical faculty of the University had commemorated the two hundredth anniversary of its foundation and the birth of the Edinburgh School of Medicine of which the Royal Infirmary, three years later, had become the necessary complement.

As the actual date of the opening of the original hospital,

the 6th August, occurred during Edinburgh's principal holiday month, the religious service was postponed till later in the year, but on the anniversary day every patient in the Infirmary and the members of the medical and administrative staffs were presented with an illuminated Commemoration Card as a souvenir of the event. On 27th November a large and representative gathering of the citizens and public bodies assembled in the Cathedral. Among those present were the Lord Provost, Magistrates and Councillors, along with representatives of those "classes and societies" from which the original members of the Board of Management of the Infirmary had been selected and which have continued to give representation throughout the years. The officiating clergy, in the unavoidable absence of the Right Rev. John White, Moderator of the General Assembly of the Church of Scotland, were the Very Rev. Charles Laing Warr, Dean of the Thistle and Chapel Royal; the Very Rev. James Harvey, Clerical Representative on the Board of the Royal Infirmary; the Right Rev. Bishop Reid, and the Rev. Thomas C. Macaulay, Chaplain to the Royal Infirmary.

The decision of the Board of Management of the Royal Infirmary to make a renewed appeal to the public in the bicentenary year was no sudden or eleventh-hour resolution, but the necessary continuation of the post-war policy of expansion that had failed to achieve its full purpose owing to the insufficient response to the appeal of 1920. A good deal had been accomplished, as has already been related, but one extension of particular urgency had been postponed —the erection of a new Home for Nurses, the construction of which could no longer be delayed.

Since the opening of the Central Nurses' Home—the "Red Home"—in 1892, the difficulty in accommodating the increased nursing staff had been temporarily and partially overcome by purchase of, or by leasing, house property in the immediate vicinity of the Infirmary or at some distance from it. As far back as 1907 houses had been bought on the east side of Archibald Place, a row of tall tenements forming one side of the short street extending from Lauriston Place southwards to the grounds of George Watson's College for Boys, (see Plan facing p. 280). At subsequent intervals other tenements in Archibald Place were purchased as they came into the market so that, in 1929, they provided accommodation for 104 nurses and 15 maids and the term " West Home " was eventually applied to this row of buildings : being contiguous to the property of the Infirmary, entrance to the Home was easily obtained.[1] In 1914 it was necessary to lease from the University at an annual rent of £85 and for a term of five years number 36 George Square, beyond the eastern boundary of the Infirmary. This house which made provision for 18 nurses was finally vacated in June 1927. In 1922, in which year 340 nurses were on the staff, the managers found it expedient as a further temporary measure to acquire in the southern district of the city Woodburn House and grounds, a mansion in Canaan Lane, Morningside which for some years had been used as a sanatorium for the treatment of patients suffering from pulmonary tuberculosis. Opened on 1st October of that year it provided accommodation for from 40 to 45 nurses, but in 1927 by the provision of a pavilion in the grounds an additional 20 were accommodated. Thus 65 nurses, while on night duty in the Infirmary, found their sleeping quarters at Woodburn, the garden, tennis courts and relative quietness of the area adding to the attraction of the Home. But the impending regulations to reduce the number of working hours of the nursing staff, then fifty-six hours per week, necessarily entailed a further numerical increase and made more accommodation imperative. A large Home in the vicinity of the Infirmary was deemed preferable as centralisation permitted of better supervision and greater economy : further, it gave facilities for providing larger and more suitable rooms for recreation and improved sickroom accommodation during temporary epidemics of illness.

After the conclusion of the war considerable anxiety began to be felt owing to the growing pressure upon the bed

[1] In 1935-36 the West Home accommodated 178 nurses and 17 maids, making a total of 195 persons.

accommodation in the hospital, returns compiled for the last eight months of 1918-19 showing an average of 606 names upon the list of patients awaiting treatment in the wards ; and this total progressively increased as, in 1922-23, the average number was approximately 1500 over the period of twelve months.[1] It seemed desirable, therefore, that further extension of the hospital should be considered with a view to preventing, if possible, a still longer list.

As the accumulation of these names was a matter of grave concern to the managers and to others, not only in 1923 but in the ensuing years, a more detailed reference to the subject at this point cannot fail to be of interest. The number of patients admitted into the Infirmary in 1922-23 was 14,239, of whom 4449 passed into the medical and 9790 into the surgical departments, the total number of beds available for their accommodation being 909. The average period of residence of patients in the medical wards was 28·81 days and in the surgical wards 18 days. As the great majority of those awaiting admission were entered for treatment in the various surgical departments, the medical cases forming a comparatively small proportion of the total, the two explanatory tables appended deal only with the former. Table A shows the number of beds available in the surgical departments at 1st October 1923, 1929 and 1936, and Table B the number of prospective patients awaiting surgical treatment at the same dates.[2]

It is evident from a study of these tables that, although more beds had provided increased facilities for indoor treatment, they had not effected any reduction in the number of those seeking admission to the Infirmary : on the contrary, the list of names continued to grow at a disconcerting rate in the surgical department to which most of the extra beds had been added. More than one suggestion has been offered in explanation. After the termination of the war

[1] No case of acute illness or serious injury was at any time refused admission, arrangements being at once made to provide the necessary beds.

[2] Beds are classified as *total* and *available*, as a number are held in reserve for occupation when wards in daily use are being cleaned, or in the event of emergencies. In 1923, total, 963, available, 909 ; in 1929, total, 1006, available, 982 ; in 1936, total, 1125, available, 1107.

economic conditions had altered considerably so that a section of the community, which had formerly refrained from

SURGICAL WAITING LIST

Table A. *Analysis of the Available Surgical Beds at 1st October 1923, 1929, 1936*

Year.	Total Available Surgical Beds.	General Surgery.	Gynæcology.	Ear and Throat Diseases.	Eye Diseases.	Total Waiting List.
						1440 Surgical 215 Medical
1923	514	348	90	24	52	1655
						2494 Surgical 415 Medical
1929	545	348	90	55	52	2909
						2971 Surgical 419 Medical
1936	605	392	90	59	64	3390

Table B. *Analysis of the Surgical Waiting List at 1st October 1923, 1929, 1936*

Year.	Total Surgical Waiting List.	General Surgery.	Gynæcology.	Ear and Throat Diseases.	Eye Diseases.	
1923	1440	504	250	608	78	
1929	2494	1370	536	507	81	
1936	2971	1608	813	469	81	

Note on Table A. In 1926, Ear and Throat Department increased by 31 beds; in 1936, Eye Department, by 12 beds; after 1929, General Surgical Department, by 56 beds; total additional beds = 99.

seeking advice in times of sickness at a voluntary hospital, was now through force of circumstances compelled to do so. With the rise in the cost of living and of medical and surgical services illness had become more expensive and many were unable to meet the increased charges. Another factor was the influence of the motor car in facilitating and accelerating the transport to hospital, from widely scattered areas, of a large number of persons acutely ill or seriously injured, many of whom in pre-war days would have been attended to at home. Therefore the vacant beds in the hospital intended for the admission of patients on the waiting list were often filled by urgent cases, many of which, such as motor accidents, required prolonged treatment in the wards. And thus each week fresh cases regarded as of less urgency were being added to the bottom of the list while many of those at the top still remained, " sacrificed to the acute conditions on the plea of urgency." [1] So the waiting list lengthened slowly but surely.

For both these purposes—more accommodation for nurses and additional surgical beds—a new site was obviously necessary as no space remained on the existing property of the Infirmary on which a Central Nurses' Home and a Surgical Pavilion could be erected.

At this stage in the deliberations of the managers a new factor was introduced destined not only to modify the form in which the bicentenary appeal was issued but to influence the future course of the development of the Infirmary. The directors of the Edinburgh Royal Maternity and Simpson Memorial Hospital, recognising the urgent need of a new and larger building, were contemplating an appeal to the public for funds. The Hospital in Lauriston Place had been giving constant service to the community since 1879, but, through lack of the necessary accommodation, was becoming less able to cope with the demands made upon it. During the war, through the pioneer work of John William Ballantyne, one of the physicians on the staff, the first Antenatal Department had been inaugurated making provision for the observation and care of the expectant mother, and still further taxing the resources of the hospital.[2]

[1] Address by Professor Sir John Fraser at the annual conference of the British Hospitals Association, Edinburgh, 18th June 1936. *The Scotsman*, 19th June 1936.

[2] J. W. Ballantyne died on 23rd January 1923.

A NEW MATERNITY HOSPITAL

With a view to considering what action should be taken the directors of the Maternity Hospital called a meeting of representatives of certain public bodies in the city—the Scottish Board of Health, the Town Council, the University of Edinburgh, the Royal Infirmary, and the Royal Colleges of Physicians and Surgeons. On 16th November 1923, a Conference took place in the Old Council Room of the City Chambers at which were discussed the necessity of a new hospital, the accommodation required, a suitable site, and the means of financing the scheme. The delegates, who were unanimous in their opinion that a hospital of at least 150 beds was required, agreed generally on the importance of erecting it in the vicinity of the Royal Infirmary so as to secure the advantages which such proximity would offer; and a suggestion was made by representatives of the latter that it might be of advantage to the Maternity Hospital if there were some form of association or affiliation between the maternity and gynæcological work of the two Institutions, in the interests of efficiency and economy. Accordingly, information was sought from the managers of the Infirmary on two points: the possibility of their obtaining the necessary site within a reasonable period of time, and the basis upon which the two bodies might cooperate.

The only area suitable for extension in close proximity to the Infirmary was the ground occupied by George Watson's College for Boys; therefore, on 4th February 1924, a special committee of the Board of Management was appointed to meet the Education Board of the Merchant Company to ascertain if the latter would be prepared to consider the disposal of the College and grounds. Thus for the fourth time in the long history of the Infirmary the Merchant Company and the managers entered into negotiations: they had done so originally in 1736 for the purchase of Thomson's Yards which had been acquired by the trustees of George Watson's Hospital as a prospective site for their school; in 1869, when the managers bought George Watson's Hospital and grounds in Lauriston Place as the site for the new Infirmary; in 1891-92 when it was desired to purchase the Junior School of Watson's College;

and now, in 1924, when the managers offered to buy the College and its playground. With the present College secure in its new situation, one and a half miles from the Royal Infirmary, it is difficult to conceive future managers requiring to negotiate with the Merchant Company for a part or the whole of their School!

Considerable delay occurred before the final settlement was reached. At first, an offer of £60,000 was put forward, but "it was felt that an advance on that sum would require to be made in order to compensate the Company for the disturbance, and the committee of the managers have already indicated that the Board might be prepared to advance their offer to £75,000 as a maximum."[1] But it was difficult for the Merchant Company to arrive at an immediate decision on so important a question as the sale of their school-buildings. They were naturally reluctant to dispose of a site which had given educational facilities to two of their schools since 1818; in that year the Merchant Maidens' Hospital had been transferred from Bristo Street to a building facing the Meadows which, in 1871, became George Watson's College for Boys, after the Infirmary had acquired its new site in 1869.[2] Nor was it easy for the Company to refuse the appeal of the Royal Infirmary burdened with its ever growing waiting-list. Nevertheless the problem of finding another site on which to erect a new George Watson's College had to be faced. In 1925, negotiations between the two parties were continued without any decision being reached, as the Merchant Company were asking for a sum of £100,000, realising that the cost of a new site and school would be considerably in excess of the price offered by the managers for the purchase of their old building.[3]

During this long period of discussion the directors of the Maternity Hospital were chafing at the delay, as more than two years had elapsed since they had called their Conference in the City Chambers. As there seemed to be an imminent

[1] Minute, Royal Infirmary, 6th July 1925.
[2] The new Merchant Maidens' School was then opened in Queen Street.
[3] Minute, Royal Infirmary, 15th February 1926.

risk that no agreement would be reached on the question of a site in the vicinity of the Infirmary, they intimated to the managers in February 1926 their intention of calling together a committee of the public bodies to report upon the situation. But a final settlement was in sight and, through the generosity of one of Edinburgh's prominent citizens, the danger of an *impasse* was prevented. For nearly a year the Infirmary had been slowly accumulating an extension fund and to this Sir John Ritchie Findlay, Bt., of Aberlour, offered to contribute £10,000 if the managers would increase their offer for the purchase of the site to £90,000.[1] This they agreed to do, at the same time intimating that the payment would be made in one sum. The terms were accepted by the Merchant Company on the condition that they secured a suitable site for their new school at a reasonable price and that the buildings should be ready for occupation before the boys were obliged to leave the existing premises, the expectation being that the Infirmary would obtain possession at the Martinmas Term, 1931.[2]

With the purchase price finally settled the managers were at last in a position to make definite proposals to the directors of the Maternity Hospital, which, transmitted in a letter dated 23rd June 1926, were as follows:—1. The erection on the acquired property of a complete maternity and gynæcological department of 245 beds, or thereby, along with an operating theatre annexe and out-patient department, and the existing gynæcological pavilion of the Infirmary to be utilised for other surgical requirements: 2. The only satisfactory method of amalgamation with the Maternity Hospital would be by absorption of it, as divided authority or management within the Royal Infirmary could not be contemplated, and that the Capital funds of the Hospital would be taken over and used towards meeting the cost of the new building, Parliamentary powers being probably necessary to legalise this transfer: 3. The name of "Simpson," intimately linked with the Royal Maternity Hospital, would continue to be associated with the

[1] Minute, Royal Infirmary, 1st March 1926.
[2] Actual possession of the property was not obtained by the Infirmary till 1932.

new building: and 4. The appointment of a Consultation Committee of the Hospital to meet the committee of the managers of the Infirmary in the preparation of the plans and for other matters. It was considered impossible to increase the membership of the Board of the Infirmary, but it was hoped that as vacancies occurred in the seats open to representatives of the Court of Contributors, places might be found for some of the directors of the Maternity Hospital.

These proposals were accepted by the directors, with the concurrence of the medical staff of the Hospital, as constituting a foundation upon which the new scheme might be constructed. The proposals embodied advantages to both Institutions. With the transference of the women from the Diamond Jubilee Pavilion to the new building, the Infirmary would be provided with approximately one hundred additional beds for the treatment of surgical patients with the expectation that the problem of the waiting list would in part be solved. They gave to the Maternity Hospital a much enlarged modern building and a central training school for the more efficient education of students of medicine and midwives; and, with the maternity and gynæcological services as one unit served by the same medical and surgical staff, and with all the advantages of close association with a large general hospital, administration and control would be conducted with greater efficiency and economy. In addition to the proposed hospital, part of the site was to be reserved for the new Home for Nurses and for accommodation of the increased domestic staff.

The Bicentenary Extension Appeal was accordingly drawn up on these lines, and the sum regarded as necessary for its completion and for the many alterations in, and additions to, the existing buildings, heating, lighting and other improvements, was estimated at half a million pounds. To quote the concluding paragraph of the Appeal, " Of this sum approximately £100,000 are required for the purchase of the site; [1] the remaining £400,000 for building and equipping the Maternity and Gynæcological Hospital of 240 beds, for the Nurses' Home

[1] The site purchased included, in addition to George Watson's College, properties on the west side of Archibald Place.

with accommodation for 400 persons, and for a number of much needed developments—for example treatment by radium —to bring the existing Institution into line with modern requirements."

Such were the conclusions arrived at in 1929, the bi-centenary year of the Royal Infirmary. Since the autumn of 1923, when some form of collaboration between the Infirmary and Maternity Hospital was first mooted, the journey had been long; several years were yet to elapse before the scheme was finally adjusted and the buildings were ready for occupation.[1]

In unrolling the pages of the past and transcribing what they disclose, the attempt has been made to chronicle, however imperfectly, the story of the Royal Infirmary and the Edinburgh School of Medicine, their origin, early development and subsequent extensions; and to show how future events justified the aspirations and the actions of those pioneers, men of vision, sagacity and determination, who, two hundred years ago, founded the hospital and the medical faculty at Edinburgh. At the beginning of the eighteenth century the demand for a hospital service for the sick and injured poor had been met by the establishment throughout the country of the voluntary hospital system. But at Edinburgh a second factor, the need for a more complete education, influenced the minds of the founders, it being their intention that the hospital should also form the necessary complement of the medical school created three years earlier: "That students in Physic and Surgery might hereby have rather a better and easier opportunity of experience, than they have hitherto had by studying abroad, where such Hospitals are, at a great charge to themselves, and a yearly loss to the Nation." Hence, following the example of Leiden where, in the seventeenth century, a hospital for clinical

[1] In July 1933 the managers found it necessary on financial grounds to revise and modify the original Bicentenary Extension Scheme and to proceed on more economical lines: the modified scheme consisted in the erection of a Maternity Hospital of 122 beds and of a Nurses' Home to provide 260 bedrooms. This alteration precluded the liberation for other purposes of the gynæcological beds in the Diamond Jubilee Pavilion.

instruction had been established in organised relation with its university, they founded the Infirmary as a correlated part of the school of medicine. Thus the Greek inspiration of Medicine, reborn at Padua and nurtured at Leiden, passed on to Edinburgh whence it spread across the seas to America and Australasia.

During a comparatively brief space of time the practice of medicine and surgery was taught in a small hired house with six beds in a narrow Close of the old medieval city, till the large hospital was built and opened in 1741 in Infirmary Street; and, in the old Town's College before its reconstruction, in classrooms " mean, straitened and inconvenient and with little to recommend them," the science was expounded to an ever increasing number of students of medicine. But the attraction of the young school was not in its buildings but in the human factor which guided and controlled its destiny. Staffed by men who regarded their duty as teachers as their primary concern in the day's engagements, a practice was established which, handed down through the years, has become the tradition of the Edinburgh School to the present day. And for two hundred years the Royal Infirmary has discharged its threefold function, " the saving and restoring to health members of society whose labours are indispensable to a State," the education of the practitioner of medicine, and the training of the nursing profession.

While the opening years of the eighteenth century had witnessed the birth of the voluntary hospitals in Britain, and in Scotland also the foundation of the medical faculties in the Universities of Edinburgh and Glasgow, the early nineteenth century was identified with the widespread development of the provincial medical schools in England and with an increase in the number of the hospital schools in London. The rapid growth of industrialism with its teeming centres of population had already created in a number of areas the demand for hospitals, in some of which medical instruction on a small scale was imparted. But it was not till the advent of the nineteenth century that these hospitals became more firmly established as centres of medical education. The Apothecaries'

Act, 1815, laid down regulations for systematic teaching and extended the authority of the Society of Apothecaries of London to grant a diploma qualifying the holder to practise outside the limited area of London, thus creating a body of general practitioners in England and Wales who were entirely independent of the Colleges of Physicians and Surgeons. Probably acting under the stimulus which the Act provided medical schools were established between 1824 and 1834 in Manchester, Birmingham, Sheffield, Leeds, Newcastle, Bristol and Liverpool, schools which, at the beginning of the twentieth century, became incorporated in the medical faculties of their respective universities. In London, the hospitals of Charing Cross, King's College and St Mary were founded and, after the creation of their medical schools, the old privately owned schools of anatomy and surgery which had been a feature of medical education in the eighteenth century eventually ceased to exist.

In the early development of more than one of the provincial schools in England, Edinburgh, through its graduates or those who had received part of their training north of the Border, exercised a formative influence. But nowhere was the Scottish inspiration more pronounced than in the foundation of University College, London, and of its medical school.[1]

During the latter half of the eighteenth and the early nineteenth centuries, Scotland and its capital had enjoyed a period of great intellectual and academic activity somewhat comparable to that of Holland in the seventeenth century. It was an epoch which had given to Europe the philosophy of David Hume and Adam Smith, and later, of Dugald Stewart and John Playfair; a period which also embraced the writings of the historian, William Robertson, Principal of the University of Edinburgh for thirty years; the poetical works of Thomas Campbell, Allan Ramsay and Robert Burns; the architecture of Robert Adam and the portraiture of Sir Henry Raeburn,

[1] Prior to the opening of University College Hospital in 1834, the students of medicine at the College received their clinical instruction at the Middlesex Hospital and at the Dispensary.

culminating in the romantic personality of Sir Walter Scott. The period also saw the birth and early career of the *Edinburgh Review* under the able and critical editorship of Sydney Smith, Francis Horner, Henry Brougham and Francis Jeffrey, and the pages of *Blackwood's Magazine* fostered a younger literary school which included " Christopher North," John Gibson Lockhart, the biographer of Scott, and the pathetic figure of de Quincey. It was an epoch also that was remarkable in the contributions that were made to science: the perfecting of the steam engine by James Watt; the discovery of carbon dioxide and the principle of latent heat by Joseph Black; the determination of the maximum density of water by Thomes Charles Hope; the recognition of nitrogen gas by Daniel Rutherford and the discovery of the function of the lymphatic system of the body by Alexander Monro, *secundus*.

In the foundation of University College, the germ of the University of London, " the strongest, single, intellectual influence was that of Edinburgh, and, from the example of the Scottish Universities, London drew many of its most distinctive features. The extended range of the subjects of university study, the lecture system, the non-residence of students, their admission to single courses, the absence of religious tests, the dependence of the professors upon fees and the democratic character of the institutions, were all deliberate imitations of Scottish practice." [1] And amongst the founders of University College were Thomas Campbell, at one time a student at Glasgow, Henry, Lord Brougham and Leonard Horner, the first Warden of the College, both former students at Edinburgh. Of the early professors in its medical faculty the majority received their training at Edinburgh, Sir Charles Bell, in the chair of physiology and surgery, Edward Turner in chemistry, Anthony Todd Thomson in materia medica, John Connolly and John Elliotson in the practice of physic, John Gordon Smith in forensic medicine and, later, William Sharpey in anatomy and physiology and Robert Liston in clinical surgery.

[1] *University College, London, 1826-1926,* by H. Hale Bellot, M.A. London: University of London Press Ltd., 1929.

RETROSPECT

At the commencement of the nineteenth century Edinburgh, like other parts of the country, benefited by the development of the Scottish industries, agriculture, the mineral resources and the woollen industry ; while the growth of the population, the expansion of the city, and the improvements in the roads and means of transport were factors which increased the demands made upon the resources of the Infirmary. From the year 1800 to 1900 the school of medicine at first occupied an even stronger position than it had done at the close of the previous century so that, by the end of the first decade, the number of students enrolling in the faculty of medicine of the University had reached 934 : although this large total afterwards declined considerably through several decades, there being a distinct reduction in the number of those entering the profession of medicine at Edinburgh, before the end of the century the numbers again increased and the students matriculating in the year 1889-90 reached the unprecedented total of 2044. Moreover, early in the period two chairs of surgery had been created in the University and a strong extra-academical school grew up, providing a valuable means of training the younger men as teachers.

Four other factors, however, during the century, had a profound influence upon the future development of the Infirmary, contributing largely to its expansion : the introduction of general anæsthesia as a means of preventing pain during operations ; the new science of bacteriology which laid the foundation of the Germ Theory of disease and upon which was based the antiseptic principle in the treatment of wounds, by which the whole field of surgery was enlarged ; the adoption of the modern system of nursing ; and, finally, specialisation in surgery and medicine. Their influence upon the expansion of the hospital was manifested in the active steps taken to acquire more property on which to erect buildings to provide the additional accommodation. In 1832, with the occupation of the old High School for surgical cases, the hospital was subdivided into medical and surgical houses, the original Royal Infirmary building opened in 1741 being retained as the medical house. The erection of a second surgical hospital followed in 1853. Specialism was first recognised in 1850 with the appointment of Sir James Young Simpson as extra-physician for diseases peculiar to women, and five years later nineteen beds, which had been reserved in the New Surgical Hospital for the treatment of diseases of the eye, were placed under the charge of an ophthalmic surgeon. In these small beginnings specialism, which was to make so many claims upon the hospital before the century closed and after, was firmly established in the old Royal Infirmary.

In due course Time inevitably laid its hand on the fabric of the old medical hospital and, after a keen controversy extending over a period of nearly five years, which excited the interest of the medical profession and the general public, the important decision was reached to build a large new modern Infirmary upon the site in Lauriston Place. With the foundation stone laid in 1870, the new Royal Infirmary was opened in October 1879. The succeeding fifty years became a period of great activity and rapid expansion, with the Infirmary on two occasions, in 1892 and in 1926, extending its boundaries by the purchase of adjoining property. A Central Nurses' Home, long delayed, was occupied in the spring of 1892 : new pavilions were constructed for special departments, for the diseases of women, a memorial of the Diamond Jubilee of Queen Victoria, and pavilions for the treatment of diseases of the eye and of the ear, nose and throat ; a new radiological and physio-therapy department and a large clinical medicine laboratory were erected on the area occupied in 1879, while the Bicentenary Extension Scheme of 1929 envisaged the erection of a Maternity Hospital and a New Home for Nurses. And so through the long period of two hundred years the small hired house with six beds had grown into a great hospital capable of accommodating 1025 patients.[1]

What of the future ! It would be idle, perhaps unprofitable in 1929, the bicentenary year, to predict what the future may have in store for the Royal Infirmary of Edinburgh. Recent legislation has made it competent for County and Town Councils to submit schemes for the reorganisation of hospital

[1] In October 1936 the total beds in the Royal Infirmary numbered 1135.

facilities and to provide treatment for sick persons residing within their area ; and to take reasonable steps to secure full cooperation with every voluntary hospital, university or medical school within or serving the area of the Council. It is possible that a new system of hospital administration may profoundly affect the status of the Royal Infirmary in the years to come.[1] Perchance the cross-roads have been reached and, in the misty haze of uncertainty, it is difficult to discern along which route, indicated by the sign posts, the voluntary hospital will travel in order to fulfil its destiny.

[1] Local Government (Scotland) Act, 1929. [19-20 Geo. 5, Ch. 25.]

APPENDICES

APPENDIX I

Table of Data indicating Expansion of the Royal Infirmary at Intervals: in 1836-37; in 1879-80; in 1928-29; in 1935-36

Selected Data.	Hospital in Robertson's Close, 1729-30.	Old Royal Infirmary, 1836-37.	New Royal Infirmary		
			1879-80.	1928-29.	1935-36.
Total in-patients during year .	35	4,164	5,315	19,889	21,568
In-patients treated and discharged during year . .	30	3,829	4,857	18,972	20,612
In-patients treated in medical wards	23	...	2,547[1]	4,743	5,536
In-patients treated in surgical wards	7	...	2,310	14,229	15,076
Available beds in the hospital .	6	373	477	1,006	1,117
Daily average number of patients	6	...	420	956	965·5
Highest number on any one day	9	...	490	995	1,019
Average stay of patients under treatment	36·9 days	...	31·6 days	17 days	17·4 days
Average stay of patients in medical wards . . .	35·8 days	...	34·5 days	26·18 days	26·04 days
Average stay of patients in surgical wards . . .	40·2 days	...	29·9 days	13·8 days	13·8 days
New out-patients in all departments	...	...	15,000	67,623	72,543
Medical and surgical Officers (honorary and salaried) .	2[2]	13	24[3]	75[3]	82[3]
Nurses and probationer nurses .	0	...	101	411	460
Annual ordinary income . .	£159, 12s. 8d.	£5,381	£21,540	£114,898	£129,020
Annual ordinary expenditure .	£97, 19s. 7⅜d.	£6727	£27,818	£143,684	£169,694
Average cost per day per patient	10¾d.	...	...	8s. 2¾d.	9s. 7¼d.
Average annual cost per occupied bed	£2, 16s.	£25	£60	£150	£175

[1] 358 fever patients are included in this total: they occupied beds in part of the old Royal Infirmary.
[2] Of the physicians and surgeons attending in rotation, one of each was on duty for short periods.
[3] This number represents the active staff: the consulting staff are not included.

APPENDIX II

MEDICAL AND SURGICAL OFFICERS

MEDICAL DEPARTMENT

Physicians-in-Ordinary

In 1729 the Fellows of the Royal College of Physicians of Edinburgh attended the Infirmary in rotation for short periods. The first physician, John Drummond, senior, commenced his visits on 6th August, and the second physician, Robert Lowis, on 20th August.

In January 1751 the managers appointed two physicians-in-ordinary to attend the Infirmary daily as from 24th June: no time limit was attached to the period of service. The College of Physicians continued to send some of their number monthly by rotation to assist these physicians.

	Ordinary Physicians	Retired or Resigned, Died[1]
David Clerk	1751	1768, died
Colin Drummond	1751	1773
John Hope professor of medicine and botany, 1761-1786	1768	[2]
John Steedman	1773	1775
Joseph Black professor of chemistry and medicine, 1766-1795	1774	1774
James Hamilton, senior	1775	1823
Henry Cullen	1776	1790, died
Daniel Rutherford professor of medicine and botany, 1786-1820; see professors of clinical medicine	1790	1802
Robert Freer appointed special assistant physician in 1790	...	1795
Thomas Spens	1802	1842
James Buchan	1824	1827
William Cullen see surgeons-in-ordinary	1827	1828, died
Sir Robert Christison, Bt. see professors of clinical medicine	1827	1832
Thomas Shortt	1828	1840
James Crawford Gregory	1828	1832, died
David Craigie	1832	1845
George Augustus Borthwick	1833	1840

[1] "Died" signifies death while in office. [2] Missing Minute Book, 1775-1788, probably contains this date.

APPENDIX II

	Ordinary Physicians	Retired or Resigned, Died
John Home Peebles	1839	1841
William Henderson	1840	1843
William Thomson	1840	1841
Robert Spittal	1841	1843
George Paterson	1841	1849
John Rose Cormack	1843	1845
Andrew Halliday Douglas	1843	1852
William Robertson	1845	1854
James Andrew	1846	1856
Thomas Wright	1849	1850
Sir William Tennant Gairdner, K.C.B.	1853	1862
appointed special assistant physician in 1851		
James Warburton Begbie	1855	1865
William Rutherford Sanders	1861	1869
see professors of clinical medicine		
Daniel Rutherford Haldane	1862	1877
appointed special assistant physician in 1858		
Robert Edmund Scoresby-Jackson	1865	1867
George William Balfour	1868	1882
Sir Thomas Grainger Stewart	1869	1876
appointed special assistant physician in 1865: see professors of clinical medicine		

Assistant Physicians are now Appointed

	Assistant Physicians	Ordinary Physicians	Retired or Resigned, Died
Claud Muirhead	1869	1876	1891
Sir Thomas Richard Fraser	1869	...	1874
see professors of clinical medicine			
David James Brackenridge	1874	1877	1892
John Wyllie	1876	1882	1897
see professors of clinical medicine			
Sir James Ormiston Affleck	1877	1885	1900
Andrew Smart	1880	1891	1906
Alexander James	1882	1892	1907
Sir Byrom Bramwell	1885	1897	1912
George Alexander Gibson	1890	1900	1913, died
Alexander Bruce	1890	1903	1911, died
Sir Robert William Philip	1890	1906	1921
see physician-consultants			
William Russell	1891	1907	1913
see professors of clinical medicine			
James Murdoch Brown	1891	...	1907
Ralph Stockman	1892	...	1897
George Lovell Gulland, C.M.G.	1892	1911	1915
see professors of clinical medicine			
Robert Fraser Calder Leith	1897	...	1899
John James Graham Brown	1897	1912	1919
Francis Darby Boyd, C.M.G.	1899	1913	1919
see professors of clinical medicine			

APPENDIX II

	Assistant Physicians	Ordinary Physicians	Retired or Resigned, Died
Robert Alexander Fleming	1900	1913	1927
Harry Rainy	1906	1915	1923, died
Douglas Chalmers Watson	1907	1919	1934
Edwin Bramwell	1907	1919	1922
see professors of clinical medicine			
Edwin Matthew	1909	1921	1934
see professors of clinical medicine			
William Thomas Ritchie, O.B.E.	1911	1922	1928
see professors of clinical medicine			
John Eason	1912	1923-	...
John Dixon Comrie	1913	1927-	...
Alexander Goodall	1913	1928-	...
George Douglas Mathewson	1919	1934	1935, died
David Murray Lyon	1919	1924	...
see professors of clinical medicine			
Charles McNeil	1919	...	1920
Andrew Fergus Hewat	1920	1934-	...
Herbert Lindesay Watson-Wemyss	1921	...	1933, died
Charles George Lambie	1922	...	1930
William Douglas Denton Small	1923	1935-	...
Andrew Rutherford	1924	...	1930, died
William Alister Alexander	1927	1936-	...
Leybourne Stanley Patrick Davidson	1928	...	1930

Professors of Clinical Medicine

In the eighteenth century the professors of medicine in the University were granted liberty to give clinical lectures on the patients in the Infirmary, a privilege, however, which was not exercised by all of them.

1st February 1748, John Rutherford, professor of medicine, commenced a course of clinical lectures.

6th December 1756, John Rutherford, Alexander Monro, *primus*, William Cullen and Robert Whytt were authorised to give a conjoint course of clinical lectures.

During the later years of the eighteenth century courses of lectures on clinical medicine were also given by the following professors of medicine :—

John Gregory
William Cullen
James Gregory
Daniel Rutherford
Francis Home
Andrew Duncan, senior

In the early years of the nineteenth century lectures in clinical medicine were given by

Daniel Rutherford
James Home
James Gregory
Andrew Duncan, senior and junior
Robert Graham
Thomas Stewart Traill

APPENDIX II

	Appointed	Retired or Resigned, Died
William Pulteney Alison	1823	1854
professor of institutes of medicine and of medicine		
Sir Robert Christison, Bt.	1832	1856
professor of materia medica		
John Hughes Bennett	1848	1874
professor of institutes of medicine		
Thomas Laycock	1855	1876, died
professor of medicine		
Sir A. Douglas Maclagan	1864	1885
professor of forensic medicine		
William Rutherford Sanders	1869	1881, died
professor of pathology		
Sir Thomas Grainger Stewart	1876	1900, died
professor of medicine		
Sir Thomas Richard Fraser	1878	1918
professor of materia medica		
William Smith Greenfield	1881	1912
professor of pathology		
John Wyllie	1900	1914
professor of medicine		
William Russell	1913	1919
Moncrieff Arnott professor of clinical medicine		
George Lovell Gulland, C.M.G.	1915	1928
professor of medicine and clinical medicine		
Francis Darby Boyd, C.M.G.	1919	1922, died
Moncrieff Arnott professor of clinical medicine		
Jonathan Campbell Meakins	1919	1924
Christison professor of therapeutics and professor of clinical medicine		
Edwin Bramwell	1922	1934
Moncrieff Arnott professor of clinical medicine		
David Murray Lyon	1924	1936
Christison professor of therapeutics and professor of clinical medicine		
William Thomas Ritchie, O.B.E.	1928-	...
professor of medicine and clinical medicine		
Edwin Matthew	1934	1936
Moncrieff Arnott professor of clinical medicine		

Physician Consultants

Physician Consultant in Tuberculosis

Sir Robert William Philip 1922-
professor of tuberculosis

Physician Consultant in Psychiatry

George Matthew Robertson 1923-1929
professor of psychiatry, 1919-1932
William Malcolm McAlister 1929-1932

Physician Consultant in Diseases of Tropical Climates

Lieut.-Colonel Edward David Wilson Greig, C.I.E. 1929-

APPENDIX II

SURGICAL DEPARTMENT

In 1729, the offer made by six Surgeon-Apothecaries, members of the Incorporation of Surgeons, each to attend the Infirmary for two months in rotation, was accepted by the managers. The surgeons were :—

John McGill
Francis Congalton
George Cunynghame
Alexander Monro, *primus*
John Douglas
Robert Hope

By regulations of 7th July 1766 and 3rd April 1769, the managers appointed four "fixed surgeons" or surgeons-in-ordinary, each to attend for two months at a time, and during the month falling to them by rotation ; the managers changed one of the four ordinary surgeons annually, electing another of the Incorporation in his place. In addition, all members of the Incorporation of Surgeons, who were willing to act, attended the Infirmary for one month in rotation. The first four surgeons-in-ordinary were :—

James Rae, Peter Adie, James Balfour, Alexander Wood

Benjamin Bell and John Bell, amongst others, were surgeons to the Infirmary during this period.

23rd December 1800, the managers elected six surgeons, the two first in the list acting as surgeons-in-ordinary for two years, to be followed in succession by the second and third pair : at the end of every second year two other surgeons were elected and placed at the foot of the list [1] : no surgeon after acting as surgeon-in-ordinary was eligible for re-election till the expiry of four years after his previous period of attendance. The old system of attendance at the Infirmary by rotation was abrogated in 1800. The six surgeons elected in December 1800 were :—

James Russell
Andrew Wardrop
James Law
Andrew Inglis
William Brown, senior
John Thomson
professor of surgery, Royal College of Surgeons

From 1803 to 1818 (inclusive), while this system of staffing was the practice of the Infirmary, the following Fellows of the College were elected to the surgical staff :—

George Bell
Sir William Newbigging
James Russell
regius professor of clinical surgery, 1803-1833
Patrick Erskine
William Wood
James Law
Alexander Gillespie
John Henry Wishart
Joseph Bell
John Gordon

[1] After the retirement of the two ordinary surgeons in December 1802, apparently four years elapsed, and not two as provided in the regulations, before the ordinary surgeons retired.

APPENDIX II

14th December 1818, system changed : six surgeons were appointed by the managers, subdivided into three classes, two consulting surgeons, two acting surgeons and two assistant surgeons, all on the *active* visiting list, the two acting surgeons being in charge of the surgical beds ; at the end of every second year the following changes were made—the senior consulting surgeon retired, the senior acting and senior assistant surgeons were promoted, and a new junior assistant surgeon was appointed.

	Assistant Surgeons	Acting Surgeons	Consulting Surgeons	Retired or Resigned, Died
James Law	...	...	1818	1820
George Bell	...	...	1818	1822
Alexander Gillespie	...	1818	1820	1824
Sir William Newbigging	...	1818	1824	1826
John Henry Wishart	1818	1820	1824	1828
Joseph Bell	1818	1822	...	1824
Robert Allan	1820	1824	...	1826, died
Sir George Ballingall professor of military surgery, 1823; chair abolished, 1856	1822	1825	1829	1855, died
Adam Hunter	1825	1826	...	1829
John Campbell	1825	1829	1832	1838
Andrew Inglis	...	...	1827	1832
William Cullen see physicians-in-ordinary	1827	...	...	1828, died
Robert Liston	1828	1829	...	1834
John Lizars	1829	1832	...	1838
John William Turner professor of surgery, 1831-1835	1829	1834	...	1835, died
James Syme regius professor of clinical surgery, 1833-1869	1833	1836	1869	1870, died
Alexander Watson	1834	1836	1840	1847
Sir William Fergusson, Bt.	1835	1838	...	1840
Sir Charles Bell professor of surgery, 1835-1842	...	...	1836	1842, died
John Argyll Robertson	1838	1840	...	1842
Peter David Handyside	1840	1840	1844	1848
James Duncan	1840	1843	1848	1853
James Miller professor of surgery, 1842-1864; in 1852 granted beds as professor of surgery	1840	1842	1850	1863
Sir Andrew Douglas Maclagan see professors of clinical medicine	1842	1848	...	1850

APPENDIX II

About this date the Consulting Surgeon is no longer on the active staff

	Assistant Surgeons	Ordinary Surgeons	Retired or Resigned, Died
James Dunsmure, senior	1844	1849	1856
Richard James Mackenzie	1848	1849	1854, died
James Spence	1850	1854	1882, died
professor of surgery, 1864-1882			
James Donaldson Gillespie	1850	1856	1871
Sir John Struthers	1853	1862	1863
Sir Joseph Lister (Baron Lister)	1856	...	1877
regius professor of surgery, Glasgow, 1860-1869 ; regius professor of clinical surgery, Edinburgh, 1869-1877			
Sir Patrick Heron Watson	1860	1863	1886
extra-acting surgeon in 1878 with beds while in the old Infirmary			
Alexander McKenzie Edwards	1863	...	1864
Thomas Annandale	1865	1869	1907, died
regius professor of clinical surgery, 1877-1907			
Joseph Bell	1865	1871	1886
John Duncan	1869	1877	1897
extra-acting surgeon 1892, with beds			
John Chiene, C.B.	1871	1878	1909
professor of surgery, 1882-1909			
Alexander Gordon Miller	1877	1882	1897
Peter Hume Maclaren	1878	1886	1901
John Bishop	1878	...	1885
Charles Watson MacGillivray	1882	1892	1907
Sir Joseph Montagu Cotterill	1883	1897	1912
Charles Walker Cathcart, C.M.G.	1884	1901	1918
Francis Mitchell Caird	1885	1903	1919
regius professor of clinical surgery, 1908-1919			
Sir James William Beaman Hodsdon, K.B.E.	1886	1907	1922
John Shaw MacLaren	1889	...	1902
Sir David Wallace, K.B.E.	1892	1908	1923
Henry Alexis Thomson	1892	...	1923
professor of surgery, 1909-1923			
Sir Harold Jalland Stiles, K.B.E.	1897	...	1925
(1898 resigned) regius professor of clinical surgery, 1919-1925			
Alexander Miles	1898	1910	1924
John Wheeler Dowden	1901	1912	1924
Archibald Adam Scot Skirving, C.M.G.	1903	1916	1928
George Lyall Chiene	1903	1922	1937
William James Stuart	1907	1923-	...
John William Struthers	1908	1924-	...
Henry Wade, C.M.G.	1909	1924-	...
Edward Scott Carmichael	1909	...	1915, died
Sir David Percival Dalbreck Wilkie, O.B.E.	1912	...	...
professor of surgery, 1924-			

APPENDIX II

	Assistant Surgeons	Ordinary Surgeons	Retired or Resigned, Died
Lionel C. Peel Ritchie	1913	...	1914, died
Denis Cotterill	1913	...	1918, died
Sir John Fraser, K.C.V.O.	1919	...	...
regius professor of clinical surgery, 1925-			
James Methuen Graham	1919	1928-	...
Alexander Pirie Watson	1919	1937-	...
Francis Evelyn Jardine	1919-	...	...
James Norman Jackson Hartley	1922	...	1926
Walter Quarry Wood	1923-	...	...
John James McIntosh Shaw	1924-	...	...
Francis Gordon Bell	1924 (Oct.-Dec.)	...	1924
Walter Mercer	1924-	...	...
William Alexander Cochrane	1924	...	...
associate assistant surgeon in orthopædics, 1932			
Keith Paterson Brown	1925-	...	...
Robert Leslie Stewart	1927-	...	...
Thomas McWalter Millar	1928-	...	...

Medical and Surgical Registrars

Alexander Lockhart Gillespie, medical	1891-1904, died
Kenneth Mackinnon Douglas, surgical	1891-1898
William Menzies Hutton, surgical	1898-1899
Alexander Dingwall Fordyce, medical	1905-1910
Edward Scott Carmichael, surgical	1899-1910

Appointments discontinued

DEPARTMENT OF MIDWIFERY

	Obstetric Physicians	Retired or Resigned, Died
Thomas Young	1756	1780
professor of midwifery 1756-1780		
Alexander Hamilton	1780	1793
professor of midwifery, 1780-1800		

The Edinburgh General Lying-in-Hospital was opened in 1793

DISEASES PECULIAR TO WOMEN AND INFANTS

	Assistant Extra-Physicians	Extra-Physicians	Retired or Resigned, Died
Sir James Young Simpson, Bt.	...	1850	1870, died
professor of midwifery, 1840-1870			
Alexander Keiller	...	1851	1861
Thomas Graham Weir	...	1857	1861
James Matthews Duncan	...	1861	1877
Sir Alexander Russell Simpson	...	1870	1905
professor of midwifery, 1870-1905			

APPENDIX II

	Assistant Extra-Physicians	Extra-Physicians	Retired or Resigned, Died
Angus Macdonald	...	1877	1886, died
Sir John Halliday Croom	1883	1886	1901 [1]
professor of midwifery, 1905-1921			
David Berry Hart	1886	...	...
Alexander Hugh Freeland Barbour	1886	...	...

GYNÆCOLOGICAL DEPARTMENT [2]

	Assistant Gynæcologists	Gynæcologists	Retired or Resigned, Died
David Berry Hart	...	1901	1906
Alexander Hugh Freeland Barbour	...	1906	1921
Robert Milne Murray	1901	...	1904, died
Nathaniel Thomas Brewis	1901	1906	1921
Francis William Nicol Haultain	1904	...	1908
James Haig Ferguson	1906	1921	1927
William Fordyce	1906	1921	1928
Benjamin Philp Watson	...	1922	1926
professor of midwifery, 1922-26			
Robert William Johnstone, C.B.E.	1922	1926-	...
professor of midwifery, 1926-			
Hugh Stevenson Davidson	1922	1927	1932, died
James Young	1922	1928	1934
William Francis Theodore Haultain	1926	1932-	...
Douglas Alexander Miller	1927	1934-	...
Ernest Chalmers Fahmy	1928-	...	...

EXTRA-SURGEON FOR THE TREATMENT OF OVARIAN DISEASES

Thomas Keith, appointed 1870, resigned 1888.

Skene Keith, appointed 1885 as Special Assistant to Thomas Keith; the appointment expired with the resignation of the latter in 1888.

DEPARTMENT FOR DISEASES OF THE SKIN

	Assistant Physicians	Physicians	Extra Physicians	Retired or Resigned, Died
William Allan Jamieson	...	1884	...	1906
Sir Norman Purvis Walker	1892	1906	1924 [3]	1925
Frederick Gardiner	1904	1912	...	1933, died
Robert Cranston Low	1906	1924	...	1933
Robert Aitken	1924	1933-	...	...
George Hector Percival	1927	1936-	...	...

[1] Sir J. Halliday Croom was appointed to the Chair of Midwifery in 1905 and took temporary charge of one ward as Gynæcologist during 1905-6.

[2] In 1898 the title of Extra-Physician was changed to that of Gynæcologist.

[3] Extra-Physician for Lupus and Sunlight Treatment.

APPENDIX II

OPHTHALMIC DEPARTMENT

	Assistant Surgeons	Surgeons	Extra-Surgeons	Retired or Resigned, Died
William Walker	...	1855	...	1882
Douglas M. C. L. Argyll Robertson	1862	1870	1895	1897
Sir George Andreas Berry	1882	1885	1900	1905
George Mackay	1889	1895	1910	1913
William George Sym	1890	1905	...	1920
Ernest Edmund Maddox	1895	...	...	1897
James Veitch Paterson	1899	1913	...	1927
Arthur Henry Havens Sinclair	1905	1920	...	1932
Harry Moss Traquair	1913	1927-	...	...
Ernest Hugh Cameron	1920	1932-	...	...
Charles William Graham	1927-	...	...	...

EAR, NOSE AND THROAT DEPARTMENT

	Assistant Surgeons	Surgeons	Surgeon Consultant	Retired or Resigned, Died
Peter McBride	...	1883	...	1903
Robert McKenzie Johnston	1890	1903	...	1906
Arthur Logan Turner	1903	1906	1921	1924
John Malcolm Farquharson	1904	1906	...	1921
John Smith Fraser	1906	1921	...	1936, died
John Davis Lithgow	1906	1921	...	1936
William Tyler Gardiner	1921	...	...	1933
George Ewart Martin	1921	1936-	...	...

VENEREAL DISEASES DEPARTMENT

	Assistant Clinical Medical Officer	Clinical Medical Officers	Retired or Resigned, Died
David Lees	...	1919	1934, died
Robert Campbell Lindsay Batchelor	1920	1935-	...

DENTAL DEPARTMENT

	Assistant Surgeons	Surgeons.	Retired or Resigned, Died
John Smith	...	1863	1888
William Guy	...	1895	1910
John Herbert Gibbs [1]	...	1903	1929
Douglas Llewellyn George Radford	1921	1924-	...
Robert Charles Scott Dow	1924	1927-	...
Frederick George Gibbs	...	1927-	...
James Morham	...	1927-	...
Herbert Moncrieff Sturrock	...	1927-	...
David Skene Middleton	...	1927-	...

[1] Appointed Surgeon Consultant in 1924.

APPENDIX II

MEDICAL ELECTRICAL DEPARTMENT

	Assistant Medical Electricians	Medical Electricians	Extra-Medical Electrician	Retired or Resigned, Died
Robert Milne Murray	...	1896	...	1901
see gynæcologists				
Dawson Fyers Duckworth Turner .	1896	1901	1911	1925
William Hope Fowler, C.V.O. . .	1901	1911	...	1926
Archibald McKendrick	...	1911	...	1926

RADIOLOGICAL DEPARTMENT

	Assistant Medical Officers	Medical Officer in Charge.	Retired or Resigned, Died
John Miller Woodburn Morison . .	...	1925	1930
William Crichton Fothergill . . .	1926	...	1928
Elsie H. Parker	1927	...	1927
John Burnett King	1927	...	1929
George Grant Allan	1928	...	1929
Elizabeth Nixon Thompson . . .	1929	...	1930

PATHOLOGICAL DEPARTMENT

	Assistant Pathologists	Pathologists	Retired or Resigned, Died
John Reid	...	1839	1841
see superintendent-pathologist			
Thomas Beavill Peacock	...	1841	1843
see superintendent-pathologist			
John Hughes Bennett	...	1844	1848
Sir William Tennant Gairdner, K.C.B. . .	...	1848	1853
Daniel Rutherford Haldane	...	1853	1862
Sir Thomas Grainger Stewart . . .	...	1862	1869
James Bell Pettigrew	...	1869	1875
John Wyllie	...	1875	1877
David James Hamilton	...	1877	1882
Sir Byrom Bramwell	...	1882	1885
Alexander Bruce	...	1885	1890
German Sims Woodhead	...	1885	1888
William Russell	...	1888	1891
William Henry Barrett	...	1890	1892
Sir Robert Muir	...	1892	1898
Robert Fraser Calder Leith	...	1892	1897
Robert Alexander Fleming	...	1897	1900
David Arthur Welsh	...	1898	1901
Stuart McDonald	1901	...	1906
Theodore Shennan	1901	1902	1914
James Martin Beattie	1902	...	1905
George Lyon	1905	...	1906

APPENDIX II

	Assistant Pathologist	Pathologist	Retired or Resigned, Died
William Elliot Carnegie Dickson	1906	...	1909
Henry Wade, C.M.G.	1906	...	1908
John Dixon Comrie	1908	...	1910
James Miller	1909	...	1920
Alexander Murray Drennan	1910	...	1915
professor of pathology and honorary pathologist, 1931-			
James Hunter Harvey Pirie	1911	...	1912
David Murray Lyon	1912	...	1919
see professors of clinical medicine			
James Lorrain Smith	...	1914	1931, died
consultant pathologist, 1913 ; honorary pathologist, 1929			
James Walker Dawson	1916	...	1919
Andrew Rutherford	1919	...	1920
Peter MacCallum	1920	...	1925
assistant clinical pathologist			
Benjamin James Ryrie	1919	...	1921
William Alister Alexander	1920	...	1924
George Buchanan	1920	...	1925
assistant clinical pathologist			
Duncan Hedley Wright	1920	...	1921
George William Marshall Findlay	1920	...	1923
Henry Thomson	1921	...	1921
Thomas Sprunt	1921	...	1922
Francis Esmond Reynolds	1921	...	1924
James Davidson	1922	1930	1934
senior assistant pathologist, 1925			
Ronald Douglas Mackenzie	1923	...	1928
Douglas James Acworth Kerr	1924	...	1928
Arthur James Cochrane Hamilton	1924	...	1924
Robert Carmichael	1924	...	1931
William Nairn Boog Watson	1925	...	1925
Thomas McWalter Millar	1925	...	1925
William Gilbert Millar	1925	1930	...
		senior pathologist, 1934-	
Herbert Reynold Morgan Richards	1925	...	1925
Angus Elrick William McLachlan	1925	...	1925
Ronald Macdonald	1925	...	1926
Ian Hyslop McLure	1925	...	1925
Alexander Millar Meek Grierson	1925	...	1926
Donald Angus MacMillan Shearer	1925	...	1925
James Maxwell Alston	1926	...	1927
George Lionel Alexander	1926	...	1927
Joseph Ryland Whitaker	1927	...	1929
Charles Frederick William Illingworth	1928	...	1930
Thomas Robert Rushton Todd	1929	...	1930

APPENDIX II–III

BACTERIOLOGICAL DEPARTMENT

	Assistant Clinical Bacterio-logists	Assistant Bacterio-logists	Bacterio-logists	Retired or Resigned, Died
Thomas Jones Mackie . . . . professor of bacteriology : honorary bacteriologist, 1929-	...	...	1923	...
William Robertson Logan . . . . clinical pathologist, 1914 : clinical bacteriologist, 1925	...	...	1929-	...
Ronald Macdonald	1926	...	...	...
John William Starkey . . . . assistant clinical pathologist, 1925	1926	...	...	1927
William Happer	1926	...	...	1926
Alexander Gorrie Paton . . .	1926	...	...	1927
Richard Norton	1926	...	...	1928
John Telfer Smeall	1927	1930- senior assistant	...	...
Robert Lees	1927	...	...	1927
Arthur Dewar Frazer . . .	1928	...	...	1928
Alistair Westland Rose . . .	1928	...	...	1929
Frank Fiddes Main	1929	...	...	1930
John Angus Burgess	1929	1930	...	1930

Extra-Bacteriologist, the senior assistant to the professor of bacteriology

APPENDIX III

OFFICIALS AND ADMINISTRATIVE STAFF [1]

TREASURERS

David Spence [2]	1730-1744
Gavin Hamilton	1744-1754
Gilbert Laurie	1754-1769
Archibald Hope	1769-1790
Henry Jardine, W.S.	1790-1818
Francis Wilson, W.S.	1819-1831
Harry Maxwell Inglis, W.S.	1831-1843
James Farnie, Treasurer-Superintendent	1844-1846, died
Alexander McDougall, Treasurer-Superintendent . . .	1846-1871
Alexander McDougall, Treasurer	1871-1879
Alexander Ellison Ross, Treasurer	1879-1880
James Spence Trainer, Treasurer	1881-1883
James Spence Trainer, Treasurer and Clerk	1883-1893, died
William Strathie Caw, Treasurer and Clerk	1893-1929
Henry Maw, Secretary and Treasurer	1929-

[1] The Tables in Appendix III have been placed as far as possible chronologically in the order in which each group of officials was instituted.

[2] David Spence, secretary to the Bank of Scotland, had acted since February 1728 as secretary to the committee appointed to call in the subscriptions to the fund being raised for the erection of the Infirmary.

APPENDIX III

CLERKS TO THE CORPORATION

Henry Balcanquhal	1730-1771, died
Robert Boswell	1771-1804, died
Alexander Boswell	1804-1836
James Hope, D.K.S.	1836-1843
Peter Bell	1844-1883

After this date the office is continued as that of Treasurer and Clerk.

MISTRESS, GOVERNESS, HOUSEKEEPER, OR MATRON

Mistress Nisbett	1729-1730
Mistress Waldie	1730-1744
Mistress Waddell	1744-1749
Mistress Paxton	1749-1754
Mistress Morison	1754-1762
Mistress Dawson	1762-1770
Mistress Elizabeth Paton	1770-1775
Mistress Mary Rannie	1775-1801
Mistress Carse	1802-1803
Mistress Barbara Hume	1803-1813
Mistress Montgomerie	1813-1818
Mistress Ann Macfarlane	1818-1839
Mistress Wood	1839-1843
Miss S. Peat	1843-1852
Miss Helen Hill Baxter	1852-1858
Miss Ann Forsyth	1859-1879

SUPERINTENDENT OF NURSES

Miss Anne L. Sidey	1866-1871

LADY SUPERINTENDENTS OF NURSES

Miss Elizabeth Anne Barclay	1872-1874
Miss Angélique Lucille Pringle	1874-1887
Miss Frances Elizabeth Spencer	1887-1907
Miss Annie Warren Gill, C.B.E.	1907-1925
Miss Ellen Frances Bladon	1925-1931
Miss Elizabeth Dunlop Smaill, O.B.E.	1931-

ACCOUNTANTS AND/OR AUDITORS

Alexander Chalmers	1744-1760
Robert Chalmers	1761-1796
James Forrest	1797-1802
James Bruce	1797-1821
Archibald Bruce	1819-1865
James M. Macandrew	1865-1891
Hugh Blair, C.A.	1891-1906
Patrick A. Blair, C.A.	1906-1917, died
William Home Cook, C.A.	1917-1927, died
Laurence Bruce Bell, C.A.	1928-

APPENDIX III

LAW AGENTS

From 1836, the year of the foundation of the firm of Hope, Mann (Todd) and Kirk, W.S., the legal business of the Royal Infirmary has been transacted by the Firm ; but since 1873 individual members of the Firm have been appointed Law Agents.

James Hope, D.K.S.	1873-1882, died
William Mann, S.S.C.	1882-1893 ,,
Charles Todd, S.S.C.	1893-1900 ,,
William J. Kirk, W.S.	1900-1915 ,,
James Arthur Hope, W.S.	1915-1925 ,,
Arthur H. C. Hope, W.S.	1925-

CLERK OF THE HOUSE

Robert McKinley	1741-1747

APOTHECARIES

From 1729 to 1747 the Surgeon-Apothecaries supplied the medicines from their shops : in the latter year the Surgeons' shop was instituted in the Infirmary "to free the Surgeons from the expense of furnishing medicines."

Mr Petrie, also Clerk of the House	1747-1750
Mr Sutherland, also Clerk of the House till 1751	1747-1752
Mr Short	1752-1758
John Shiells	1758-1765
Robert Reid	1765-1767
Robert Jardine	1767-1770
James Maltman	1770-1775
missing minute book, 1775-1788	
Mr Miller	1784-1803
George Wilson	1803-1805
William McDonald	1805-1828
George M. Murray	1828-1829
George McCulloch	1829-1832
Alexander Hamilton	1832-1834
Samuel Shortridge	1834-1838
John Brown, M.D. see House Governor	1838-1839
Alexander McDougall[1] see Treasurer-Superintendent	1839-1863

[1] Alexander McDougall combined the duties of Apothecary with those of Treasurer-Superintendent till 1863.

APPENDIX III

DISPENSERS

H. P. Laurence	1863-1866
Douglas D. C. Menzies	1866-1867
P. Gowan	1867-1869
Alexander Gunn	1870-1877
William H. M. Barclay	1877-1878
Charles Hunter Stewart	1878-1882
Charles Arthur	1882-1895
Thomas Alexander	1895-1926
see Registrars	
Gordon Perrins	1926-

CHIEF PORTERS

John Forbes	1742
John Taylor	1742-1755
John Brown	1756-

dates of resignation of John Brown and appointment of James Grant are contained in missing minute book

James Grant	-1818
Frank Beatton or Beattie	1818-1823
Udney Marshall	1823-1831
Philip Phillips	1831-1838
John Macnab	1839-1841
Robert Blackie	1841-1854
John Tait, Porter and Gardener	1855-1863
Alexander Blaikie, Porter and Gardener	1863-1865
Peter Robin, Porter and Gardener	1866-1870
Alexander Kiel	1871-1887
David Ramage	1887-1899
William Smith	1899-1920
Alexander Strathdee	1920-

CHAPLAINS

Rev. Mr Willis	1756-1759
Rev. Mr Gillis	1759-1769
Rev. James Milne	1769-1771
William Sprott, preacher	1771-1774
Samuel Macnight, preacher	1774-
missing minute book, 1775-1788	
Rev. Charles Ochiltree	1794-1809
Rev. James Porteous	1809-1832
Rev. Andrew Buchanan	1832-1838
Rev. Robert Drummond	1839-1843
Rev. Alexander Shand	1843-1844
Rev. James Laurie	1844-1851
Rev. James Brotherston	1851-1854
Rev. James Hamilton [1]	1854-

[1] Rev. James Hamilton held office as chaplain, 1854-1885.

APPENDIX III

William Mackenzie, missionary	1854
William Mackenzie, missionary, Surgical House	1855-1856
Rev. James Hamilton, chaplain, Medical House	1855-1856
Rev. James Hamilton, chaplain, Surgical House	1857-1870
Rev. William Strauchon, chaplain, Medical House	1857-1869
Rev. James Hamilton	1871-1885
Rev. James Greig	1885-1890
Rev. William Aitken	1890-1901
Rev. Robert Henderson	1901-1923
Rev. Thomas C. Macaulay	1923-1934
Rev. Peter Lockhart	1934-

HOUSE GOVERNOR AND CHIEF APOTHECARY

John Brown, M.D.	1838-1839, died
see apothecary	

SUPERINTENDENT-PATHOLOGISTS

John Reid, M.D.	1839-1841
see pathological department	
Thomas Beavill Peacock, M.D.	1841-1843
see pathological department	

From 1843-1871 see office of Treasurer-Superintendent

SUPERINTENDENTS

Deputy Surgeon-General Charles Hamilton Fasson, I.M.S.	1871-1892, died
Surgeon Major-General Stewart A. Lithgow, C.B., A.M.S.	1892-1899, died
Colonel William P. Warburton, C.S.I., M.D.	1899-1911
Lieut.-Colonel Sir Joseph Fayrer, Bt., R.A.M.C.	1911-1924
Colonel George David St Clair Thom, C.B., A.M.S.	1924-1935, died
Lieut.-Colonel Alexander Dron Stewart, C.I.E., I.M.S.	1935-

REGISTRARS

Alexander Moir	1867-1869
D. B. Bain, G. H. Aitchison	1870-1872
John Davidson	1873
John S. Mackay, M.A.	1873-1874
Frederick McMahon	1874-1879
Walter J. Smith	1874-1889
R. Frank Rand	1879-1881
Thomas Alexander	1890-1894
see Dispensers	
Benjamin Coppock	1895-1904
W. F. Scott Craig	1904-1934
Duncan McNeill	1934-

APPENDIX III–IV

CASHIERS

No official recognition of this office prior to 1878.

James Spence Trainer	1878-1880
see Treasurers	
William Strathie Caw[1]	1887-1893
see Treasurer and Clerk	
Benjamin Johnston Hodge	1893-1922
James Williamson	1923-

STEWARDS

John Macpherson	1879-1920
Andrew Whyte	1920-

CLERKS OF WORKS

William Thorburn	1901-1911
R. R. Mill	1911-1920
Thomas W. Turnbull	1920-
appointed Master of Works, 1924; appointed Architect and Master of Works, 1929	

ORGANISING SECRETARY FOR SUBSCRIPTIONS

Russell Paton	1906-

LADY ALMONERS

	Assistant Lady Almoner	Principal Lady Almoner	Retired or Resigned, Died
Miss E. Alice Callender	...	1924	1927
Miss Helen Young Watt . . .	1925	1928-	...

APPENDIX IV

Section 94, Edinburgh Corporation Act, 3 & 4 George V. 1913

POWER TO ALTER DATE OF ANNUAL MEETING OF COURT OF CONTRIBUTORS AND ELECTION OF MANAGERS

When in any year the first Monday of January is a public holiday the annual meeting for the election of managers and the annual meeting of the General Court of Contributors of the said Corporation may be held on any day between the first and seventh days of January in such year, both days inclusive, and may be adjourned to such other day either within or beyond that period as the meeting may determine,

[1] W. S. Caw appointed a junior clerk in Treasurer and Clerk's department in December 1880.

and when in any year the said annual meetings are to be held as herein provided on a date other than the first Monday of January, then in that event such date shall be fixed by the General Court of Contributors at their annual meeting, or any adjournment thereof, in January of the previous year and shall be duly advertised at least a fortnight before the date fixed as aforesaid, and any business transacted at a meeting fixed as herein provided shall be as binding and effectual as if transacted on the day prescribed by the said Royal Charter and Act of Parliament. Provided that if the said General Court of Contributors fail to fix the date for the next annual meeting as herein provided, the date may be fixed by Resolution of the Board of Managers at any ordinary meeting of managers in the previous year, but not later than the first meeting of managers in the month of December of the previous year. Provided further, that any omission to advertise the date of a meeting fixed as hereinbefore provided shall not invalidate anything done at such meeting when held.

APPENDIX V

Section 8 of the Edinburgh Corporation Order Confirmation Act, 1919

Power to Increase the Number of Managers from Twenty-one to Twenty-six

. . . the numbers of the Managers of the Royal Infirmary of Edinburgh shall, from and after the first Monday in January 1920, be twenty-six of whom twenty-one shall be appointed in the manner provided by the said Edinburgh Royal Infirmary Act, 1870, and the remaining five members shall be appointed in the manner following, that is to say :—

One Manager by the Miners' Association of Fife and Kinross ;
One Manager by the Miners' Association of Mid and East Lothian ;
One Manager by the Coal and Shale Miners' Associations of West Lothian ; and
Two Managers by the Edinburgh and District Trades Council.

Except as altered by this Order the whole of the provisions of the Edinburgh Royal Infirmary Act, 1870, as amended by Section 94 (Power to alter date of annual meeting of Contributors to the Royal Infirmary of Edinburgh) of the Act of 1913, shall apply to the appointment of Managers of the said Royal Infirmary of Edinburgh.

APPENDIX VI

Section 35 of the Edinburgh Corporation Order Confirmation Act, 1930

Power to Increase the Number of Managers from Twenty-six to Twenty-eight

35. (1) Notwithstanding anything contained in the Royal Charter granted by His Majesty King George the Second of date the twenty-fifth day of August one thousand seven hundred and thirty-six incorporating the Royal Infirmary of Edinburgh or in the Edinburgh Royal Infirmary Act 1870 or in the Order of 1919 the number of the Managers of the Royal Infirmary of Edinburgh shall as from the first Monday in January next after the holding of the Annual General Meeting first referred to in Subsection (2) of this section be twenty-eight of whom twenty-six shall be appointed in the manner provided by the said Edinburgh Royal Infirmary Act 1870 and by the Order of 1919 and the remaining two Managers shall be appointed by the Association known as the League of Subscribers to the Royal Infirmary of Edinburgh (hereinafter in this section referred to as " the said League ").

(2) The two Managers to be appointed by the said League as provided for in the immediately preceding subsection shall be so appointed at the Annual General Meeting of the said League to be held in the month of November next after the commencement of this Order and at the Annual General Meeting to be held in each following year and they shall hold office as Managers from the first Monday of the month of January next after their election until the first Monday of the month of January following.

APPENDIX VII

The Edinburgh Royal Infirmary Act, 1870

Section 11. The agreement made between the Company of Merchants of the City of Edinburgh, the governors of George Watson's Hospital, and the Corporation, for the sale to the Corporation of the lands and buildings belonging to the said hospital, dated the twenty-eighth day of February eighteen hundred and seventy (a copy of which agreement is set out in the schedule to this Act), is hereby sanctioned and confirmed as between the parties thereto;

and the said governors, with the consent and concurrence of the said Company, may execute conveyances of the said lands and buildings in favour of the Corporation, which shall be valid and effectual ; but nothing in this section, or in any such conveyance contained, shall prejudice or affect the right, title, estate, or interest of any corporation or person other than the said Company of Merchants, the said governors, and the Corporation.

Section 12. The Corporation may, for such purposes as they see fit, sell either at gross prices or in consideration of annual payments by way of feu duty or ground annual, or partly in the one and partly in the other of those modes, or may let on lease, the whole or part of the lands and buildings now belonging to and occupied by them, and such part of the lands and buildings acquired as aforesaid as are not ultimately required for the purposes of the Corporation, except the lands in which they are only to acquire a right of servitude for making the drain or sewer authorised by this Act, and may also sell such feu duties or ground annuals.

Section 14. Provided always, that if any persons or corporations who have subscribed and paid to the said committee any money for the erection or improvement of buildings on or in connection with the lands now belonging to and occupied by the Corporation, and who have not already consented to or acquiesced in the application of such contributions towards the acquisition of the new site authorised by this Act, and the erection of the infirmary buildings thereon, shall apply to the Corporation for repayment of such contributions on or before the first day of November next after the passing of this Act, the Corporation shall repay to such persons or corporations the amounts so contributed and paid by them respectively, so far as the same shall have been paid over to the Corporation by the said committee of subscribers.

Section 15. The Corporation may appropriate and apply in and towards the purchase of the lands and buildings which they are by this Act authorised to acquire, and the erection of new hospitals and other buildings necessary and convenient for the purposes of the infirmary, and the construction of the said drain or sewer, and the other purposes of this Act, any moneys which are now in their hands, whether accumulated capital or annual proceeds, and any moneys which they may receive by way of consideration for the value of the existing infirmary site and buildings, or for the feu duties or ground annuals reserved by them in respect thereof, and also any moneys which shall be paid to them by the said committee of subscribers, and any moneys which have been or may hereafter be contributed by other corporations and individuals for the purposes aforesaid.

APPENDIX VIII

Extracts from the Rules of the Court of Contributors relative to Membership of the Court, Attendance at Meetings, and the Privilege of Voting at Meetings

1. The qualification necessary for membership of the Corporation and of the General Court of Contributors (hereinafter referred to as "The Court") shall be as set forth in Section 16 of the Edinburgh Royal Infirmary Act, 1870.

2. A List of Contributors qualified to be members of and to vote at meetings of the Court shall be prepared in each year by the Treasurer and Clerk[1] of the Infirmary (hereinafter referred to as "The Clerk").

6. A contribution which bears to be the joint contribution of two or more persons named shall, when the amount contributed when divided by the number of persons named is sufficient to qualify each contributor, be taken to have been contributed in equal proportions by the individual persons named. If the names of the persons jointly contributing are not stated, the Clerk shall ascertain from the joint contributors by which person or persons and in what shares the amount is contributed.

7. For the purposes of these presents the word "person" shall be taken to include Private Firms or Partnerships, Corporations, Joint Stock Companies, Associations, Societies or other collective bodies.

8. No subscription given in the name of a "firm and employees" or of an "individual and employees" shall carry with it the right to membership of the Court.

9. Any contribution received from a Private Firm, Partnership or any other body mentioned in Rule 7 hereof shall be taken to be contributed wholly by such body, unless it be accompanied by a detailed statement by the party remitting the same, giving the names and addresses of such persons as shall have contributed during the year in which the contribution is given, the amount necessary to qualify in terms of Rule 1 hereof.

21. All persons attending a Meeting of the Court shall, if required, give their names and addresses with the name and address of the member he represents, as provided in Rule 23 hereof, in order that

[1] The designation "Treasurer and Clerk" has been altered by resolution of the Managers to "Secretary and Treasurer."

the same may be checked against the List and Supplementary List of members.

22. Only members of the Court and the representatives provided for in Rule 23 shall be entitled to take part in the proceedings of the Court, and vote on any motion before the Court.

23. For the purposes of Rules 21 and 22 the following Rules in regard to representation of members of the Court shall apply :—

(*a*) A Private Firm or Partnership, being a member of the General Court may be represented at a Meeting of the said Court by any partner of the Firm or Partnership, or by any person authorised in writing by the said Firm or Partnership to represent it at said Meeting.

(*b*) A Corporation or Joint Stock Company, being a member of the said Court may be represented at a Meeting of the said Court by any person authorised in writing by the Corporation or Joint Stock Company to represent it.

(*c*) An Association, Society or other collective body, being a member of the Court may in like manner be represented by any person authorised in writing by the Association or Society.

30. In the cases provided for in Rule 23 hereof where a member of the Court is represented by a partner of a firm, director or other authorised person, such representative shall in addition to his own name and address state also in full the name and address of the member of Court whom he represents.

31. A person attending the Meeting as representing a member in terms of Rule 23 shall, if he is also as an individual a member of the Court, be entitled to separate votes, one as an individual and one as representing such member, but such votes shall be recorded on separate copies of the printed list.

35. No proxies shall be received, and each vote shall be tendered personally by the member or his representative at the Meeting.

INDEX

INDEX

INDEX

INDEX

INDEX

INDEX

INDEX

INDEX

INDEX

INDEX

INDEX

INDEX

INDEX

INDEX

INDEX